THE DIET TRAP

THE DIET TRAP

*Your 7-week plan
to lose weight—
without losing yourself!*

PAMELA M. SMITH, R.D.

LifeLine
Press

WASHINGTON, DC

First paperback edition 2001

Library of Congress Cataloging-in-Publication Data

Smith, Pamela M.
      The diet trap : your seven-week plan to lose weight without losing yourself / Pamela Smith.
      p.cm.
      Includes index.
      ISBN 0-89526-209-6
1. Weight loss. I. Title
RM222.2.S6228 2000
613.2'5—dc21   00-029895

Published in the United States by
LifeLine Press
A Regnery Publishing Company
One Massachusetts Avenue NW
Washington, DC 20001

Visit us at www.lifelinepress.com

Distributed to the trade by
National Book Network
4720-A Boston Way
Lanham, MD 20706

Printed on acid-free paper
Manufactured in the United States of America

10 9 8 7 6 5 4 3 2 1

Books are available in quantity for promotional or premium use. Write to Director of Special Sales, Regnery Publishing, Inc., One Massachusetts Avenue, NW, Washington, DC 20001, for information on discounts and terms or call (202) 216-0600.

To my daughters, Danielle and Nicole
May the truth of who you are—beautiful masterpieces created
with purpose and promise—keep you forever free
of the diet trap and any snare of life.
Loving you is food to my soul.

CONTENTS

ACKNOWLEDGMENTS

I am forever grateful to so many people who have made The Diet Trap *a living reality.*

Special thanks to those at Regnery and LifeLine Press who helped fire my passion to help others "just say NO" to the diet teachings of our day—Jeff Carneal, Harry McCollough, Harry Crocker, and Al Regnery. And to Marji Ross, Jennifer Azar, Marja Walker, Nancy Bryan, Erica Rogers, and Tom Freiling for investing their incredible gifts into creating a worthy vessel to carry the message.

To Traci Mullins, my forever friend and visionary editor, who encourages me, gently guides me, resists redundancy, and makes writing fun and fulfilling. It has been a freedom walk for us both.

To my loving family—Larry, Danielle, and Nicole, my mom—and to the Martins, Phillips, Smiths, and Hensleys—for being my best cheerleaders and replenishers.

To all of my awesome clients whose life experiences, the hurdles and the victories, have shaped *The Smart Weigh* and laid the foundation for *The Diet Trap*. Thank you for your unwavering commitment to never diet again!

To Joe Lee, for believing that good food that's great for you can taste great too—and for entrusting your health to *The Smart Weigh* principles. You are an inspiration.

PART ONE ■ DIETS MAKE YOU FAT

CHAPTER 1 ■ Diet Mania

Sometimes when we're stuck with a locked door in front of us there's a key hidden under the mat, or a window open on the side of the house.

—ANONYMOUS

For JoAnn, the moment of truth came when she couldn't button her favorite size-8 skirt. Ever since hitting her mid-thirties she had known that a little extra weight was creeping on. But that day, a "little" became depressingly close to "a lot." When she finally weighed herself, JoAnn, a thirty-nine-year-old mother of two, couldn't believe she had gained twenty-three pounds—as much, all told, as when she delivered her first baby.

Where did all those pounds come from? And when? Oh, JoAnn was aware that she'd been expanding—but she had blamed that on her lack of exercise, on not playing tennis because of a knee injury. She just needed to tone up. Or maybe she should go on a "serious" diet—at least half of her friends were doing that.

For Mike, weight had always been a major battle. He was a pudgy, stocky kid who never seemed to grow out of his baby fat. The family nickname for Mike was "Beefy King," a name that somehow followed him to school. Throughout his early teens, the extra weight was a nuisance that he hadn't really done much about, except to try to wish it away. That is, until he started playing football.

Then his bulk served him well. It helped "Beefy King" rise to be the starting linebacker for his high school team. It also landed him a scholarship to college. Mike played to great acclaim for three years, but then came the knee injury that took him out of the day's game, and ultimately, out of football. That's when his weight really ballooned—and that's when he first tried serious dieting.

That was fifteen years ago, and Mike has been on close to fifteen diets since. He's done Herbalife, protein shakes, Fit for Life, Butterbusters, Jenny Craig, even a hospital fasting program, to name just a few. And he's always been pretty successful—as long as he was "on it"—and especially if he was exercising hard to boot. But he can't stay "on it" forever. He gets the "misery factor" weight off, gets distracted or hurts his knee again, and then he's right back to eating and drinking whatever, whenever, and quits exercising. Worse, he always gains back more than he lost.

But as Mike sat before me, his diet history was only part of the story. The bigger issue was that he'd been hospitalized over the previous weekend with chest pains, and extensive testing had revealed a coronary artery that was 90 percent blocked. Blood tests measured his cholesterol at a dangerous 270, with a low level of protective HDLs.

Mike's moment of truth had come: He now *had* to lose weight, but in a different way from how he ever had before. Now he had to change his lifestyle permanently in order to lower his cholesterol, strengthen his body, and hopefully reverse the blockage without surgery.

Mike came to me because he just didn't know what to do. In the past, either diets he'd tried had failed him or he had failed at them. Deep down he knew they had all been unhealthy. But was it possible to lose weight, keep it off, and restore his health at the same time?

Susan had some of the same questions. Her fit-and-trim appearance was the envy of all her friends. They assumed it was easy for her; she must just be naturally thin. They never really saw her eating; but then, she was always a bit tired, but who wouldn't be with a schedule like hers?

What Susan's friends didn't know is that staying thin wasn't "natural" or easy for her, and never had been. They didn't know that she kept pictures of herself at a plump age of twelve on the refrigerator and bathroom mirror to remind her of what she never wanted to look like again. And she hadn't backtracked—but it had taken a lot of working out and a lot of dieting.

And I do mean diet. Susan sat with me and ticked off her dieting history. A bout of mono served as her first "diet" at age thirteen and gave her enough of a boost to show her she *could* be thin, and that she liked it—*a lot*. It also showed her that starving was her best bet for weight loss. But headaches stopped that several years ago. So she turned to her own version of every popular diet to come down the pike.

It started with protein shakes in college, then Fit for Life, then a vegetarian diet, then a no-fat diet.... Susan wouldn't just go "on" the various diets, she would adopt them as a way of life. What she ate depended on which diet she was on at the time.

It was the confusing array of new high-protein diets that brought her to me, seeking my direction on which one would be best for her, a vegetarian, to boost her immunes and keep her weight down. She ended her story with, "I'm so tired, and I get sick so easily, so I'm thinking the high-protein diet might be good for me, but is it what I need?" She was too weary to decide on her own anymore.

But it was the letter I received from Brenda that summed up the dilemma, confusion, and entrapment of a nation:

Pam,

What *am I doing wrong? I try to eat the right foods and I exercise, but my weight is higher than it's ever been. At fifty-two, I weigh forty pounds more than I did at thirty-two. Sure, I know it's been a stressful number of years. There's been work to do, a family to tend to, spiritual needs, emotional demands. It's hard to be "good" all the time, but I've never been what I'd consider a big overeater. So why do I seem to gain weight so easily?*

Diets are not the answer for me—I've gone on enough of them through the years, and I know better. I've probably lost a sum total of 200 pounds, but I've gained back 210! Yet I have to admit, going on a crash diet is so tempting to me right now. Especially one of the high-protein/low- or no-carbohydrate ones that EVERYONE seems to be on. I've read some of the stuff—and have seen shows from Oprah! *to* 20/20 *to* Larry King Live. *I'm so confused—maybe eating carbohydrates is the problem. I know they're good for you and will probably make you live longer—but will they make you live longer* fatter?

I watch my friends who are on the hot diets eating steak cooked in butter and loading up on bacon and eggs, and I think, "How can people eat that way?" Yet, they are losing weight—no doubt about it.

Pam, I don't know what to do. Maybe we're supposed to weigh more as we get older. Maybe our Baby Boomer struggle is to try to hold tight to some image of our youth—and have it enshrined in thinness. Or maybe that's a cop-out, and I'm just giving up. I'm so confused. Can you help me make sense of all this?

Brenda

Millions of Americans are crying out just like Brenda. They want a thin and healthy body, but that body seems to be an impossible dream.

More than 120 million people each year report going on a weight loss diet. And, on any given day, about one-third of all adult women (30 million!) are desperately trying to lose weight, searching for the magic diet or workout that will catapult them to their ideal body.

They try everything to lose weight, no matter what the cost: high-protein diets, high-carbohydrate diets, food-combining diets, expensive weight-loss programs, drinks, potions, pills, herbs, spas, fasting, and feasting. And they do lose weight—some lose quite a lot. But the vast majority also gain it back, and with a vengeance—most with more than they lost, and most, with more fat than they started with. Many more simply fail to lose any weight at all.

The puzzle is this: How come one person can go on a diet, get rid of fat, and keep it off easily, while *nine* others get caught in a never-ending chain of disappointing diets that lead to despair and defeat? The odds are exactly that overwhelming—nine to one—that people who have lost weight on a diet will gain it back within a year. In fact, follow-up records of virtually every diet program indicate that one-third to one-half of dieters gain back even more weight than they lost.

THE AMERICAN WEIGH?

No doubt about it: Dieting is a national obsession—and problem. The United States is by far the fattest country in the world; the prevalence of overweight people has increased by 20 percent in twenty years. In 1962, 12.8 percent of Americans were obese; in 1980 it was 14 percent. Now, 22.5 percent are obese and more than 50 percent are overweight. On average, we eat 7 percent more calories than we did twenty years ago. Even the nation's children are pudgy; 25 percent—one quarter of them—are overweight. A 1998 Harris Poll found that 76 percent of adults were heavier than recommended for their height and body frame. In the late seventies, that figure was only 46 percent. The latest estimate is that 97 million Americans are overweight and most of them want to lose the excess poundage. Even more of them go on a diet each year, whether they need to or not.

How is all this weight gain possible in a country that spends billions each year on attempts to slim down? The U.S. Department of Agriculture surveyed American eating habits a few years ago and determined that only 12 percent of us have a healthy diet. And making a change—any change—is tough. Some have become so discouraged that they do nothing at all regarding their weight. A major poll in 1998 found that although 58 percent of Americans wanted to lose weight, only 46 percent were seriously trying. Why try again—only to fail?

This was where Sandy was when she came to see me for nutritional counseling. She started our meeting with "I'm forty-something and feel as if I've been fighting a war against my body for forty-something years. I think I've tried every diet created. I've swallowed pills, taken shots, and eaten carefully formulated foods and powders. I've fasted and drunk protein shakes. I've prayed and been prayed for. I've spent untold amounts of money on weight-loss programs guaranteed to work. And they do work. Actually I can lose weight quite easily—but not nearly as easily as I can gain it back!"

Sandy's most recent diet had resulted in a rapid loss of sixty-five pounds—down to the thinnest she'd ever been. She had been motivated by the invitation to her twenty-five–year high school reunion, and with dieting helping her to feel thin and beautiful, she had walked proudly through the door. Unfortunately, she broke the diet that night and continued to eat and overeat the rest of the weekend. As with any fad diet, Sandy gained back five pounds almost immediately. Then came a vacation, followed closely by Christmas. She gained back the entire sixty-five pounds within five months.

That was a year ago. Sandy finally mustered up the gumption to try again—and started the Carbohydrate Addict's Diet after seeing the book's authors on a number of TV talk shows. She lost fourteen pounds in four weeks. But then Thanksgiving arrived, and she broke the diet—but just for that one day, of course. And now, three weeks later, Sandy was sitting across from me, having already gained back the full fourteen pounds. She was desperate.

Sandy's story could be the story of countless numbers of discouraged people just like her. A measure of our discouragement is how we suspend our good sense and do some pretty outrageous things, falling for some incredibly ludicrous schemes to lose weight. Americans spend $40 to $60 billion a year on the diet and weight-loss industry—and that dollar figure is increasing every year. The desperate search for *how to do it*—this time—usually ends with a headfirst fall into a new diet plan or scheme, or a revisit to an old (failed) one.

Yes, diet mania is alive and well today—even though statistics show again and again that diets never have and never will be effective on a long-term basis. Diet programs abound, complete with lots of advertising and many faithful followers armed with before-and-after pictures. There is a virtual weight-loss smorgasbord from which to choose our next diet: celebrity authors, diet doctors, model spokespersons, multilevel product plans in mall kiosks—even at churches. More than just a weight-loss game alone, there are diets to combat hypoglycemia, diets to prevent aging, diets to cure chronic fatigue and arthritis. There are high-protein/low-carbohydrate diets and low-protein/high-carbohydrate diets—sometimes written by the same author!

Diets and their teachings bounce us back and forth like pinballs between this and that. They get cycled and recycled. As soon as one generation forgets the worthless and dangerous diets of the past, out comes a "new-and-improved," "revolutionary" version with a new name. Many of these deceptive diets have been used and overused so much that they've even been accepted as good nutrition. We're bombarded with mixed messages. On the one hand, we hear the depressing statistics about diets being ineffective, unhealthy, about their even making us fatter. On the other, those before-and-after pictures in advertisements and infomercials seem too good to ignore.

This is the essence of the diet trap: We are sucked dry by life, fall headfirst into overeating and unhealthy choices, and are seduced into the newest diet that will show us how to regain control of our weight, our image, and our lives. But the diet ends up controlling us instead. Our hopes are misplaced, our road a dead end. For most of us, no amount of dieting or exercise will give us the physique of models and movie stars—it's an unattainable goal.

But exercise and better nutrition *are attainable.* Anyone can improve his or her health by exercising and eating well, even if that person doesn't become thin. Losing weight can be good for a person, but only if it's done in a healthy way. A lot of people, despite dieting, weigh more now than they ever have. Is it what they eat? Partly. Is it heredity? Yes, that's also important. But the secret to permanent weight loss lies elsewhere—it is being set free from the diet trap and embarking on a lifestyle of wellness. Until we are ready to go beyond dieting and look at the real issue—the way we live—then fatigue, unhealthy living, overeating, and being overweight will continue to have a powerful grip on our lives.

DESTINED FOR FAILURE

I've always proclaimed that the word "diet" is the original four-letter word. Think about it: The very word is spelled D-I-E-T, just a letter away from the word *die*. And that's how you feel when you're on a diet—as if you are going to die! This is one big reason why diets are bound to fail.

Diets are all about denial—focusing on what you can't eat. The temporary deprivation cries out for a nice reward. Going "on" a diet to go "off" the diet, being "good" to be "bad," eating "legal" foods only to "cheat"—all this leaves us exhausted, unhealthy, and usually unsuccessful. People feel guilty about eating unhealthy "bad" food. Yet their biggest nutritional mistake is not what they *do* eat; it's what they *don't* eat. They don't choose nourishing foods, and they don't eat the right foods in the right balance at the right time. Their eating is sporadic and erratic until, driven by hunger and low blood sugar, they choose the very foods they are struggling to avoid. Even when their diets are high in protein, if whole carbohydrates are lacking, the nutritional imbalance ultimately brings failure.

Physiologically and in some ways psychologically, dieters are no different from people who are starving. Like water and air, food is necessary for life. Obsessive behavior over weight and dieting creates all sorts of havoc that even health care professionals don't fully understand. For example, normal eaters will decrease their food intake after a high-calorie meal. Yet, in one study, when dieters were given just one high-calorie meal, they immediately felt the diet was over and began to overeat, even to gorge. The dieting had put them into a state of deprivation that triggered a physiological and emotional drive to eat, and overeat. Their metabolism, moreover, had moved into a "store" rather than "burn" path, so that what they ate was much more damaging. How many times has that happened to you?

It's happened to me a lot. Like many of you, I grew up with dieting as my second language—a bona fide member of the Dieting
Generation. And with good reason: I inherited a tendency toward
being overweight and had a family filled with compulsive overeaters
and obesity. By the time I was eleven I had already gone on my first
diet, an awful grapefruit and poached egg diet (it was called the
Mayo Clinic diet, but did not originate there—nor has any stamp of
approval from this respected medical and research institution ever
been given). Was I overweight at the time? Not really. But I was
growing and at the start of menses, and my body shape was changing. My hips simply didn't conform to the popular "Twiggy" look of
the day. Add to that an unhealthy dose of fear about my family's obesity problems, and I fell headlong into the diet trap.

I lost weight at first. But, sadly, I regained it—more than I had
lost. It was the classic story: I lost five pounds only to gain that five
and raise it three. The next year, on the next diet (five days of
spinach and orange juice!), I lost ten pounds, and quite quickly
gained fifteen. The pendulum was swinging higher and wider each
year with each new diet. All the dieting was doing was leaving me
a malnourished mess, yet weighing more and more. I spent half of
my time discouraged and depressed—and the other half overeating
to compensate.

In the last semester of my senior year at Florida State University,
I got a wake-up call. I was anxious to graduate and take on the world
of fashion design and marketing. I needed a class to fill a core
requirement for my chosen field and stumbled on a class in nutrition. I was on one of my many diets at the time—lose-five-pounds-
in-five-days-for-a-weekend-beach-party crash diet. It was straight
out of the newest diet book on the block, *Dr. Atkins' Diet Revolution*,
and it was working great! I had actually shown a loss of twelve

pounds in seven days! It was miraculous... and definitely the way I was going to eat for the rest of my life.

But then, sitting in this nutrition class in the early seventies, I was amazed to learn of the damage I was doing to my body by following this diet and all the others, by my naiveté and drive for thinness at any cost. And, like all crash dieters, I was paying a high price—poor health, mood swings, and a body that was yo-yoing between fat and lean. I was an "expert" dieter, but I didn't have a clue what I was doing. While taking the course, I began to understand that I knew precious little about health. I had not been taught—I had only been mentored by diet doctors and gurus who had become successful by selling quick ways to lose weight, not telling the truth about caring for the *whole* body.

After an emotional seesaw and much deliberation, I changed my major to nutrition. It was the first thing in my life that I really felt passionate about—I had to help others learn what I was learning and break free from the diet trap right along with me. That decision changed my life—and changed my dieting ways. I never went on a diet again.

WHOLE-BODY WELLNESS

As I learned more about nutrition and began to take care of my physical body, I was able to lose weight and, for the first time, gain health and energy. My nails became strong and long, my hair was shiny and full, my eyes were clear and sparkling. I no longer got headaches every day, nor did I sit on the cliff-line of depression. I could think clearly—even studying was less of a chore. I grew in understanding of why I did what I did, and why I didn't do the things I wanted to do when it came to self-care and healthy eating.

I have now been living this life of wellness and teaching it for twenty-two years. Throughout my years of nutritional and behavioral counseling, people have come to me seeking a quality of life filled with energy and well-being. Many people have knocked on my door because they want to lose weight for good. Some need to manage stress better. Some want more energy. Others arrive very ill, in need of a nutritional plan to control serious disease—even to save their lives.

I started my nutrition practice as a Registered Dietitian for a progressive hospital's oncology unit—working with very brave patients and their families to fight their cancer with every means available. These challenging days led me into private practice working with people seeking wellness, helping them to get well and live well today, while focusing on preventing the diseases of tomorrow.

Early in my practice I sensed that, like my dieting college self, most of my clients needed simple nutritional education and guidance. They needed to be led beyond the cultural diet deceptions and myths to a true understanding of holistic health and nutrition. Rather than finding out what they *shouldn't* eat, they needed to learn what they *should* eat, when to eat, and how to balance their intake in a way that would benefit their bodies. My clients needed to learn how to break away from the typical American eating style while still living a normal lifestyle. And they needed to learn the vital part food plays in their well-being.

Different from the run-of-the-mill physicians and programs, I worked with my clients in a very focused, time-intensive manner. The foundation of their lifestyle changes was individual and practical. In 1985 I developed *The Smart Weigh*—a seven-week plan of practical education and lifestyle direction. Since then, over 12,000 people have followed the program—and hundreds of thousands more have adopted the principles found in my books: *Eat Well-Live Well*, *Food for Life*, and *The Energy Edge*.

The first step in *The Smart Weigh* plan was a lifestyle assessment and blood work profile that helped me to learn about a client's health and weight history, eating and self-care patterns, and current nutritional status. From this information I could develop an educational and meal plan to fit within a person's lifestyle and preferences. Weekly sessions and consultations helped the person to adopt the newly learned principles and adapt them into habits.

As my clients put these principles into practice, most succeeded in achieving their goals: more energy, leaner bodies, weight loss and management, lower cholesterol, and stress resiliency—all direct benefits of the new way of eating and living. They began to learn how to maintain those goals for life. Their success was contagious, and the principles of *The Smart Weigh* overflowed to their friends and family.

And so, I offer you too a word of hope: *The Smart Weigh*—and its principles revealed in these pages—provides a plan for nourishing your body with the right foods at the right time, and for dealing with what's eating you. It will allow the healing and repair—the natural ability to lose weight that is scripted into every cell of your body—to flow through your being. It works because, quite simply, it's how we were created. Whatever our need of the moment—losing weight, gaining weight, controlling overeating, getting well—the goal is to learn how to get our body working for us and with us.

In this book, I have tried to break down a complex subject into seven simple principles. These principles are expressed in my *Smart Weigh* plan in Parts 3 and 4. They will equip you to plan your own proper balance of nutrients at each meal, according to the foods you like, and to develop a lifestyle that will propel you towards your goals.

If weight loss—even weight gain or just maintenance—is what you are seeking, I want to help you attain it. But I'm not interested just in weight management, or your hormones, or your heart, or your gut—I'm interested in your *whole* body and soul. Change in one area shouldn't have to compromise the vibrancy of another. Just the opposite. That's why the information you will receive from this book is different from most. It's not a tunnel-vision view toward one goal at the expense of all others. Rather, it is designed to help you achieve whole-body wellness.

NO QUICK FIXES

The amount of personal pain among those striving to be something they cannot be is enormous. It impacts everything they do, everything they see. The effects of the stress and depression are impossible to evaluate.

Perhaps for you it's not so serious, it's just time to get in control of your waistline and back into last year's shorts. Sure you know that a healthy, lower-fat eating plan may be the right way to lose weight, but you don't really have a serious weight problem—you just need a quick fix! People that have a real problem with weight and overeating need to focus on long-term answers. But a slew of *New York Times* best-sellers are delivering quick results to people all around you. And, if they didn't work, they wouldn't be flying off the shelves, right?

Right. They *are* working; they *do* deliver quick results. But are they wise? A fast-acting diet is not your answer, whether you have eight pounds to lose or eighty. But you do need an answer, and that is why I've written this book.

Diets are confusing and robbing us of our health, wealth, and wellness. In a day when health care costs are immobilizing our country's economy, we see a huge segment of our population selling U.S. health to fad diets and diving headfirst into disease.

I say *ENOUGH*! It's simply time to clear the confusion—to cast a vote for new ways and a new weigh. It's time to get freed from the diet trap—for life.

CHAPTER 2 ■ The Top Seven Diet Myths

Don't think you are necessarily on the right track just because
it's a well-beaten path.

—ANONYMOUS

Afriend swears that by cutting out all wheat from her diet she
dropped ten pounds almost instantly. Another woman over-
hears her, tells her friend, who tells her coworkers. One of them
sends it out to his Internet address book... and that's how diet
myths are born.

Unfortunately, buying into half-truths about weight loss is as
dangerous as jumping out of a plane with an unchecked parachute—
and no sky-diving lessons.

This is the boring, unchangeable truth about losing weight: *A
pound of fat equals approximately 3,500 calories. If you eat 500 fewer calories a day, at the end of a seven-day week, you can lose a pound. If you exercise away another 500 calories a day, together with cutting your calorie
intake, you could lose two pounds of fat by the end of the week.*

Anyone who tells you that you can lose more fat than this is misleading you—whether they intend to or not. Even if you could, it
would be dangerously unhealthy. Oh sure, the scale can go down a
lot quicker than one to two pounds a week on a fad diet—that's
what makes them so attractive. But the extra pounds being stripped

away are simply the fluid being temporarily purged from your cells and the muscle mass that follows. Not the fat. (I'll explain all this in detail in Chapter 3.)

The bottom line: A human baby produces a certain number of fat cells, depending on genetics and how he or she is fed. The baby never loses these cells, and the body can add more if overfed for an extended period of time. It appears that the more fat cells we have, the hungrier we feel; they are continually signaling the brain to feed them. If we drastically cut our food intake by going on an unbalanced fad or semistarvation diet, our bodies slip into famine mode. Our metabolism slows down, using fewer calories than usual for the same activities, putting our fat cells into the "store" mode. This is why there are plateaus in dieting (which occur in even healthy, sensible weight loss). The body is working hard to maintain weight for survival. It is also why weight is regained so quickly when the diet is over. The body reads that the time for feasting is here, and it had better "stock up" fat in the cells to prepare for the next famine.

WHO DO I BELIEVE?

One reason it may be so easy to accept diet myths is that health and diet advice is always changing. If you believe every sensational headline, it can seem that way.

Most of us simply don't like sound nutritional advice. In focus groups people complain that the advice makes them feel guilty, angry, and confused. They don't want to take the time to keep track of a diet and are confused over nutritional guidelines: a food that is praised today may be trashed tomorrow. That accusation is understandable. A nutritional message is sometimes difficult to decipher and to follow. For example, consumers tend to interpret "low fat" as meaning "no fat," an unachievable—and undesirable—standard.

Getting 25 to 30 percent of your calories from fat is considered a sensibly low-fat diet by mainstream nutritionists—but to many fat-phobic teens, it is a fat gorge.

What is unchangeable is how changeable medical science is. It's constantly evolving and growing, and so of course the medical advice is constantly being modified. Reliable advice must be based on good science, and good science means continuing research that utilizes ever more refined methods for arriving at the truth. Diet myths remain the same year after year because they are based on wishful thinking, not on solid research. So untruths can stick, year after year, and even become public health beliefs. We'll explore all these myths, truths, and half-truths thoroughly in the next chapter, but for now keep in mind these warning signs of a bad diet.

WARNING SIGNS OF A BAD DIET

1. FORBIDDEN FOODS. Any diet that restricts or cuts out whole food groups is guaranteed to cause problems. Not only will the deprivation lead to binges; it cuts out exposure to essential nutrients and nutraceuticals (pharmacological agents in food that are vital for vibrant living). Although choices need to be made wisely, all types of real food fit into a healthy diet.

2. VERY LOW CALORIES. A normally active woman trying to lose weight should consume no fewer than 1,500 calories per day. A normally active man trying to lose weight should consume no fewer than 1,800 calories per day.

3. SPEEDY RESULTS. For healthy, permanent weight loss, you should aim to lose no more than one to two pounds per week.

4. NO EXERCISE. A healthy weight loss plan should encourage at least thirty minutes of moderate-intensity exercise four to five days per week.

5. INFREQUENT MEALS. It's best to eat before you get intensely hungry. For most people, that's at least every three to four hours.

Here is a brief rundown on some dieting myths that have become mainstream beliefs about nutrition in our culture.

MYTH NO. 1:
High-protein diets help you drop pounds fast!

REALITY: If you're on a high-protein plan that limits carbohydrates, you may appear to lose weight more quickly because your body is dumping a lot of water weight. This happens for three reasons. First, you are cutting out sweets and refined starches. They are triple threats—loaded with fat, sugar, and calories (more on this later). Second, when total carbohydrate intake is low, the body must turn to the stored carbohydrate supply (known as glycogen) for energy. Since these molecules are bound with water, the water is released to provide fuel when the glycogen stockpiled in the muscles and liver is burned. And third, excess protein, unlike carbs, must pass through the kidneys, which need to draw additional water from tissues to flush out the protein waste products. So all that water you excrete shows up on the scale as lost pounds. But that loss is temporary, as you'll see the moment you return to your normal eating habits.

And of course, high-protein fare holds risks and dangers. Diets heavy in animal protein—meats, dairy, even poultry—are linked to higher incidences of colon cancer, kidney disease, and osteoporosis. A lot of evidence exists showing that the body has to work extra hard to process the protein that it doesn't need, and those waste products open the door to disease. That's a big concern when considering the current popularity of high-protein diets. An even bigger concern is robbing your body of precious whole carbohydrates that more than twenty years of research have proved to prevent disease and promote wellness and longevity.

Read more about these deceptive high-protein diets on page 30.

MYTH NO. 2:

Carbohydrates pack on the pounds.

REALITY: You can gain weight by eating carbohydrates *only if you overeat them.* Whole-food carbohydrates in the least processed form—harvested grains, fruits, or vegetables that have been prepared without destroying their nutritive value or fiber—are vital fuel for your body. These complex carbohydrates are broken down slowly during digestion, gradually and steadily releasing glucose into the system to be burned. But refined carbohydrates—complex carbohydrates that have been stripped of their fibers and most of their vitamins, minerals, and phytochemicals, such as white bread and pasta, crackers, and cookies can add to your weight by creating chemical gymnastics in your body that may increase your appetite and your craving for fuel. Refined carbohydrates break down quickly during digestion and are almost immediately released into the bloodstream to be metabolized—leaving your body's efficiency on a high/low roller coaster.

Whole-food carbohydrates can actually aid in weight loss because their fiber satisfies you longer—a sure way to curb cravings. In addition, fiber-filled foods are nutrient-rich, contributing to overall body wellness. But the simple truth is that when you exceed the amount of calories your body needs to maintain your weight, everything is fattening. The portion size is often your biggest enemy. It may be wise to measure what you eat against the recommended servings—and serving sizes.

Read more about low-carbohydrate diets on page 30.

MYTH NO. 3:

Eating certain combinations of food helps you lose weight.

REALITY: This concept does only one thing: it helps to sell diet books. The body has a very efficient digestive system, and no matter what combination of foods you consume, it will disassemble them naturally and digest them equally. The digestive system is not a trash compactor! What goes in first doesn't have to be digested before what follows. In addition, proteins and carbohydrates are primarily digested in different spots anyway—they don't interfere with each other's breakdown. Eating them together does not cause weight gain or gas, unless you are eating large quantities of fat and refined starch. Avoiding one and eating the other at a meal just throws off the balance of nutrients, forces dehydration, and makes the scale artificially drop. If the diet eliminates even more foods with important nutrients, such as dairy products (which provide valuable calcium), the ensuing unbalanced eating can be even more hazardous to your health.

Read more about deceptive food-combining diets on page 44.

MYTH NO. 4:

To drop pounds, simply cut all fat from your diet.

REALITY: Not only is this statement untrue, following the advice can actually backfire on the would-be dieter. An insufficient intake of fat not only throws hormones out of whack, but also appears to slow metabolism (how many calories we burn per minute to fuel our essential bodily functions). Drastically low fat intakes also appear to turn on the appetite thermostat for fat by triggering the release of the fat-craving hormone, galanin. Taking in a moderate amount of fat is actually more effective in speeding weight loss than banishing fat altogether.

Low-fat diets became a big nineties fad when people started replacing fat with highly refined, high-sugar/fat-free products, and lots of them. The truth is, the road to health and weight management is not paved with fat-free brownies. "Eat anything as long as it's fat free" is no more healthy or smart than "eat anything as long as it doesn't contain carbohydrates."

Read more about the dangers of no-fat/high-carbohydrate diets on page 42.

MYTH NO. 5:

You don't have to exercise to lose weight.
REALITY: Actually, it is possible to lose weight by following a sensible diet and limiting calories without working out. But it's not a good idea. Records of dieters show that weight loss is maintained only when a routine of exercise continues after the calorie limitation has ended. In addition, exercise helps to preserve and build lean muscle mass during the weight loss, and more muscle leads to boosted metabolism, even when the body is at rest. What's more, exercise is simply good for you, head to toe.

MYTH NO. 6:

You can lose weight safely and effectively by using weight-loss drugs, herbal supplements, and "superfoods."
REALITY: You've seen advertisements promising that you can lose weight without changing what you eat one single bit. *You can even eat more!*—and do it all, even build muscle—with *no exercise!* Why, basically, you can lose pounds while you sleep. Of course, the question of the day is, Where does it go? Are your sheets greasy when you wake up in the morning?

The lose-it-while-you-sleep hype has become a $6 billion-a-year business. Herbal supplements and power drinks for weight loss and energy are readily available in health food stores and even some gyms. They are widely used by bodybuilders and athletes, and recommended by trainers, friends, and multilevel marketers alike. Metabolife, Thermadrene, Blue-green Algae, Chromium Picolinate, Fat Trapper, Exercise in a Bottle, and DHEA are just a few of the popular products being hawked, and multilevel plans offer scads more. The products seem so natural, so safe, so *quick*, but most people aren't aware that some can have serious repercussions—and can even kill you.

It would be hard not to have heard about the Fen-Phen or Redux craze and fall for them. Those are just a couple of the many drugs still coming down the pike to help in the weight-loss battle. Many more medications will follow. But because they are drugs—with risks right along with potential benefits—they shouldn't be a first choice! Prescribed weight-loss drugs should be used only if you are likely to have eminent and serious health problems as a result of your weight—not just appearance problems. And they should only be used as part of an overall program that includes long-term changes in your eating and physical-activity habits.

MYTH NO. 7:
If a certain food tastes good, it's more than likely bad for you; and if it's good for you, it's going to taste like cardboard.

REALITY: Healthy eating is not a prison made of rice cakes! But if you feel this way, you have a lot of company. In a Gallup Poll commissioned by the American Dietetic Association, 56 percent of adults surveyed said they no longer found eating pleasurable because of their worries about fat, cholesterol, carbohydrates, and calories. Nearly half said they believe the foods they like are not good for them.

This may be why another public opinion survey in 1999 showed that although diet and nutrition is important to 85 percent of American adults and getting enough exercise is important to 84 percent of adults, only 41 percent feel they are doing all they can to achieve a healthy lifestyle. An unwillingness to forego favorite foods was the main reason cited for not doing more to achieve a balanced diet.

This myth is simply that—a myth. Eating well is not about giving up all the foods you love, it's about opening the door to a whole new world of fresh, flavorful, and fun foods that bring your body natural energy and healing.

THE BIGGEST MYTH OF ALL

The biggest myth of all is that fad diets work for the long term. Yet, convincing a disciple that his or her newest cure is doomed to failure is difficult at best. Body logic and nutritional science are no match for a good diet salesperson or convert especially after the first rush following the rapid water loss.

The truth is that all of these diets do work, for the short term. They show quick results on the scale. Believe me, you *will* lose weight on *any* diet that cuts your calories below what you burn. No matter how seductive the claim of the diet—NEW! MIRACLE! STRAIGHT FROM EUROPE! GROUND-BREAKING! REVO-LUTIONARY!—add up the calories and you'll see that you are losing weight for one reason: you are consuming fewer calories than before. Although you may be "allowed" by your diet to eat "as much as you want" of certain high-calorie foods—eggs Benedict (without the muffin), fried steak and gravy—there is a limit to how much you can eat for long. The fat fills you up, and you cut calories without counting them. But after you stop the diet, watch out! Because of the imbalance your body is left in, you don't have to eat more than before to gain back the pounds.

Forgive me, but let me say it one more time (and several more times throughout this book!): When you lose weight quickly on any fad diet, it's only because the diet has manipulated your carbohydrate and protein intake to cause quick dehydration. And that's only for the first two weeks. If you continue to lose more than one to two

HOW TO CREATE YOUR OWN FAD DIET

(Excerpted from www.faddiet.com)

NOTE: This is especially effective if you have a doctorate degree in something obscure like genealogy. That way you can call it the "Dr. Scardsmayo Diet." Follow this up with a book, and you'll be rich.

Here are the basic ingredients you will need to create your own fad diet:

1. A book that lists the nutritional values of every food under the sun.

2. A good idea about what foods the grocery store carries (so that you can include those it doesn't).

3. A bag of chips (you'll need a snack while you work).

4. No nutritional knowledge whatsoever.

5. A picture of someone who was slim five years ago, but is now larger. The larger person has to own an outfit that is at least ten years old.

6. Pick a promised weight reduction. Most people don't think they can lose more than four pounds per day, so keep it a little less than that, but be positive. Also, put an official sounding disclaimer in there for good measure. Here are some examples:

   ■ Lose up to 12 pounds in 3 days! (Actual weight loss ranges from 8 to 12 pounds depending on the person, their metabolism, and the digestibility of the potassium manganate encountered.)

   ■ I lost 13 pounds between Monday and Thursday and you can, too! (My experience may not be yours; however, I am a very average person who has never excelled at anything.)

   ■ Follow Dr. Jingleheimerschmidt's program and get down the pounds! (Consult a doctor before starting Dr. Jingleheimerschmidt's program, especially if you ever experience shortness of breath when climbing more than eight flights of stairs.)

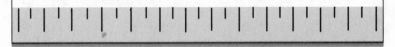

pounds per week, it's because the diet is turning for fuel to your muscle mass as well as fat. Although your body fat will be burned, you are losing a great deal of lean body tissue as well. This is because muscle is a more readily available fuel than fat, and when the body is being starved of carbohydrate energy, it turns to the most efficient source—protein, not fat.

The truth is that the only desirable kind of weight to lose is fat, never muscle. And the best way to restrict calories and control appetite is not by being tricked into it, but by learning how to eat to meet the demands of your body with the proper supply. Losing weight should really be considered "releasing weight," because you sure don't want to *find* the weight that you've lost!

Losing weight is best accomplished through a "leaning down" process that comes from a balanced intake of nutrients. Smart weight *release* occurs only when you (1) burn more calories than you take in, (2) fan the flame of your metabolism by eating strategically and exercising, (3) crack the code of the fat storage mechanism to put your body into a "burn" rather than "store" mode, and (4) change your perspective about the way you eat and live. To be set free from the diet trap, you must throw out your old belief systems and learn to separate fact from fiction.

I compare going on a fad diet to using throat lozenges for a strep throat infection. The throat pain you are soothing and the redness you might be reducing are symptoms of the real problem: a dangerous infection. It will persist, even become life threatening, until treated properly with antibiotics. Similarly, weight issues need to be addressed with *real* answers, not with temporary, feel-good, look-great-on-the-scale measures.

A BETTER CHOICE

The best diet? One that focuses on real foods that you like and can live with, one that is generous in complex carbohydrates, moderate in lean proteins, and light on fat. Eat small, balanced meal portions often throughout the day, drink water, and exercise.

Unlike the diet designers you may have followed or been taught by in the past, I emphasize eating, not starving or manipulating the body. The emphasis is not just on what to eat, but on how and when to best stabilize body chemistries, boost the metabolic burn, handle stress, and release your full energy. *The Smart Weigh* is a week-by-week building plan that enables you to function close to your peak in seven weeks: thinner, more fit, and equipped to continue on that positive road to your goals—for life.

Remember this: *You don't need to learn how to diet; you need to learn how to eat in a healthy way.* The strategies in the pages that follow will cut through controversies and diet teachings; they will change your perspective about the place of food, exercise, and rest in your life; and they will greatly enhance your understanding of your body.

You can take charge, feel better, have abundant energy from morning till night, and look more radiant and healthy. Forget the "miracles." Save your money, your time, and maybe even your life—do it *The Smart Weigh.*

Let's start by taking a closer look at the popular diet schemes of today. Armed with a thorough understanding of why they are dangerous and ultimately ineffective, you'll be able to protect yourself from being seduced by their empty promises.

CHAPTER 3 ■ Six Weight-Loss Schemes to Avoid

There is no right way to do a wrong thing.

—ANONYMOUS

S o what are the most popular destructive weight-loss schemes of our time? The variety is endless—all protein, or all carbs; all liquids, or all grapefruit; all eggs, or all cabbage soup. At times, it seems that the wackier the diet, the more the American public swallows the theory. It makes some people (the authors, diet businesses, or investors) very rich, while a lot of other people (those who follow them) get hurt. Any diet that focuses on one food group at the expense of others is unhealthy at best, downright dangerous at worst.

All quick weight loss diets boil down to being variations on six main themes (a.k.a. schemes) of deception: (1) the high-protein/low-carbohydrate diet; (2) the high-carbohydrate/low-fat diet; (3) the semistarvation diet; (4) the food combining diet; (5) the blood or body type diet; and (6) the "lose it while you sleep" diet. Many of these weight-loss schemes have come back from the seventies like bell-bottoms, just under a different name or new packaging. All work, *quickly*, by the same mechanism—throwing the body into a state of imbalance. This promotes sudden weight loss primarily from dehydration.

All fad diets are based on nutrients, not on foods. Specifically, fad diets are based on a manipulation of carbohydrates, protein, or fats. On any of these diet schemes, 10 percent of your body's fluid weight can be lost in just two weeks—which, depending on your weight, can fulfill the sensational promise—"Lose twenty-five pounds in twenty-five days!" If you weigh 210, it's not difficult to lose fifteen pounds in fourteen days. Even after the first two weeks, these diets will continue to make the scales go down (for the short term) by eating away at your valuable lean muscle tissue, which weighs more than fat. Over time, the waste products from your tissue breakdown will depress your appetite, so you'll continue to lose weight because you are eating less.

But the moment you "cheat" or stop the diet, the tide turns. Your body's survival mode turns your appetite on *high*, releasing galanin, a brain hormone that regulates your body's desire for fat. The higher your galanin level, the higher your craving for high-fat foods and the more fat you will store. You don't even have to gorge to regain weight; your sluggish metabolism will do that for you. Since you are burning calories at a slower, less efficient rate, a little overeating goes a long way. And sadly, the weight you gain back is water and fat, not muscle.

Years of this kind of dieting will leave you in terrible shape. With each loss/gain cycle, the percentage of lean muscle mass decreases and the percentage of fat increases. Eventually, you begin to deposit fat in new places, and finally diet yourself into a pumpkin shape! And your body will make it harder to lose weight each time you try, because your slower metabolism (due to the body's higher fat percentage) takes on a life of its own.

The reality is that your metabolism can be your greatest ally... or your worst enemy. If you've been an on-again, off-again dieter, the dieting itself could now be making you fat. Why? Because for every pound of fat you gain, your body burns just two calories a day at rest compared to an average of fifty calories for each pound of muscle. So if you lose five pounds of muscle mass on the latest high-protein/low-carbohydrate diet only to regain it as fat, you're burning 240 fewer calories a day. That's bad news for your body and your weight. And that's without considering the hazards and side effects of the fad diets themselves.

And the hazards are many. On an unbalanced diet, you do lose— you lose your health, your energy, your time, and your money. What you gain back is your weight—in spades. While being fat is not automatically the big problem in health, especially if you are fit, major studies have found that "yo-yo dieting" is downright bad for you. In a study of 11,000 Harvard graduates, researchers found that weight cycling adversely affects longevity. Rapid weight loss from extreme dieting has been shown to result in everything from high levels of blood cholesterol, decreases in memory and mental performance, irritability, depression, and altered reaction time, including deficits in hand-eye coordination that led one study to conclude that "driving while dieting" is hazardous!

Sure, you can lose ten pounds in ten days, shocking your body into dehydration and muscle cannibalism. But at the same time you also put a deadly strain on every organ in your body: your heart, liver, gall bladder, kidneys, and pancreas included. You can shed pounds—and shave years off your life.

How many diets do we have to go through before we figure out we've been misled, and that we're missing the real issue? Diet promoters need a new gimmick with the start of each new diet season, and you've got to give them credit for the job they do. It's not easy to come up with a dieting "revolution" every year! It's not easy to build a book around an old story, retold. But the real issue is not even touched, and it's the issue of our souls. For whatever reason, when life leaves us hungry and empty and looking for a quick fill, the bait is set for the diet trap. And then, when this doesn't fill the hole or slim the body, our wounded beings start looking for the next quick cure of body and soul.

THE SCHEMES UNMASKED
High-Protein/Low-Carbohydrate Diets

High-protein/low- to no-carbohydrate diets are like nuclear bombs—they really work, because they devastate everything. But they seem like such a dream—and a wonderful dream, at that. Eat bacon, steak, and butter to lose weight! After years of being steered toward a healthier intake of grains, fruits, and vegetables, finally a diet to cause meat-lovers to rejoice: cut out carbohydrates, eat high-fat protein (and a lot of it), and you'll lose weight. Voila!

Oh, there's a trade-off: none of those comfort foods like pasta, bread, or potatoes—and certainly no dessert. Oh, and there's one more trade-off: evidence that the odds of getting heart disease and cancer increase hasn't changed a bit. Such foods increase work for our kidneys, promote stones, and thin bones, increase gout, raise blood fats, and shorten life span. And because the lost weight comes back with a vengeance, these diets make us fat, fatter, and fatter still.

Today's protein-praising diets echo the popular regimens of the seventies. The big diet schemes then were six: *Dr. Atkins' Diet Revolution*, Dr. Stillman's *Quick Weight Loss Diet* (I lost my hair on this one!), Dr. Tarnower's *Scarsdale Diet*, the *I Love New York Diet*, the *Drinking Man's Diet* (I was grounded for a month on it), and Dr. Taller's *Calories Don't Count Diet*. Then along came protein powder diets: the *Cambridge Diet* and the *Last Chance Diet*. They are all marketing spins, twists, and turns, and hugely successful—at least for the companies behind them.

Atkins came back (with a NEW program, of course!), and a lot of other voices have joined the high-protein/low-carb choir: Drs. Michael and Mary Ann Eades are promoting *Protein Power*; H. Leighton Steward and company are touting *Sugar Busters!*; Richard and Rachel Heller are championing *The Carbohydrate Addict's Diet.* These diet books are seducing the public with almost unlimited amounts of meat, cheese, eggs, cream, and butter, while strictly limiting portions of carbohydrates such as grains, legumes, even some healthy fruits and vegetables.

The arguments that fuel these weight-loss schemes are based in half-truths that sound very convincing to the average person who isn't educated in nutritional science. Basically, they claim that when we ingest carbohydrates, our body turns them into sugar, stimulating the pancreas to release the hormone insulin, which accelerates the conversion of calories into fat. When we restrict or eliminate carbs, advocates say, our body will burn stored fat for energy and we'll lose weight.

Reality

Calling the latest fad diets high-protein may be somewhat of a misnomer. The average low-carbohydrate/high-protein dieter gets a whopping 50 percent of his or her calories from *fat*, upping the ante for long-term disease risk. This type of diet—high-protein; high-fat—has been linked to higher incidences of colon cancer and kidney disease. Many researchers have accumulated a lot of evidence showing that the body has to work extra hard to process protein that it doesn't need, and the waste products produced open the door to disease. The more protein you eat, the greater the risks.

Questions have also arisen about the link between eating too much protein and developing the bone-weakening disease osteoporosis. This may be because calcium, essential for strong bones, is drawn from the body along with excess protein in the urine. As protein intake increases, the amount of calcium excreted in the urine increases as well. This can be a problem if your calcium intake is low.

And, of course, skewing your diet toward protein is apt to lead you away from other important sources of nutrients, particularly plant-based foods and all their myriad of vitamins, minerals, and phytochemicals. Again, it's not just what you *are* eating, it's what you *aren't* eating that's the problem. Don't necessarily think of protein as the bad guy in the fight to lose weight; it's critical for metabolic boosting power. And studies have shown that it's better at suppressing hunger than carbs or fat, so eating enough of it (15 to 20 percent of your total calories) will help you stick to a reduced calorie meal plan when the going gets tough. And taking in protein with carbohydrates helps to regulate blood sugars. But packing in proteins at the expense of carbs can ultimately result in sluggishness and walk you right through the door of disease.

Researchers at Brigham and Women's Hospital and Harvard Medical School in Boston report that women who consume two to three servings of whole grains per day by eating foods such as whole wheat bread, oatmeal, or popcorn, reduce their risk of heart disease by almost 30 percent. By eating a sandwich with two slices of whole wheat bread (instead of just eating a hunk of meat), a woman will get the two servings of whole grains she needs to protect her heart. This, of course, would not be allowed on a high-protein/low- or no-carbohydrate diet.

As I've mentioned earlier, if you're on a high-protein plan that drastically cuts carbohydrates, you may appear to lose weight more quickly because your body is dumping a lot of water weight. Carbohydrates enter the body in the form of food—either in simple structures that are easily and quickly digested, or in more complex forms that require more time. Complex carbohydrates (starches) must first be broken down to short-chain molecules, and then those molecules and disaccharides (the food sugars) are further broken down to the monosaccharides glucose, fructose, or galactose, all of which are absorbed into the bloodstream as sugar. Fructose and galactose are absorbed a little more slowly and evenly than glucose, which serves as the body's prime fuel to the brain, lungs, and central nervous system. The body needs sufficient carbohydrates to maintain a certain level of glucose in the blood. To ensure an easily accessible supply of glucose, the body stores glucose in the muscles and the liver as glycogen.

If you are eating insufficient carbohydrates, these glycogen stores are broken down and converted to needed glucose. Glycogen molecules are bound with water, which is released as fuel when the glycogen is burned. Once the glycogen

ANOTHER PROTEIN DANGER

Data collected over a fourteen-year period from over 88,000 women enrolled in the Nurses' Health Study indicate that women who eat large quantities of beef, pork, or lamb may be at higher risk for non-Hodgkin's lymphoma (NHL), a cancer of the lymph system. Eating larger quantities of trans-unsaturated fats, as found in margarine, partially hydrogenated vegetable oils, and baked goods, also appears to be associated with a greater risk of that cancer.

After adjusting their analysis for age and other risk factors, the researchers found that women who had a main meal of beef, pork, or lamb daily were more than twice as likely to develop NHL than those who had such meals less than once a week. Women who consumed more trans-unsaturated fats were more likely to develop NHL than those who ate little of this type of fat.

The researchers noted that the major findings from this study are consistent with nutritional guidelines for other chronic diseases, such as colon cancer and heart disease. These findings appear to be "one more reason to eat right," reducing red meat and trans-unsaturated fats, and increasing fruits and vegetables in the daily diet.

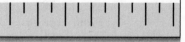

reserves are used up, the body will turn to muscle protein to synthesize glucose for vital body functions. It turns first to muscle rather than fat tissue because the body's fat stores cannot be converted to necessary glucose. Fat can be used as an energy source, but not to aid the functions of the brain or central nervous system, and it is also less desirable because only 10 percent of fat can be converted to energy compared to protein's 48 percent. The remaining components have to be excreted as waste products. At this point the metabolism begins to slow down to protect your valuable muscle mass, and the body becomes very efficient at functioning on less fuel. As your metabolism slows, it's a no-brainer to figure out why the weight comes back, surely and steadily, the minute you deviate from the diet.

What about the role of insulin? Eating food (in some cases, even just seeing or thinking about food) will signal the brain to release insulin into the bloodstream. Insulin is a hormone produced by the pancreas that is necessary for carbohydrate metabolism. It is the "key" that unlocks the body's cells to allow sugars to enter the cells and be burned for energy. Insulin influences the way we metabolize foods, determining whether we burn fat, protein, or carbohydrates to meet our energy needs—ultimately determining whether we will store fat. It's true that after eating carbs, insulin levels rise and allow the unused carbs to be stored as fat or glycogen, but that's only part of the equation. Several hours after eating, insulin levels fall and the stored fat or glycogen is released from the cell and used for energy.

Insulin is vital to well-being; but an overproduction of insulin can create an imbalance associated with weight gain, high blood fats, high blood pressure, and even insulin resistance, a precursor to diabetes for those genetically inclined. An overproduction of insulin and insulin surges occur when the system is hit with a calorie over-

SO WHY DOES BREAD MAKE YOU FAT?

Does it? A guy at the office swears he dropped pounds just cutting out bagels. Your neighbor insists that bread makes her bloated. Your sister won't go near any bread at all; she's determined that she's allergic to it—or to wheat.

Bread has a bad rap. But it's not the guilty party; at least, not *all* types are. Bread is a great source of energizing complex carbohydrates and is loaded with heart-healthy fiber and essential vitamins and minerals. A typical slice is low in fat (1 to 2 grams) and can contain 2 to 3 grams of fiber. But the term "bread" is a catch-all word, including calorie-packed high-fat items like muffins, biscuits, and croissants. And any bread can become a fat trap if you slather it with high-fat spreads like butter and cream cheese.

You can see that all bread is not created equal in calories—or nutrition. Any bread made from plain white flour can call itself "wheat" bread, but only those that list "100 percent whole wheat" (having whole-wheat flour as their first ingredient) are high-fiber, healthier breads. Breads that are made from whole-wheat flour naturally contain fiber, vitamins B6 and E, folic acid, copper, magnesium, manganese, zinc—and forty-one other nutrients. Again, these vital nutrients are processed out of white flour, and even though most bread is "enriched," only thiamin, niacin, riboflavin, iron, and folic acid are added back.

Take a look at these numbers:

BREADS	Calories	Fat
croissant	300	17
doughnut	280	12
toaster corn muffin	120	12
bagel	250	2
English muffin	140	2
1 slice whole wheat bread	70	.5

TOPPINGS (per tablespoon)		
butter	99	10.5
margarine	90	10.5
regular cream cheese	90	9
fat-free cream cheese	10	0

By the way, although many popular diet books would have you believe the world has a wheat allergy, it is an extremely uncommon allergy. Only 1 to 2 percent of adults suffer from any kind of food allergy, and wheat allergies are rare. The symptoms are not what is often listed on "allergy checklists" (bloating, lethargy, cravings); the symptoms of a wheat allergy are severe: hives, swollen lips, difficulty breathing. Gluten intolerance, also know as celiac disease, causes the body's immune system to attack the small intestine as if it were an invader. This condition is still rare, affecting just one-half of 1 percent of the population.

load—eating too much at one time—and when the body accumulates fat weight. The fat-stuffed cell is resistant to insulin, meaning
that as people gain fat weight there are fewer active insulin receptors on the cell—and those don't work as well. Essentially the over-
stuffed fat cell locks down, preventing fat from being burned. And
the more fat you gain, the more insulin the body produces to force
those insulin receptors into action. The more insulin, the easier it is
to gain weight.

This explains why weight gain can often seem like a runaway
train: the more you gain, the easier it is to gain. But this whole cycle
of elevated insulin and insulin resistance can be turned around.
Healthy weight loss (losing body fat) promotes the creation of new,
more efficient insulin receptors. And insulin levels can be lowered
through eating small, frequent meals, exercising, and preventing
nutrient overload (not eating too much at any one time).

The fad diets that promise weight loss by lowering insulin levels
are based on a faulty theory: that high levels of insulin cause a rise in
fat weight. In fact, it's the other way around: excess fat causes insulin
levels to rise. If we overconsume calories beyond what our body can
burn for energy or store as glycogen, the energy will be ushered into
the fat cell to be stored as fat rather than into the muscle to be burned
as fuel. Overconsuming *any* form of calories will result in fat storage.
There is no scientific justification for the claim that healthy people
who eat foods high in sugars will automatically gain weight.

It's true that some foods, such as refined carbohydrates, can contribute to weight gain by igniting chemical gymnastics in the body
that may increase appetite and spark cravings. And because refined
carbs are calorie-dense (few nutrients but lots of calories), they can
seem to "turn to fat." When refined carbohydrate intake is combined with a high intake of saturated fats, the ensuing dual mecha-

nism promotes fat storage: by suppressing the lipoprotein lipase enzyme which decreases the muscle cell uptake of energy. In a nutshell, when the calories that come from sugar-laden foods (often fat-laden as well) add up to more than the body can burn at the moment, calorie (or energy) storage occurs. This will be in the form of glycogen (stored glucose) until those stores are filled; the remaining energy will be converted to fat and stored that way.

Diet gurus, and even some scientists, still advise that carbohydrates in the diet are not ideal because any carbohydrate will make blood sugars and insulin levels rise. Much of this research comes from the study of the body's glycemic response to food—the impact that food choices and consumption have on blood sugar levels. Further research continues to reveal that certain foods, particularly refined carbohydrates, do cause a quicker rise in blood sugars than others, and a corresponding rush of insulin. But this can be avoided simply by choosing a different (whole) form of carbohydrate.

Carbohydrates have gotten a bad rap because they're all lumped together. But all carbohydrates are not created equal. The *types* of carbohydrates (and proteins and fats) chosen and the timing and the balance of when they are eaten is the key to healthy weight loss and maintenance. By choosing to eat right foods in the right balance at the right time, the metabolism is activated and blood sugars can be stabilized—and you get the sure reward of appetite control and weight management.

To live well and manage our weight we need a different way of eating—certainly different from that of the typical American. Although most of the world's population eats a high-carbohydrate diet based on whole-food staples such as rice, corn, fish, millet, soy, beans, and bread, not so the developed countries. In developing countries, carbohydrates may still contribute up to 70 to 80 percent

TOP 20 SOURCES OF CARBOHYDRATES IN THE AMERICAN DIET*

1. potatoes (mashed or baked)
2. white bread
3. cold breakfast cereal
4. dark bread
5. orange juice
6. banana
7. white rice
8. pizza
9. white pasta
10. muffins
11. fruit punch
12. Coca-Cola
13. apples
14. skim milk
15. pancakes
16. table sugar
17. jam
18. cranberry juice cocktail
19. french fries
20. candy

SOURCE: Dr. Simin Liu, Harvard University School of Public Health

*These data represent the findings of the Harvard Nurses' Health Study

of a person's calorie intake, but in Canada, the United Kingdom, Australia, and the United States, carbohydrates typically contribute only 40 to 45 percent of the calories consumed—and most of those are refined. Fats make up the rest of the calorie equation.

Let's face it: Our twenty-first century diet is too high in calories, saturated fats, and refined carbohydrates, which are digested and absorbed too quickly (causing a high insulin demand), and are too low in the right kinds of essential fat and whole foods that are absorbed slowly and evenly (allowing a proper insulin release). To make bad worse, our lifestyle is filled with stress, inactivity, and fad dieting, and sparse on exercise, rest, and self-care.

The key to burning excess fat is *not* simply to eliminate or restrict carbohydrates, but to restrict *all* forms of calories while keeping the body mentally and emotionally balanced and physically well nourished. This is best done with a restricted calorie plan that provides the right balance of carbohydrates, protein, and fats. Many weight-loss plans, in attempting to control glucose and insulin levels, will cut all carbohydrate intake drastically. That's because it's easier and quicker than educating people on the healthier approach of choosing carbohydrates and fats wisely throughout life.

A second reason people lose weight on high-protein diets is that excess protein, unlike carbs, must pass through the kidneys, which need to draw additional water from tissues to flush out the protein and fat waste products produced by abnormal fat metabolism. One of these waste products is ketones, produced from an abnormal breakdown of fat for energy, and they are a very inefficient energy source. They accumulate in the blood and lead to ketosis, a dangerous state of imbalance which causes the body to excrete valuable sodium and potassium. This can result in abnormal heart rhythms and further dehydration, which shows up *quickly* on the scale as lost pounds. During ketosis the body also retains uric acid, which can trigger gouty arthritis, gout, and kidney stones. The circulating ketones can also cause bad breath, frequent urination, interrupted sleep, constipation, nausea, general edginess, and lightheadedness.

Finally, there is that sneaky calorie restriction that explains any true weight loss from a high-protein diet: the high fat intake that accompanies the protein makes you less hungry, so you eat less. If you're cutting out sweets and refined, nutrient-empty, often high-fat foods, if you're eliminating high-calorie desserts, candies, chips, and baked goods, then chances are good you'll drop pounds and feel much better. The tendency to binge-eat is controlled as well because—think about it—are you really as likely to binge on steak or scrambled eggs and bacon as you are on ice cream, pizza, or brownies? It's not the magic of eating protein that's working as much as the elimination of calorie-packed junk foods. These changes are also what spark the dramatic short-term drops in cholesterol and triglycerides that you hear about. Blood fat levels do not miraculously drop because of eating high-fat proteins; they drop because of not eating refined flours and sugars.

Although you could live a lifetime without sweets and white breads, you won't live long or well without the healthy forms of carbohydrate; no one can sustain a diet without them. Eventually, your cravings win over but rather than steering you toward healthy brown rice, carrots, oats, or broccoli, you fall headfirst into nachos and chocolate chip cookies. This is not because you are weak, bad, or lack willpower; it's the way you were created. Your body is compensating when these diets self-destruct. It's not about your strength or your weakness; it's about survival.

But wait! Most people on these diets will tell you that they don't plan to avoid healthy whole grain carbohydrates and fresh fruits and vegetables for life—just until they lose a few pounds and tame this weight monster. *Then* they'll go back to healthier eating. Unfortunately, research, diet history, and human nature are not on their side. Studies show that after even a short stint with these diets, people rarely go back to healthier eating. And they cling to the erroneous belief that carbohydrates are their enemy. When they regain some of the fluid weight as quickly as they had lost it, it only seems to confirm that the fad diet was right: carbohydrates must be the problem. The crime about such teaching is that a distinction is not adequately made between healthy carbohydrates and unhealthy ones.

The Bottom Line

High-protein–high-fat/low- to no-carbohydrate diets *work* for short-term weight loss through (1) dehydration, (2) muscle breakdown, (3) cutting out calorie-laden sweets and refined starches, and (4) sneakily lowering your calories by keeping you somewhat nauseous and turned off to "all the protein and fat you can eat." These diets are also the *most* effective for weight gaining—go on one, lose a bit, and then regain in spades. What you don't regain is your muscle mass and your health.

WHAT ABOUT *THE ZONE*?

A diet book I am often asked about is *The Zone* by Barry Sears, Ph.D. We'll discuss it here with high-protein/low-carbohydrate diets, because that's what most people think it is. The truth is, it's not. It is *not* one of the dangerous fad diets revived from the seventies; rather, it is a carefully controlled low-calorie diet (the plan allows the average woman only 1,200 calories per day) with an extreme focus on getting an exact "balance" of carbohydrates (40 percent of daily calories), protein (30 percent of daily calories), and fat (30 percent of daily calories). *The Zone* made "40-30-30" a catchphrase among those who subscribe to Sears's claims.

Sears's program was a refreshing breeze for me when it was first released—finally a diet book had hit the best-seller list that actually discussed the need for a balance of protein *and* carbohydrates. It was quite a bit lower in healthy carbohydrates than I was comfortable with (40 percent of calories, compared to the needed 60 to 65 percent), but I was thrilled to get a national spotlight on the need for people, including athletes, to consume the dynamic duo of carbs and proteins. Although higher in fat than I recommend, it's actually a lower-fat plan for most Americans who are taking in 34 percent of their daily calories in the form of fat. If someone were going to go on a "diet," I would prefer they choose *The Zone*.

But the medical and scientific communities have criticized the claims made by Sears for the diet, rather than the diet itself. He puts the total blame for the fattening of America on high-glycemic carbohydrates that stimulate an overproduction of insulin. His remedy goes like this: just eat in the "Zone Blocks" (with the exact balance of 40-30-30 carb, protein, and fat) and you can prevent insulin surges and burn more fat.

Critics say there is no real evidence, just Sears's undocumented claims that excess insulin is the *main* factor in weight gain. The fact is, weight is gained simply because more calories are consumed than burned, regardless of where those calories come from. Sears practically flaunts the lack of traditional scientific proof in support of his run-away best-sellers, *Enter the Zone* and *Mastering the Zone*. Instead, he uses anecdotal accounts as the basis for his theories.

I believe that the body's hormonal response, including insulin surges, does play a part in weight gain, and controlling such surges plays a part in weight loss—but it's certainly not the whole picture.

High-Carbohydrate/Low-Fat Diets

In the early eighties, coming off the high-protein diet atrocities of the seventies, health authorities all over the world began to do research on the value of high-carbohydrate/low-fat diets and to make recommendations. Many people wisely heeded the advice—but they started replacing the fat in their diets with highly refined, high-sugar-and-starch, fat-free products, and lots of them. At the same time that fat-free products were flying off the shelves, the average intake of fat rose by 6 percent. Result: weight gain.

The road to health and weight management is not paved with fat-free brownies and white pasta. This "eat anything as long as it's fat-free" approach was no more healthy or smart than "eat anything as long as it doesn't contain carbohydrates." Once again, a pendulum swing resulted in an ever-fatter America, led by diet programs such as the Pritikin Program and the Duke University Rice and Fruit Diet of the early eighties, followed by Susan Powter's *Stop the Insanity!* in 1993. Even Dr. Dean Ornish's lifestyle plan for heart disease reversal, if used as a casual diet for weight loss and not a carefully planned lifestyle change, can become a high-carb/low-fat nightmare. Often, in the zealous effort to slash all vestiges of fat from the diet, the high-quality protein intake gets slashed as well. Why eat a healthy ounce of low-fat cheese with an apple, when if you ate the apple alone you would get no fat at all? True, no fat—and no body-building protein.

Now, the pendulum is certainly swinging back, with protein-pushing books renewing false hopes that there is an easy, painless way to lose weight and not feel hungry. And carbohydrates are once again becoming public enemy number one.

Reality

If you've been caught on the pendulum swing and are hitting the wall right now, you need to know the truth. *You DO need protein AND fat—and you need carbohydrates, too!* Protein is the main component of the brain, muscles, blood, hair, nails, and connective tissues. Without it, your body cannot be beautiful, nor can you be healthy. Protein is needed to churn out enzymes for digestion and cellular reactions, hormones for living and loving, and the antibodies to ward off illness. You cannot be healthy and lose fat weight without adequate protein and adequate calories.

Even fat is essential to your good health—and weight loss. It is needed for hormone production, lubrication, the absorption of certain vitamins, and much more. It is necessary for healthy weight loss because a moderate intake of fat triggers the production of cholecystokinin, a hormone that helps you feel satisfied. A low intake of fat or a drastic fat loss will produce the galanin hormone that turns up your appetite thermostat for fat. Galanin is released when the body breaks down body fat (as it does in dieting), when the diet is high fat (over 30 percent of calories), or when several hours have passed between meals allowing a fall in blood sugars or insulin levels. Eating more frequently, eating less fat (20 to 25 percent of calories), and eating low-fat protein lowers galanin production. The fact is, you cannot be healthy, nor can you lose weight, without fat.

But carbohydrates are needed as well to protect the protein you eat from being wasted as an energy source. Carbohydrates are also needed to protect the health-giving benefits of its fiber and nutrients and its role in regulating blood sugars. Carbohydrates play a critical role in meeting your body's energy needs and activating your metabolism.

Of course, as mentioned, a high-carbohydrate/low-fat diet also poses problems if the avoidance of fat is taken to such an extreme that the protein baby is thrown out with the fat bath water. This kind of regime so robs your body of essential proteins that it throws off your fluid balance, dehydrates your tissues, tears down your muscle mass, and handicaps the immune system. For a while the scales may look great, but the body begins to looks terrible—inside and out.

The Bottom Line

All nutrients—carbohydrates, proteins, and fats—are vital for living well, and equally vital for healthy weight loss. Losing weight by drastically cutting fat, and sometimes protein, too, is not only difficult, but it also sets up the dieter for malnutrition and a boomerang swing back up the scale. Fat-free does not guarantee that it's good for you!

Food-Combining Diets

Food combining is a concept dating back to the nineteenth century—and one that has been disproved since its first day out of the chute. Food combining is based on the ill-founded notion that the body's digestive tract, as mentioned, is designed like a trash compactor: what goes in first has to be digested before what comes in later. This bogus theory claims that if carbohydrates come in after proteins, which take longer to be digested, they will sit "atop the heap" and putrify, letting off gas and causing metabolic paralysis.

Harvey and Marilyn Diamond's bestseller *Fit for Life* has been hawking the "trash compactor" notion since the eighties, warning us by the millions not to combine proteins with carbohydrates or we will get fat, bloated, and gaseous. It is based on a meal plan of fruit only in the morning, carbohydrates only at lunch, and proteins only at dinner—never ever eating carbohydrates with proteins.

The Beverly Hills Diet of the seventies, now back in a "new" version for these diet-manic days, was another plan that promoted the idea of eating only one food at a time (like pineapple all day) so various combinations wouldn't "clog" the intestines. It recommends eating fruit by itself and never eating protein with carbohydrates in order for food to be properly digested and not stored as body fat.

During the first ten days on the diet, only fruit is permitted; on day eleven carbohydrates and butter are added; on day nineteen, protein is added. And, of course, fatty treats are permitted.

In the nineties, Suzanne Somers came out with *Suzanne Somers' Get Skinny on Fabulous Food.* So many flaws in this book, so little space to uncover them! Now not just blasting thighs, but blasting balanced, healthy eating as well, the "Somersizing" seven-step program forces you to avoid certain foods (potatoes, corn, bananas, nuts, and olives, to name a few) and to eat other foods in specific combinations (proteins and fats separately from carbohydrates, for example). In the absence of scientific proof to support her theories, Somers says simply, "It works." She also dismisses the U.S. Department of Agriculture's Food Guide Pyramid because "it will make you look like one." Cute, but not true.

Reality

Get Skinny is a rigid and often impractical diet for people whose days are already overloaded. The diet is also very low in calories, which are simply fuel for living, not evil fattening agents. Any diet that contains fewer calories than the number you are consuming now will help you to lose weight, but you don't have to pay $24 for a book or conduct self-experiments with unproved nutrition theories to do that.

As for the theory that the digestive system is like a trash compactor... no way. The biochemical reality is that your body has a very efficient digestive system, and no matter what combination of foods you consume, it will digest them equally in their most efficient site for digestion. Proteins are primarily digested in the stomach, carbohydrates in the small intestine.

What about eating protein only once per day? Although you need to keep your fat intake within safe limits, failing to balance your carbohydrate and protein intake will prevent you from using the protein you do eat in an optimal way. Remember this: You can't store protein; it's a use-it-or-lose-it nutrient. If you don't get enough of it, you will lose your strength and well-being.

The Bottom Line

Any diet that manipulates your intake of carbohydrates and proteins will result in weight loss—but not in a healthy or long-lasting way. Diets based on food combining rely on extremely limited meal guidelines and are not based on any scientific evidence. Besides, such an unbalanced eating plan can be even more hazardous to your health. Basing a life eating plan on erroneous information about the biochemistry of the body is risky business—no matter how effective or lovely the salesperson.

Semistarvation Diets

The Cabbage Soup Diet, the Grapefruit Diet, "power shake" meal replacements, fasting programs... all are seductive to the dieter because they're easy. No need to make choices, no need to have to think. Just eat the starring food of choice—and eat it in abundance. But, because there is a limit to just how much grapefruit or cabbage you can get down before you feel nauseous and bloated, you limit

WHAT ABOUT THE *WEIGH DOWN DIET?*

Gwen Shamblin's popular *Weigh Down Diet* is difficult for me to discuss because I've seen this program help many people come to terms with their overeating—and their true hunger. I have watched people come into new and deep places in their relationship with God through the small group from which this book sprang. Any small group whose members are earnestly and honestly seeking to let go of hurtful habits and self-reliance and embrace the grace of their Creator will produce tremendous spiritual fruit.

The diet plan Shamblin recommends is the problem. It sends shivers down the collective spine of those from the medical and science community because it completely disregards years of research about how to feed the human body for wellness. Although we all need to get in touch with the true needs of our soul and not be controlled by *anything,* feeding our body is about much more than fatness versus thinness. It's caring for our body as something precious. The Bible encourages believers to care for the body as a temple, and not be anxious about anything. It does not teach that we are to ignore the basic principles of how we were created.

Rather than eating just what you "feel" you need or want—and being thrilled to lose weight on a half bag of peanut M&Ms or a plate of biscuits and gravy—learn to eat to bless your body with nutrients that give you energy and fortify your health. You can eat almost any food, if the amounts are small enough, and still lose weight. But "dieting" on candy bars or one meal a day has its price: low energy, fuzzy thinking, and being deprived of the foods that keep you well. Truly, no food should be forbidden or labeled as "bad"—but I will not encourage you to eat foods that are nutritional disasters just because you can. The fact is, you *can* learn to recognize your true need to eat and how to stop when satisfied. But those body signals can only be trusted when you are meeting your body's needs with regular meals, avoiding overeating, and getting plenty of exercise.

Learning how God designed your body for wellness and following these principles is not bondage. A person who is in serious financial difficulty must go to the root issue and examine his or her "love of money" and his or her dependence upon it. But to truly thrive, he or she must go a step further and learn how to budget and manage money. So it is with the person who wants to overcome overeating. It is important to identify the place of power you've given food, dieting, and body image in your life; but then you need to learn how to manage it—for life.

If you have had great success with the *Weigh Down* plan, I rejoice with you. But I encourage you to begin to transition gently to healthy eating, following documented scientific principles that reveal the miracle of our creation.

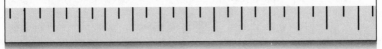

calories to a dangerous semistarvation level. The vast lack of nutrition has other limits as well—there's a limit to how long you can stay on these diets because they make you sick. Five to seven days is the average limit and enough to take off that promised five pounds. It's water, of course, but it feels as if you'd really been successful.

Each day of a typical seven-day program usually has specific foods that must be eaten, including potatoes, fruit juice, many vegetables, beef, tuna—even ice cream on some. Each day is carefully crafted to be extremely low in calories (less than 1,000 per day), complex carbohydrates, proteins, vitamins, and minerals. You can bet you'll feel lightheaded and weak, and notice a decreased ability to concentrate. Even if you love the particular food at the center of the plan (some people love cabbage!), this diet just isn't worth feeling weak and disoriented—and getting malnourished—for the sake of quick weight loss that won't stay lost once you begin eating normally again.

Reality

When it comes to calories, how much is too little? Less than your body weight times ten—so, less than 1,300 calories for a 130-pound woman. Results of four national surveys show that most people try to lose weight by eating 1,000 to 1,500 calories a day. But, overall, cutting calories to fewer than 1,500 (if you're a woman) or 1,800 (if you're a man) usually doesn't allow enough food for you to be satisfied in the long term. Eating fewer than 1,500 calories also makes it difficult to get enough of certain vital nutrients, such as folic acid, magnesium, and zinc.

Your body, created to survive, interprets long hours without enough food as potential starvation. To prepare for the long haul, the metabolism slows down dramatically so as not to burn much valuable muscle. So what does the desperate-to-lose-weight dieter do in response? Cuts calories even more. I've seen far too many people cut their calories to below 500 calories per day, and although they are losing their health, they can't lose the weight they want.

Slashing your calorie intake too drastically can slow your metabolism so drastically that it can take up to a year to normalize. That's why you gain back weight so quickly after stopping this type of diet. After starvation, even a return to healthy eating will cause your body to store the calories as fat. What comes off will come back on... and on... and on. Contrary to what you may think, in a starvation state when no carbohydrate is available your body turns first to muscle mass for stored energy and later to your fat stores.

As for fasting, going without all food in order to lose weight can be just as damaging for the overweight person as a binge of eating. Although there is a proper place for fasting and prayer in our spiritual lives, starving in order to lose weight or to even "cleanse the body" has a more mundane motive, and is without the protection of grace! Starving will certainly achieve quick weight loss, but as seen in concentration camps during the war, what you lose is primarily water and muscle weight. This may look great on the scale, but it will look terrible on your body.

The Bottom Line

Fasting, single-food diets, and low-calorie meal replacements aren't the key to long-term weight control and better health—nor is eating whatever you want whenever you want but only half a portion. The only good news about extremely low calorie diets is that people often go off of them quickly—they simply feel too awful to stay on them. Don't rely on dangerous semistarvation diets to lose weight quickly. Instead, learn how to eat.

Blood and Body Type Diets

The newest wave of fad diets base their logic on even stranger theories than insulin resistance or food combining. Take Peter J. D'Adamo's book, *Eat Right 4 Your Type,* for example. This is a particular "favorite" of mine because it is genius-born—it promotes a completely undocumented theory that blood type is a sign of your predestined eating pattern. The diet is therefore tailored to your specific blood type. Here's the theory: If you are type O, like the majority of people, then you were descended from hunters and therefore should eat lots of meat and lots of fat. Gatherers, on the other hand, have type A blood and should be vegetarians and cook a lot. D'Adamo also sells special vitamins for each blood type.

The Body Code, by Jay Cooper, divides dieters into warriors, nurturers, communicators, and visionaries. Nurturers, in addition to eating lots of fruits and vegetables, no doubt do most of the cooking.

Dr. Abravanel's Body Type Diet and Lifetime Nutrition Plan (also known as the Caveman Diet) allows you to eat only what Stone Age people ate. This diet came from the proposition that everyone falls into one of four body types—thyroid, pituitary, adrenal, or gonadal—depending on body shape, food cravings, and other personal traits. Tests within the book with questions about food cravings, personality, cellulite, and sleeping patterns help you identify which is your dominant gland. These glands, the claim goes, are at the root of every weight problem; they trigger cravings for wrong foods and are overstimulated by the foods you crave, thereby slowing down your metabolism and causing you to gain weight.

Once you've identified your body type, you must follow that type's specially tailored diet—eat foods that suppress your "problem" gland while avoiding foods that stimulate it. If you are a thyroid type, you should be eating two eggs for breakfast every morning and hard-boiled eggs for snacks, but restricting all fruit. If you are a pituitary type, you should *never* eat dairy products, but cooked hamburger would be a great snack. The big drawback of this diet is if you discover that you are a gonad. Gonads can eat only uncooked food.

Reality

The role glands play in regulating body weight is an extremely complex process that could never be remedied by an unbalanced and nutrient-deficient diet. And there is *zero* documentation showing that blood type affects your metabolism one iota. The truth is, cutting out whole food groups not only sets you up for failure, but also for malnutrition by limiting your intake of important vitamins and minerals. Furthermore, suggestions such as "waiting as much as six hours between meals to maximize fat burning" may help to cut calories, but it will also cause blood sugar levels to plummet, leaving you fatigued, irritable, and craving sweets—and your glands or blood type won't have a thing to do with it!

The Bottom Line

The real secret behind any weight-loss success in these diets is the extreme calorie restriction of each diet—too low to meet nutrient needs but low enough and unbalanced enough to allow quick fluid loss and muscle breakdown. Don't fall for a plan just because it sounds new, individualized, scientific, and complicated.

Lose-It-While-You-Sleep Diets

You've probably heard the radio personalities flooding the airwaves—particularly to the teens and twenty-something crowd—promising health and weight loss in a capsule, powder, or herbal brew. It sounds so easy. And these herbal supplements and power drinks promising weight loss and energy are readily available in health-food stores and even some gyms. They are widely used by bodybuilders and athletes. They are recommended by trainers, friends, and multilevel marketers alike. They seem so natural; they seem so safe. But most people aren't aware they can have serious repercussions.

How to be a savvy user of the myriad of alternative therapies and dietary supplements on store shelves is a vital question, yet a difficult one because it's so hard to check out the science behind the products. They all sound so good, so helpful. There's chromium picolinate, the fat-burner favorite a few years back. Then there's Fat Trapper and Exercise in a Bottle, claiming in infomercials to prevent your body from absorbing dietary fat (eat all the cheeseburgers and fries you want!) and to increase the activity of muscle cells (no exercise required!) so that you can quickly burn the fat that's already been stored. And who hasn't heard of Metabolife, an herbal brew sold in mall kiosks and over the Internet. It has been touted as everything from a safe herbal diet aid to a brain and energy booster (a.k.a., herbal speed). Natural, safe, and quick is the ad's message, but natural, dangerous, and quick may be closer to reality.

Then there's DHEA, or dehydroepiandrosterone—the nineties darling for anti-aging and weight loss. It's a steroid hormone that is produced in abundance by the adrenal glands during youth and early adulthood. Blood levels of DHEA fall considerably as people grow older (production of DHEA starts to decline in the late twenties and dwindles to about 5 to 10 percent of its peak level by age eighty), so the claim is that supplementing with DHEA will remedy the actual cause of middle-age spread. You haven't gained weight because of doing something wrong, but you can lose it by doing something "right"—taking DHEA. The health risk of DHEA could be great: One danger related to its use in men could be an increase in the risk of prostate cancer. In women, DHEA has been linked with a possible increase in the risk of breast cancer.

It's not just the "natural" supplements that abound with promises to do your weight loss for you. Now a whole new generation of prescription drugs are coming down the pike to help in the weight battle. Heard of Meridia (sibutrammine), the new player on the diet pill scene? There's also Zenical (Orlistat), the medication that works in the intestines by blocking the absorption of approximately 30 percent of the dietary fat consumed. About one-third of users experience unpleasant side effects (such as severe gas, loose stools, and anal leakage). But if it helps with weight loss, the prevailing question seems to be "How do I get a prescription?"

Reality

Do all these products that promise to "do the work for you" *really* do the work for you? Fat chance. Only if you believe in magical thinking. When it comes to herbal and supplement brews, powders, and drinks, the ingredients just haven't been shown effective in significant, healthy weight loss. You lose time and money, but you won't lose weight unless you follow the low-calorie eating plan included with the product.

But what's worse than losing time and money? Losing your health, or your life. Anne Marie Capati didn't tell her family she was taking potentially dangerous herbal supplements to lose weight. Life was a happy whirlwind for the Manhattan fashion designer and mother of two. She was exercising with a personal trainer and working on losing weight, keeping her blood pressure under control. Then, on October 1, 1998, Capati collapsed at her gym while working out with her trainer. She died of a stroke that night.

Anne Marie, it was discovered, had been taking a variety of herbal supplements including Thermadrene, a supplement loaded with ephedra, an ancient herb that stimulates heart rate and the central nervous system. Ephedra is found in many products and under many different names like Ma Huang, Ephedrine, Herbal Fen-Phen, Ultimate Xphoria, and others. Anne Marie was pumping drugs— that she beleived to be safe—as well as iron, and it killed her.

Although the FDA has linked ephedra-containing dietary supplements to more than eight hundred reports of adverse health effects, cases of muscle destruction, and forty-four deaths since

WHERE TO GET HELP

What is good nutrition? Whose answers should you listen to? The average American may have a difficult time telling you, because most of his or her health information comes from the media. A recent study found that 80 percent of women polled relied on the media as their primary source of nutrition information.

You may expect me to tell you that the very best source for accurate nutrition information is, of course, a nutritionist. I won't. Although I am one, the term *nutritionist* is the most meaningless one in medicine. The National Council Against Health Fraud ran a thirty-two–state survey of nutritionists listed in the Yellow Pages. Nearly half had questionable degrees, claiming to be doctors of nutri-medicine (say what?), food counselors, or certified nutritionists—all of which are meaningless titles without qualifications. The institutions from which they "graduated" sounded reputable, but weren't. Diploma mills abound—from which your dog or cat can get a doctorate degree as easily as you can for $1,000 cash or $1,200 with a credit card.

If you want reliable nutritional advice—someone to help you sort out reality from fiction and hope from hype, the person who physicians turn to when they need help with a nutrition issue—turn to a registered dietitian, or R.D. Those are my credentials. R.D.s are nutrition specialists who have bachelor's and master's degrees along with a completed residency/internship. They may even have medical degrees, and they must complete continuing education from accredited programs.

1993, they're still on the market. Reported side effects have included abnormal heart rhythm, seizure, stroke, psychosis, heart attack, and hepatitis. But America is still swallowing these herbal threats by the millions.

Just a few of the other weight loss supplements that are life-threatening are *Stephania*, also called magnolia (this herb has caused kidney disease and resulted in kidney transplants and dialysis in Europe); *Germander* (long-term use can lead to kidney damage and has allegedly been linked to a death); and *Kombucha tea* (an "herbal tea," also called mushroom tea, kvass tea, kwassan, and kargasok, which is really a colony of yeast and bacteria; it can cause liver and other organ damage, gastrointestinal upset, and has been linked to a death).

The ingredients in Fat Burners (chromium picolinate), Metabolife, blue green algae, Fat Trapper, and Exercise in a Bottle have not been scientifically proven to be effective, but numerous health concerns have been raised about the harm they can inflict. Many dietary supplements stress the "natural" quality of their products, which many misconstrue as meaning safer and better. But, as already discussed, this is not always the case.

So how do you sort out fact from fiction from outright fantasy amid the swirl of information about vitamin and nutritional supplements? Quite simply, you need to learn what's known about supplements and what's not. You need to learn who needs a supplement and who doesn't. And you must become familiar with critical safety issues in what has become a largely unregulated industry.

Prescribed weight-loss drugs should be used only if you are likely to have serious health problems caused by your weight. You should not use drugs to improve your appearance. Prescribed weight-loss drugs, when combined with a healthy diet and regular physical activity, may help some obese adults lose weight. But before these medications can be widely recommended, more research is needed to determine their long-term safety and effectiveness.

The Bottom Line

Anything you put in your body has the potential to harm you, as well as help you. Anything you swallow—whether labeled "natural" or not—can act as a drug in your body, bringing side effects and health risks, including death. When it comes to losing weight, the only natural choice is eating well and exercising. You *don't* lose it while you sleep. You have to do your part.

SPRINGING THE TRAP

With countless diets, programs, and products promising to help you shed pounds, it should be easy. But as any veteran dieter knows, it's hard to lose weight. And it's even harder to keep it off. That's why fad diets continue to entrap us.

The medical evidence for the six diet schemes we've discussed is flimsy or nonexistent, but you can find an "expert" somewhere to support almost every one. Even diets that have been widely criticized by the medical community retain their vocal adherents. It is clear that as long as happy dieters and supportive "professionals" keep appearing on talk shows, people with eating problems are going to be suckers for diets that let them eat pork rinds.

After reading so much about the hidden and overt dangers of dieting, you may be immobilized by a sense of hopelessness about weight loss. Perhaps you're even thinking that it's smarter and safer to stay overweight.

Of course, my vote is for you to choose long-term health. That means choosing to lose weight if you need to, but *not* by dieting.

Instead, learn to live in a way that releases you from the diet trap forever and unleashes your body's natural ability to lose weight and feel great.

Even if you've been on a hundred diets, you can reverse the damage—beginning this very day. The question is not, "What have I done to myself?" by becoming caught in the diet trap. Rather, it is, "What can I do differently for myself now?" The secret lies in cracking the code for weight loss and whole-body healing.

PART TWO ■ CRACKING THE FAT CELL CODE

CHAPTER 4 ■ Overweight or Overfat?

The doctor of the future will give no medicine, but will interest his patient in the care of the human frame, in diet, and in the cause and prevention of disease.

—THOMAS A. EDISON

Before you set a goal for weight loss, you have to become objective about your weight, which is *very* difficult. You can't exactly trust the mirror—and you sure can't get a good reading from a scale.

Traditionally, "overweight" has been defined as weighing more than the weight listed for your age and height in a weight table. But that doesn't account for differences in body composition. Athletes, for example, are often "overweight" by weight table standards because of a large frame or muscle development. But they aren't overfat. And body fat, not weight, is what concerns health. The key to successful, healthy weight loss is to lower your percentage of body fat, not to lose pounds of muscle and water as a result of a quick-weight-loss diet.

You lower your percentage of body fat in two ways: by (1) losing fat, and (2) building muscle. The problem with using a scale to measure your progress in these two areas is that, pound for pound, muscle weighs more than fat (each pound of muscle is surrounded by four pounds of water) yet takes up only one-seventh of the space. Heavier, yes, but smaller and tighter. If you gain a pound of muscle, the scale goes up. That's why only your "body feel," your appearance, and a body fat measurement can tell you the whole story.

Again, the question is not, *Are you overweight?* but, *Are you over-fat?* It doesn't really matter if you're losing weight on the scale unless you're also losing fat. The key to body fat analysis is having fat estimated by a trained professional using a reliable method, such as skinfold measurements, infrared interactance, bioelectrical impedance, or underwater weighing. But none of these methods will give you better than a ballpark figure. The older you are or the more fat you're carrying, the less reliable the measurement may be. Nonetheless, if you are serious about wanting to lose only the right kind of weight, it would be a wonderful benchmark. Your area's YMCA, health club, wellness center, or hospital can direct you in getting an accurate body-fat test.

CAN YOU BE FIT AND FAT?

Other than clothes not fitting well, is excess weight really a problem? We assume that all obesity translates into health problems, but this is not necessarily so; not all overweight people are destined to be sick. It has been estimated that 10 to 20 percent of overweight people are not "disease prone." They may not feel tip-top but they are not necessarily more apt to be ill than those who are slim.

A vital observation, however, is this: Those who "eat themselves fat" are less healthy than those who are genetically predisposed to being overweight. And *gaining* weight is even more of a problem than *being* overweight.

Another critical fact: Even if you're slender as a stalk, a sedentary lifestyle can endanger your health. Studies have shown that thin people who aren't physically active are nearly three times more likely to die young than heavy people who exercise regularly. One

BODY MASS INDEX

Another measure of your weight and health status, more accurate than the scale, is your body mass index, or BMI. This is your weight and your height factored together.

TO CALCULATE YOUR BMI:

STEP 1: Multiply your weight in pounds by .45. (For example, if you weigh 150 pounds: 150 x .45 = 68)

STEP 2: Multiply your height in inches by .025. (For example, if you're 5′6″ (66 inches): 66 x .025 = 1.65)

STEP 3: Square the answer from Step 2 (1.65 x 1.65 = 2.72)

STEP 4: Divide the answer from Step 1 by the answer from Step 3 (68/2.72 = 25)

If you use the metric system, your BMI equals your weight in kilograms divided by your height in centimeters squared.

YET ANOTHER WAY TO FIGURE YOUR BMI:

Multiply your weight by 703 and divide the result by your height in inches. Then divide that result again by your height.

In June 1998 the U.S. National Center for Health Statistics defined being overweight as having a BMI of 25 or more. For a woman of average height, 5-foot-5, that works out to 150 pounds; for the average man, 5-foot-10, it's 176 pounds. Obesity is defined as a BMI of 30 or more—180 pounds for a woman at 5-foot-5, 209 pounds for a man at 5-foot-10. This isn't a perfect formula because it could appear to be high for a healthy body builder or for adolescents not yet at their mature height.

The problem with BMI as an evaluation of obesity is that the measure doesn't really tell you directly about body composition. It's better than weight alone because it adjusts for height, but it's not as good as knowing how much of that weight is fat versus muscle.

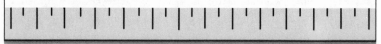

study conducted by the Cooper Institute for Aerobics Research in Dallas tracked 25,000 men and 7,000 women for eight years. Those who were the least fit based on treadmill response were twice as likely as the others to suffer fatalities from heart disease—no matter how much fat they carried. Thin, unfit men fared far worse in health matters than heavy men who were fit.

This research is compelling enough to put forth the opinion that it may be better to be overweight and active than thin and sedentary.

We can't assume that everyone who's overweight overeats. Being overweight actually stems from the interaction of several factors, genetics being one. Those who are predisposed to obesity may have a problem with leptin, a hormone released by the fat cells to signal the brain to stop storing fat. Either because they produce a defective version of leptin, or because their brain cells don't respond properly to the leptin signal, their fat-controlling mechanism is genetically flawed. Yet, their body may also be better equipped to handle the excess weight. But for the normal person who overeats unhealthy foods and exercises too little, excess body fat often contributes to cardiovascular diseases, several cancers, and numerous other medical disorders, including high blood pressure and diabetes.

A recent four-year study of more than 40,000 nurses, ages forty-six to seventy-one, linked even moderate excess weight to a greater risk of dying early. Losing just 5 to 10 percent of body fat was found to help reduce blood pressure, improve triglyceride and cholesterol levels, reduce sleep apnea symptoms, and cut the risk for joint problems such as osteoarthritis. This large-scale study suggested that the best weight for a woman at middle age was whatever she weighed at eighteen plus ten pounds. For every 2.2 pounds of weight she gained above this, the study showed, the risk of suffering a heart attack rose by 3.1 percent.

TAMING THE WEIGHT MONSTER

Clearly, the best course is to nip weight gain in the bud. Even a ten-pound gain is worth paying attention to. It's easier to tame the weight monster while it's small.

That's what Sherri wanted to do when she came to see me. Sherri just couldn't seem to get control of her seesaw eating—sometimes good and sometimes horrid. She wasn't particularly heavy; but she had battled the same ten pounds for so long that the battle itself seemed to have taken on a life of its own.

Sherri's day starts early, and ends late. She starts the day as a wife and Mom—but with an ailing mother in town, she ends up being daughter as well. She quickly turns into chauffeur for the school car-pool—which she does most mornings so that someone else can pick up the kids while she's at work in the afternoon. She then drives straight to work, which is a tense hour-long commute. At work she starts to spin more plates—creative ones, deadline ones, management ones, political ones, friendship ones—and then she comes home to yet more. Her life is filled with "gotta dos"—gotta do that report, gotta make that meeting, gotta get the kids here or there, gotta get dinner, gotta get that gift, gotta call Mom, gotta exercise, gotta pay bills, gotta lose weight.

Sherri described herself to me this way: "I feel like one of the kid's juice boxes that has about twenty straws stuck all over the place. I've been sucked dry—the box has caved into a vacuum. I'm operating on nothing—and feel just the same—nothing. I've got too much to think about to feel anything." Sherri's churning, spinning thoughts were wearing her out as much as her schedule was.

Bouncing like a pinball between an obsessive-compulsive drive for a beautiful body and a chronic lack of self-care, Sherri was battling a cycle of unhealthy eating, high stress levels, and depleted energy supplies. She would come home many nights, sucked dry, and—just for the energy to get dinner for the kids—grab a bag of chips and diet soda. Then a few doughnuts, then some cookies—and then the leftover macaroni and cheese from the kid's plates. Afterward, she'd sit down with her husband for a mindless meal. Most nights, she'd fall asleep on the couch at 10:00 and then wake up to drag herself to bed. If she was lucky, she could sleep till 2:30 or 3:00 AM, only to wake with a start of anxiety and be unable to get back to sleep. She'd finally get up and eat something—cheese, chicken, chips, anything. Then she'd catnap the rest of the night and turn off the 5 AM alarm—exhausted.

Turns out that Sherri didn't really eat that much, and the high-fat, sugar-laden foods she loved weren't the only trouble spots in her eating style. The biggest problem was the lack of routine in her eating. She might go all day with little or no food, other than the occasional doughnut grabbed at a morning meeting (she *loved* doughnuts!) and a continuous intake of coffee and diet soda. She typically ate only one "meal" a day—nonstop grazing from the time she got home till she fell into a coma on the sofa.

Because Sherri didn't seem to have time for anything, even to notice how bad she really felt, she would drown out the "I'm so tired" message with sugar, caffeine, and comfort foods. But that would only last for a while, usually until her weight would soar up seven or eight pounds. Then she couldn't stand the way she looked anymore, and felt others were noticing, she would hit bottom and start on a new diet. She had been on four different diets since January 1, and this was only April.

"I do great on diets," Sherri admitted. "It's the one time I focus just on me." Telling words. Sherri knew that diets—any diet—

worked really well for her. "I lose weight and feel great in just days!" But then the inevitable crisis, and after she had stoically starved for a few weeks, Sherri would blow it in one weary night. Then the whole cycle would begin again. She finally conceded, "I just feel like I'm killing myself with my diets, and my failures are making me crazy."

Sherri was truly caught in a trap, but her weight was not the real problem. It was a *life* trap, and her way of eating and dieting was the glue keeping her stuck.

Sherri exemplifies a classic pattern I see every day in counseling. She is a creative television producer, successful in all she puts her hand and mind to—except in the area of eating and taking care of herself. Like so many others, she has tried diet after diet, only to succeed and then fail. She never resolved her underlying problems or educated herself about how the human body was designed to function optimally. She was drowning in a tidal wave of stress—and was turning to food to keep her afloat. Food was being used to meet needs it was never designed to meet. She was feeding her soul with junk food—and it just didn't fit the bill. Every diet, followed by every failure, had her in the vice grip of the diet trap.

THE STRESS RESPONSE

Sherri is not alone in her fight against the tidal wave of stress—and the erratic eating and weight gain that often accompanies it. Nearly nine out of ten Americans say they experience stress every day and high levels several times a week. One in four complains of high stress levels every day.

Stress is as difficult to treat as it is to understand. That's because stress means different things to different people. Our reactions to life events vary from person to person; what frazzles me may challenge and inspire you. Most people refer to life's challenges as *stress*, when in fact those are *stressors*.

Stress can result from good things as well as bad; from the joy of a wedding celebration to a major loss like the death of a loved one; from minor irritations like losing car keys or a major one like a traffic jam. Research shows time and time again that it's not the number of stressors in one's life that affects health and well-being, but our response to the situations. The body's response is the actual "stress," and it comes from within.

Your body was designed to cope with the stresses you encounter in life. You were created with a "stress tracking system" that is intricately programmed to seek and find stress signals. This "stress sensor" (the pituitary gland in our brain) is much like radar equipment and is constantly on the lookout for what appears to be danger to your survival. When this master gland picks up stress signals, it sends a hormone messenger to your body's adrenal system (located near the kidneys) to prepare you to fight the present danger, or flee to escape it.

These chemical messages set in motion the symptoms of stress. They cause a shift of the chemical balance deep within your system, triggering reactions that slow down the metabolism and other bodily functions (such as digestion). The stress hormones, adrenaline and cortisol, prime your body for action, causing blood to pool in your muscles and fluid to gather in your extremities. Your heart beats faster, your blood pressure rises, your breathing rate increases, and your muscles tense up. Proteins are converted into sugar, which causes insulin levels to surge and your blood sugar to fluctuate wildly. The roller coaster ride your blood sugar takes in response to stress affects your energy levels, mood, concentration, appetite, and cravings.

This "fight-or-flight" response—this surge of chemical reactions—may have helped our early ancestors to survive when facing grizzly bears, but when our twenty-first century bodies think traffic jams, deadlines, financial pressures, or relationship struggles are modern-day grizzlies, the chronic stress response can wear us down and lock down our metabolism.

The key word with any kind of negative stress is *chronic*. All the adaptive mechanisms wired into us by our Creator were intended as a short-term alert/alarm to prepare us to flee or do battle, and to help us recover once out of danger. But today's bodies are exposed to chronic, unresolved stress, and almost never have a chance to recover and break out of the fight-or-flight reaction. When the body is exposed to the same stress again and again with no stress release, energy stores are depleted and the body begins to show signs of damage—with a metabolic slow-down and fatigue being the cardinal symptoms. Being stuck in stress causes chemical surges which can result in headaches, backaches, sleep disturbances, anxiety, depression, arthritic pain, asthma, gastrointestinal upsets, skin disorders—along with weight and eating problems.

Nothing fuels appetite like chronic stress—and nothing puts the body into the fat storage mode more quickly. Whether or not we eat more when under stress, the stressed body does more damage with what comes in than the nonstressed body. There may be other forces at work as well; for example, when a lack of self-care (sedentary lifestyle, sleep deprivation, poor eating habits) is combined with states of imbalance (illness, hormone dysfunction, depression, or worry), the fat cell stays locked in a "store" rather than "burn" mode. While we are waging war against our body, our fat cells are looking out for our survival. And a chemical imbalance occurs that slows our metabolism. The problem is not only what we are eating, but what the fat cells are storing away. The fat cells become stockpiled with unused energy, and the cells lock down.

The good news is that we all have more power than we realize to take charge of our body's stress response. But most of us just don't recognize the stress warnings, nor how they keep us caught in the diet trap.

GET YOUR BODY WORKING FOR YOU

In order to achieve a harmonious balance within your body and soul and tap into the reservoir of metabolic power and healing within, you must begin by righting the wrongs of your body and getting it to work for you rather than against you. This doesn't just happen when you go on one more diet or try to "be good." It begins when you change the way you live and eat. It requires an understanding of how your body works and what habits you have acquired that either release the natural flow of energy from the cells or lock it down.

To break out of the diet trap, you have to get beyond the weight issue. Weight problems are but a symptom of an ailing and stressed lifestyle. You must focus on the here and now of life.

Start by assessing your day: How do you feel when you wake up in the morning? How much energy do you have? Do you often experience physical or emotional rises and falls throughout your day? Are there times when hunger or cravings seem to overtake you? How do you satisfy that hunger? What logjams are blocking your total well-being?

The good news is, you don't have to push or drag through each day. You *can* have abundant life; you *can* take charge of your wellness, your energy level, and your weight. And you *can* be set free from the life traps of poor eating, stress, too little rest, and too little exercise. You are free to be well; you need only to choose to eat well of the food that gives life: physically, emotionally, and spiritually.

The bottom line goal: Even if you don't lose weight, adopt health-promoting living habits. Losing weight might not guarantee you a longer life, but being active, eating differently, and heading off more weight gain *will* make you healthier. Whatever your need of the moment—weight loss, controlling overeating, embracing self-care, regaining health and energy—the key is to get started and get strong, one step at a time.

CHAPTER 5 ■ Releasing Your Body's Natural Ability to Lose Weight

Good health has more to do with everyday behavior and habits than with miracles of modern science. Prevention is far superior to cure!

—ANONYMOUS

Weight gain is not inevitable for men or women—nor is it inevitable if you have a genetic proclivity. If you have been gaining weight—or been unable to lose it—it's probably because your fat cells are responding in a survival mode. Fighting them with a fad diet only locks them into metabolic slowdown. That's why the only way to manage weight permanently is to forego dieting and begin to live in a new and natural way that unlocks the exit door to your fat cells so they can start releasing fat again.

Getting your body working for you and shedding excess pounds *is* within your control. The key is learning and practicing the seven secrets of *The Smart Weigh*—strategies for staying fit and fueled and getting your body working for you with optimal fat-burning capability.

THE SECRETS OF *THE SMART WEIGH*

S: Stoke your metabolic fire
E: Equip yourself for stress release
C: Cultivate a positive perspective
R: Regulate your blood sugars
E: Equalize your brain chemistry
T: Take charge of your appetite
S: Strengthen your immune system

These methods will unlock your fat cells and restore the balances of your body and soul. They are not vague or complex, nor are they startling discoveries. They are simply keys to the real issues of weight management—to meeting real needs with real answers. In Chapter 11, I'll help you convert these secrets into specific action steps over a seven-week period. Once you get in the habit of living *The Smart Weigh,* you'll be free from the diet trap once and for all, and your natural ability to lose weight will blossom.

SECRET NO. 1:
STOKE YOUR METABOLIC FIRE

It's not the calories taken in but the calories burned that count—and your metabolism makes all the difference. Remember, your metabolism is the chemical process that converts food to energy and is measured by how many calories you burn per minute for body functions—both voluntary activity and movement, and automatic, involuntary functions like breathing, heart beat, digestion, and blood circulation. The largest amount of calories used (70 percent) are those burned to maintain this basic body function.

At a cellular level, our metabolism is activated by a balance of supply and demand: a supply of optimum fuel and oxygen to the cells for energy metabolism, and a demand from the body systems for energy. As I explained earlier, a combination of factors—especially our stressful lifestyles and lack of self-care—causes our fat cells to lock down, slowing our metabolic rate to a snail's pace, which results in fats being stored rather than burned for energy. This "cocooning" is the result of constant stress and not nearly enough energy supply to meet the needs.

While a calorie is a calorie, your metabolism can increase or decrease (burn or store those calories) depending on your eating patterns. The body was designed to slow itself down to protect against energy deficits. As a result, erratic eating patterns keep our metabolism locked in low gear, storing away every meal as if it were our last.

Think of your metabolism as a campfire that requires fuel to burn, and air to fan the fire's flame. A campfire dies down during the night and must have wood added in the morning to begin to burn brightly once more. Without being "stoked" with new fuel, the spark turns to ash—there's nothing left to burn.

Similarly, your body awakens in a slowed-down state. If you don't "break the fast" with breakfast and continue to feed it through the day to meet your body's demand for energy and boost your metabolic system, your body turns to its own muscle mass (not fat) for energy and slows down even more, conserving itself for a potentially long, starved state. Then, when the evening eating begins, most of that food will be stored as fat because the body isn't burning energy at a fast rate; the fire has gone out. The food you eat, after long hours without, is like dumping an armload of firewood on a dead fire.

Regardless of the number of calories consumed when we do eat, the body can use only a small amount of energy, protein, and other nutrients quickly. The rest is thrown off as waste or stored as fat. Eating the American way robs the body of vital nutrients for the remaining twenty-four hours—until the next feeding frenzy. We not only go wrong in how much we eat or what we eat; we also eat entirely too much at the wrong time. The vast majority of us get most of our calories after six o'clock in the evening—too much too late.

Starving for Nutrition

To burn the calories you consume—to metabolize them into energy, rather than store them as fat—requires nutrients. These vital nutrients are the vitamins, minerals, and phytochemicals found in foods. Certain nutrients are considered essential for the metabolism because they act as catalysts for calorie burning. The B-complex vitamins, magnesium, and zinc are important examples. (We'll talk more about them in Chapter 6.) Also important is chromium, found in whole grains, which helps to transport glucose through the cell membranes so that it can be burned for energy. Iron is also vital because it delivers oxygen inside the cells, "fanning the flame" of calorie burning.

Many people may be getting plenty of calories, but not enough of the nutrients to help metabolize those calories and activate fat-burning potential. Or, their metabolisms may be so slow because of chronic stress that they cannot burn the calories effectively. Either way, you've got a fat-storing crisis.

Living life in the fast lane (and often, the fast food lane) means that food choices are often based on convenience instead of nutrition. That not only means a junk food diet, but a *junk diet*: lots of calories, lots of fat, lots of sodium, lots of sugar—all promising energy on the run. But the energy runs out and ends up slowing down, not speeding up, our metabolism.

The classic junk diet is notoriously low in the nutrients that provide for consistent, long-lasting energy. We are more apt to eat fries than baked potatoes, ketchup than tomatoes, and drink orange soda instead of orange juice. And so most of us are deficient in the vitamins and minerals that would keep our metabolism working in high gear.

But we *can* choose to eat well and eat often. To preserve muscle mass and burn fat while losing weight, your best bet is to eat balanced meals and snacks of whole carbohydrates and low-fat protein, evenly distributed throughout the day. This, in combination with eating an adequate amount of calories, is the most important step you can take to unleash your body's natural ability to lose weight.

To activate your metabolism and get your body working for you, you need to *eat*: (1) eat early, (2) eat often, (3) eat balanced, (4) eat lean, and (5) eat bright. Read more about strategic eating in the next chapter.

Fanning the Fire's Flame

Eating strategically is one of the best ways to increase your metabolism, and exercise is a close second. Yet, research shows that most people with weight problems not only eat too much, too late, but exercise too little. And remember: Controlling your intake of food is not an alternative to exercise, nor is exercise an alternative to healthy eating.

Not only does exercise help you to burn the calories you take in better; it also serves to build muscle mass. And that's another weight-control secret: To rev up your metabolism and burn fat, *use*—don't lose—your muscle. Building new muscle through strength training is one of the best ways to reverse the metabolic slowdown of midlife and stressful living. The more lean muscle mass you can preserve, the bigger "engine" you'll have in which to burn calories.

Now, does what you've always heard about the importance of

exercise make more sense? You can boost your metabolism, lose body fat, and gain muscle mass by doing some type of aerobic activity for thirty to sixty minutes at least four times a week. No time? Break up your workouts into shorter bouts throughout the day. Reports show that squeezing in even ten-minute spurts of activity throughout the day yields results. Add in a workout with free weights, exercise bands, or a Nautilus machine twice a week, or take advantage of the humdrum tasks that have to be done anyway by doing them with vigor. Haul the garbage cans to the curb yourself and rejoice when you carry that laundry basket up and down the stairs! Even though regularly scheduled aerobic exercise is best for losing fat, any extra movement boosts the metabolism and burns calories better. Start parking at the far end of the lot, or make several trips up and down the stairs instead of using the elevator. Even foregoing such automated gadgets as remote controls and garage door openers can make a metabolic difference. (Read more about the benefits of movement in Chapter 7.)

Taking Care of Yourself

You might be wondering, *Where am I going to get the energy to do all this extra moving and working out? I can barely keep my pace as it is!* You're not alone. Not only are many of us living in metabolic lock-down as a result of our lifestyle choices, we're living in an energy crisis as well. The very things that result in a slowed metabolism produce the energy deficit, too. One of these factors is sleep deprivation. You'll read more about the power of restful sleep in Chapter 9.

Sleep is the repair shop of the body; without it we cannot be healthy or even happy. Sleep deprivation actually becomes a profound stress to your body, contributing to fat cell lock-down. Research shows that missing just one night of restful sleep can cause a surge of stress hormones to circulate through your body, weakening your immune system and causing a metabolic slowdown. Conversely, replenishing sleep and time-outs can equip the body for stress release. Again, it's how we were created.

Breathing is another normal body action that can either release stress—or actually cause it. You can't help breathing, but you can help yourself breathe better. Deep, slow, oxygenating breaths are one of the simplest things you can do to relieve stress, activate your metabolism, and keep control of yourself in any situation.

Yet in times of stress, we tend to breathe in a panicked way—rapid, shallow, or deep, heaving breaths—each breath robbing the bloodstream of the right amount of oxygen to take to the cells to fan the metabolic fire. You can think of this kind of stressbreathing as suffocating your blood cells—which signals the release of even more stress hormones. The more stressed and tense you are, the higher your brain's demand for oxygen, yet the shallow breathing that accompanies stress decreases the oxygen intake and transfer. It's a vicious cycle that takes your breath away! The good news is that learning to breathe in a relaxed way immediately defuses the stress response. (Read more about the healing benefits of focused breathing in Chapter 8.)

Drinking adequate water is another critical element for activating your metabolism and total body health. Because your body is comprised primarily of water, every cell in your body relies on this "one-of-a-kind" beverage to dilute biochemicals, vitamins, and minerals to just the right concentrations so that they can be used in energy metabolism. The body also depends on water to keep the blood at the proper fluid concentration to effectively transport these nutrients and other substances from one part to another. Blood volume actually decreases and "thickens" when you are dehydrated, meaning that the heart has to work harder to supply your cells with needed oxygen. And remember, oxygenated blood is essential for an activated metabolism—to fan the flame for fat burning. A slow-burning metabolism is a symptom of dehydration.

By now you're getting the picture: activating your metabolism is really just a matter of moving into better self-care. That means treating yourself well by eating right, drinking enough water, exercising and strengthening your body, breathing deeply, and getting rest. The opposite behavior—a lack of self-care—is the recipe for fat storage.

SECRET NO. 2:
EQUIP YOURSELF FOR STRESS RELEASE

I serve as a wellness and nutrition coach for a number of professional athletes, particularly those in the National Basketball Association and Women's National Basketball Association. I also have an opportunity to work with corporate "athletes," high-on-the-ladder executives who are under similar performance demands and pressure. But I work with many more *life* athletes—people like you and me with stresses and demands from all of life's arenas: emotional, relational, financial, physical.

Like the pros, we life athletes have an individual "court of life" in which we are expected to perform day by day with perfection, endurance, and stamina. Like basketball players, we, too, have daily "fouls" committed against us, and we are continually stepping up to the "line"—flanked by team players and opposing forces alike. We are charging full steam ahead in life with too much to do and too few resources to do it with. So we become drained emotionally, spiritually, and physically. It's a stressful way to live, and we need a different level of fueling and fitness to rise up to the continuous levels of stress.

That's where strategic eating and living comes in, with a focus on timing, balance, and variety. Just as your body is designed to work for you nutritionally, it is also designed to survive, even thrive, amidst the stresses of daily life. As important as it is to identify how stress affects us, learning how to defuse life's stressors is even more critical. For once the body picks up a stress signal and interprets "danger," chemical reactions tell the body to go into a conservation mode. This includes three predictable physical responses that clearly affect the whole being.

(1) THE BODY'S METABOLISM SLOWS, storing excess energy in the fat cells for fight or flight. This metabolic slowdown explains part of the quick weight gain that often accompanies stressful times. The slowdown affects energy as well, throwing a person into the fatigue ditch.

Gastrointestinal function is also hit through increased secretions of gastric acids and improper movement of food stuffs through the digestive tract. This means constipation for some; gastritis, ulceration, diarrhea, spastic colon, or Irritable Bowel Syndrome for others. Those prone to increased acidity often have difficulties "facing food" when stressed; they keep a low-grade "queeze" at all times and are prone to a vicious "the less I eat, the worse I feel, and thereby the less I eat" mode.

(2) THE BLOOD SUGAR DIPS, stimulating an appetite for high-calorie foods that will provide needed energy. As the blood sugars fluctuate, energy and moods drop, but appetite soars. Yes, there is a physical reason for getting tired and cranky in stressful times. And, yes, there's a physical reason for craving M&Ms (compounded with strained emotions asking for food to tranquilize the anxiety—after all, *stressed*, spelled backward, is *desserts*).

(3) THE BODY RETAINS EXCESS FLUIDS, keeping the system lubricated

and hydrated for the survival defense. Blood pools in our muscles and extremities, and we store the fluids in the extra poundage in our abdominal area, making us feel bloated and sluggish.

All in all, a stressed body is a rotten place to live—and for some of us it's a 365-day-a-year residence. Some days we face intense, crisis-oriented stress. But some of us live with a level of day-to-day stress that makes us feel chronically out of control to some degree. Chronic stress takes a particular toll on the body because, though it fluctuates in intensity, it never really goes away.

Strategic eating and drinking, exercise, proper breathing, and adequate rest will enable you to stand strong even with a particularly heavy stress load.

The Value of Eating Well

Strategic eating strengthens our barricades against attack and feeds our stress-fighting army. When it comes to righting the fat-storage mechanism of stress and having all the metabolic burn you want and need, eating the right foods at the right time is the bottom line.

Unfortunately, when stress comes in the front door, wise eating often goes out the window. "Quick and easy" takes precedence over nutritious—which leads to fatigue. The more fatigued we get, the less we exercise. The less we exercise, the more fatigued—and stressed—we become.

Although we know that healthy eating and exercise would make a world of difference, they seem like more time-robbers and add to our already long list of "shoulds." If this sounds familiar, try transforming "shoulds" to "coulds." Take charge of what you *can*. As the body's metabolism slows, properly timed and balanced eating can gear it up. When the stress chemicals produce more gastric acids, smart eating can neutralize the acids and stabilize digestive function.

As the blood sugars fluctuate more wildly, the right foods at the right time can keep them even. When the body retains more fluids, adequate protein and fluid intake helps restore proper fluid balance.

Strategic eating keeps your body actively metabolizing the nutrients you eat. In addition, it energizes you for exercise and allows for more restful sleep, both of which further equip the body to alleviate stress.

The Power of Exercise

Exercise is a sword that cuts away at the negative symptoms of stress—a powerful offensive weapon in the war against stress.

Aerobic exercise simulates the physical exertion in the fight-or-flight chemical reactions that occur in the body under stress. It prompts the release of endorphins, powerful stress-busting chemicals. Working somewhat like morphine, endorphins tell the body that it is no longer in danger. You defeated or outran the grizzly bear! You took control of the challenging situation; it no longer controls you.

When you hit a tennis ball, your body thinks you've had your fight. When you walk, your body thinks you are fleeing your present danger; ballroom dancing tells your body that you're waltzing away from the threat. Even laughing is an exercise that contains great stress-busting power—it tells your body that the stress is nothing to fret about. It can't be life-threatening if you can laugh.

Nothing can replace exercise; it is the key to a positive response to stress. This is why exercise is considered nature's best tranquilizer. Exercise just thirty minutes—it can even become your quiet time in the midst of a busy life, a time when you can see the stress through a different lens.

Ironically, when life is most stressful, when we have the least

amount of time to exercise, rest and reflect, eat well, or find anything to laugh about, is when we need those things most. Taking
charge of our bodies is one thing within our control, even in the
midst of situations that feel very out of control. We can respond as
victims or victors.

SECRET NO. 3:
CULTIVATE A POSITIVE PERSPECTIVE

A positive mental attitude is a vital spoke in the wheel of wellness—
and critical in successful weight loss. In contrast, a negative attitude
saps our well-being and aims us toward just what we expect: the
worst.

There is both spiritual and scientific wisdom behind having a
positive attitude; it is imperative that we set our eyes and our belief
on the good things of life. The wisdom behind this is that our mind
is a magnet and we gravitate toward what we think about most. We
move straight toward whatever we have our eyes on.

Have you ever noticed how often automobile wrecks involve tele-
phone poles? When a car is running off the road, there is much more
open space to go toward than there are poles to hit. Yet they are
what the driver sees, and they are what the driver hits.

If I continually grouse that nothing ever works for me, that there
is never enough time, that nobody cares for me, that only tough
things come my way, then I will attract more of the same. Because
my eyes are only on my lack, I will overlook opportunity, refuse
offers of help, and continue to propel myself into emotional and
spiritual bankruptcy.

I have observed that if a person consistently concentrates on what he
doesn't have, he will get less and less of what he wants. If we focus on
what's wrong, we never find what's right. Alternately, the people who

are continually rejoicing in what life gives them, and are always looking for and expecting the best, lead active and fulfilling lives. Those
who have the most beautiful lives are those who value life highly.

I'm not suggesting that all the answers to life's problems come
simply through "the power of positive thinking," but I do believe
that a positive perception goes beyond our circumstances. True joy
stems from deep within our souls and flows from our spiritual connection.

Attitude Lifters

Pessimists blame every setback on their personal flaws or on how
rottenly the world treats them, and they feel that nothing they do
can make it better. It's a state of mind with huge metabolic
impact—the negative "I'm gonna go eat worms" response weakens
the immunes and locks down the metabolism. Happiness and success—even in weight loss—will be elusive.

Cultivating a positive, optimistic attitude—the belief that you
can take charge of your choices and influence your circumstances—
protects you against sagging spirits and a lagging metabolism by
protecting you against the stress hormones that accompany hopelessness. Try these ten tips to bolster your self-image and lift up your
attitude:

(1) PAY ATTENTION TO YOUR SELF-TALK. A negative perspective and negative self-talk become a habitual thought pattern, and it's a hard
habit to shake—particularly when it's focused on our own body
image. We can be our own worst enemy or our own best friend. It's
all revealed in how we talk to ourselves. It's amazing how often we
put ourselves down throughout the day—and it's time to stop! We
need to replace the negative thoughts with positive ones. It's much

like giving our mind and soul a healthy dose of weed and feed—weeding out the negative belief system, and feeding the one that allows us to thrive.

Next time you catch yourself making critical comments, fight back by immediately complimenting yourself and marveling at how specially you were created. Turn a phrase like, "No one could like anyone as fat as I am," into a positive statement like, "I am liked and respected by others because of who I am. Beauty is an inner quality that comes from caring about myself and about others, not from my weight on the scale."

You may choose to eat well and exercise, but it will not make you a more wonderful, likable person. And believing that you already *are* that wonderful, likable person is what begins the process of lasting change.

(2) SEE THE WORLD REALISTICALLY. It's common to compare ourselves to people in magazines or movies, but this is almost guaranteed to make us feel inferior. Realize that envy is a mental state with no payoff. It is human nature to feel sure that others are happier than you are. But the better you know the people you envy—whether the wealthy, the famous, the celebrities with gorgeous partners—the more you will realize their facades hide the same worries, hassles, and sadnesses we all face.

If you must compare yourself to others, look at the real people around you. They come in different shapes and sizes, and none of them is airbrushed or highlighted. Rather than studying pictures in magazines or listening to celebrity talk, read articles or books about uplifting subjects that can raise your spirits.

(3) RECOGNIZE YOUR SPECIAL QUALITIES. Make a list of all your positive qualities, not including your physical traits. Are you kind? Artistic? Honest? Good in business? Do you make people laugh? Post your list near the mirror or some place where you'll see it every day.

(4) PUT YOUR BODY BACK TOGETHER. Most of us with negative body images have dissected our bodies into good and bad parts. "I hate my thighs and bottom." "My backside is okay, but my stomach is fat and my arms are flabby." Reconnect with your body by appreciating how it all works to keep you going. Try a daily routine of stretching; the fluid movements are great for getting in touch with your body that is so wonderfully made.

(5) REMEMBER THE KID INSIDE YOU. Give yourself permission not to be perfect. Inside all of us is the kid we used to be—the kid who didn't have to be perfect and worry about everything (or shouldn't have had to!). Give yourself a break. Place a photo of yourself as a child in your bedroom or at your desk at work so you can see it each day and remember to nurture yourself and laugh a little. Spend time with children as well—they are wonderful reminders of how playful and fun life should be.

(6) PEPPER YOUR DAYS WITH SMALL PLEASURES. Big changes won't make you positive or happy permanently. Negative, unhappy people who win the lottery are no happier a year after they win. But every little thing you enjoy gives you an immediate mood boost. Example: Walk in the park, concentrate on a hobby, or take time off to spend an afternoon with your kids.

One step toward being kind to your body, and inevitably yourself, is to indulge yourself with healthy pleasures. Get a massage, take a long, hot bath, use lotions that smell good, treat yourself to a manicure or a pedicure or go hit some golf balls. It makes a positive statement to your inner self—that you're worth it!

(7) ENJOY YOUR FOOD. Eating is pleasurable. So enjoy it! Food gives us energy and sustains life. Don't deprive yourself or consider eating an evil act. Don't make any food a "forbidden fruit." Focusing on what you shouldn't do and what you shouldn't eat only sets you up for failure. The negative behavior or food becomes an obsession—and it's only a matter of time before you fall headfirst! If you allow yourself to enjoy food, and eat more often, you'll be less likely to overeat. And your body won't feel bloated and uncomfortable.

(8) THINK YOURSELF HAPPIER. When a bad mood overcomes us, a slip-up becomes a life sentence of being no good; a bad hair day becomes an "I've always been so ugly" week.

The good news is that it's possible to reverse this negative outlook by becoming aware of it and working to change it. The next time something happens that puts you into a funk, make a mental list of what's going right. You didn't get that desperately needed raise? Oh well, you have lots of friends, and your boyfriend and your dog love you. If a friend forgets to call you at an appointed time, don't be bitter or stay mad. Replace the negative thoughts with happier ones like "Maybe he/she had an emergency" or "Everyone forgets."

(9) BE ACTIVE. Movement and exercise can make you and your body feel terrific! Not only does exercise help boost your mood, it stimulates your muscles, making you feel more alive and connected to your body. Exercise also distracts you from negative feelings and forces you to concentrate on your breathing, stamina, and physical power. By the time you've completed your workout, your negative feelings are likely to be less intense or even replaced by a positive sense of accomplishment.

(10) THRIVE! Live well—whatever that means for you. Living well according to a strong value system will help you feel better about who you are and how you look. Whenever a problem seems daunting, take action. Define your goal, then plan specific steps to get there. Every "hopeless" situation you turn around this way will make you a more positive person.

You are a unique, amazing person—don't forget it! A healthy, *happy* life can be yours.

SECRET NO. 4:
REGULATE YOUR BLOOD SUGARS

Our blood sugar level is one of the more powerful influences on our well-being, our ability to lose weight, and our appetite. From a chemical perspective, regulating our blood sugar level is the most effective way to release our fat-burning capacity.

When our blood sugars are up and even, but not too high, we are brimming with energy and vitality and our appetite is in control. When the levels are bouncing widely and wildly, our energy, mood, memory, clarity of thought, and overall performance is apt to rise and fall along with them.

Blood sugar levels normally crest and fall every three to four hours, and even more often and intensely when your body is stuck in the stress response. As sugars fall, so will your sense of well-being, energy level, concentration, and ability to handle stress. Your body will need about half an hour to convert what you eat to energy, so waiting to eat until you're cranky and starving doesn't help immediately. If you've starved all day, the drop in sugars will be a "free fall," leaving you weak, sleepy, dizzy, and *hungry*. There's one thing that doesn't fall with blood sugars, and that's your appetite. As the blood sugars crash, the body sends a chemical signal to the brain's appetite control center, demanding to be fed. And your cells are screaming for a quick energy source—not broccoli or cauliflower, but chocolate chips or Reese's Peanut Butter Cups!

Too much sugar and refined carbohydrates is a drain on anyone's energy metabolism, and a serious one for people with sensitive blood sugar responses. Once a person who is sensitive to the rises and falls

ARE YOUR THOUGHTS AND FEELINGS MAKING YOU SICK?

Intriguing research is affirming that chronic insidious thoughts of doom and feelings of hopelessness or unforgiveness can affect the immune system. For instance, doctors at the University of Ohio have shown that significant anxiety can actually lower several of the immune factors in your bloodstream. Other studies suggest that a negative state of mind can increase the risk of infection from a cold or virus, or even more serious diseases.

Medical researchers in California, Florida, and North Carolina have found that chronic worry, irritability, and unresolved anger may increase production of hormones that are responsible for reducing the body's ability to fight disease and can lead to high blood pressure and heart attack. In another study on people with diabetes, a negative state of mind that develops into depression has also been shown to trigger an adverse physiological response, driving up blood glucose and insulin levels and promoting weight gain. How it does this is not yet properly understood; however, it is theorized that the brain chemistry that accompanies these emotions and thought patterns alters levels of the hormone cortisol, which can worsen insulin resistance and lead to heart disease and other killer diseases from the lowered immune response.

in blood sugar has eaten, his or her blood sugar rises quickly, very quickly if the person has consumed a refined carbohydrate with a high glycemic index (one that is fast-released into the bloodstream as glucose). And that's the problem: what comes up quickly will quickly come down. These quick bursts of energy can ultimately cause fatigue and stimulate appetite by creating a drop in blood sugar due to the insulin surges that result. Remember, insulin levels rise in response to the higher blood glucose level that moves the sugar into the cell to be processed. The insulin does so by opening muscle cell doors wide to usher in the glucose that is to be burned for energy. But if you've consumed more calories than you can use at that time for energy, the insulin ushers the calories into the fat cells to be stored as fat. If you're also overloading on fat, those fat cell doors swing open wider still.

Everyone responds poorly to a high glucose load, but some respond worse than others. To estimate how blood sugar will be affected by eating, the glycemic potential of food has been established to show whether a food will raise blood sugar levels dramatically and quickly (fast release), moderately (quick release), or just a little (slow release). The glycemic rating of pure sugar is set at 100, and every other food is ranked on a scale from 0 to 100, based on its actual effect on blood sugars. Carbohydrates that break down quickly during digestion have the highest glycemic values—the level of glucose in the blood increases rapidly when these foods are eaten. On the other hand, carbohydrates that break down slowly, releasing glucose gradually into the bloodstream, have low glycemic ratings. The fast-releasing carbohydrates will be ranked with a glycemic index of more than 70, quick release carbs rank between 55 and 70, and slow release carbohydrates are given a rating below 55. The higher the number, the faster the blood sugars rise.

When the blood sugar rise is fast, the insulin released into the bloodstream is abundant. The high insulin level will outlast the sugar burst, taking more and more sugar into the cells and dramatically dropping the blood sugar levels to a less-than-desirable level. The result is that the person soon feels spacey, unable to concentrate, weak, sleepy, anxious, sweaty, or dizzy. The quick drop in blood sugar will also trigger a craving for more carbohydrates, the essence of what is termed sugar or carbohydrate "addiction." (If you suspect you may be strongly reactive to sugar level swings, read more in "Out of the Sugar Trap" on page 310.) In addition, the higher levels of circulating insulin stimulate the storage of fat in the cells and inhibit the burning of fat as energy. This is why eating evenly and wisely will keep blood sugar and insulin levels in check and enable the body to burn fat and release optimal energy.

The need to stabilize blood sugar and insulin levels is one area in which I do agree with the pop diets of today: One of the most important things you can do when it comes to losing weight is to control your body's hormonal response to food. But there isn't just one hormone to worry about (insulin), nor is the answer as simple as just cutting out or severely limiting all carbohydrates or sugar, or restricting carb choices to those with a low glycemic potential. The

FOODS LOW ON THE GLYCEMIC INDEX

Some foods produce a lower glycemic response than others—meaning that they result in a lower insulin surge—and are considered smart choices for day-by-day eating, especially for those seeking stable blood sugars and lower insulin levels. I consider those foods with a glycemic index ranking under 55 to be the better choices.

BETTER CHOICE GRAINS
Oats
Barley
Buckwheat
Uncle Sam's Cereal
Kellogg's Bran Buds with psyllium
Bulgur
Long Grain Brown or Basmati Rice
Tortilla
Whole wheat or artichoke pasta
100 percent stoneground
    whole wheat bread
Whole grain Pumpernickel bread
Whole wheat Sourdough bread

BETTER CHOICE LEGUMES
Chick Peas
Kidney Beans
Lentils
Navy Beans
Soybeans (the best!)
Peanuts

BETTER CHOICE VEGETABLES
Carrots
Corn
Green Peas
Lima beans
Sweet Potatoes
Yams

BETTER CHOICE FRUITS
Apples
Apricots, dried
Small Banana
Cherries
Grapefruit
Grapes
Kiwis
Mangos
Oranges
Peaches, fresh or canned in own juice
Pears
Plums
Tomatoes

fact is, when you eat *anything*, your blood sugar goes up. How fast and how much depends entirely on the food, the amount, the combination, and your own physiology.

The information regarding the glycemic response of food and the body's resulting chemical response are not just a theory or based on preliminary results of research. It is fact, the documented, confirmed results of many studies that have been published by medical and scientific journals around the world. Most of the popular diet plans and books written in the past decade have addressed the hormonal response to food and attempted to solve it in different ways, but the attempts are almost always knee-jerk reactions causing pendulum swings. Cutting out all carbohydrates is not the answer, because all carbohydrates are not the problem. It's the unbalanced diet that's the problem: refined carbohydrates are being eaten to excess, and the excess calories are being stored as fat.

The key to long-term weight loss and maintenance is to get plenty of carbohydrates—but make them whole and don't overload. Their intake needs to be balanced with low-fat proteins. Eating the right proteins increases your level of glucagon, another hormone that works to lower your insulin level. If you eat lunches that are high in refined carbohydrates but low in protein, you will throw off the glucagon–insulin balance and may find yourself feeling tired and craving sweets in the afternoon. It's a normal physical reaction. So keep your metabolism, fat burning capacity, energy, and concentration *up,* and appetite and cravings *down,* throughout your day by eating small amounts more often.

SECRET NO. 5:
EQUALIZE YOUR BRAIN CHEMISTRY

Our brain is amazing. It weighs slightly more than three pounds and has about 100 billion nerve cells. It conducts our life with every breath we take and every bit of food we eat.

You may not be aware of how much your appetite and satiety, your thinking, your memory (particularly short-term memory), and your moods depend upon your brain chemistry. During the past twenty years, science has learned that our sense of well-being is delicately controlled by a powerful group of chemicals in the brain called neurotransmitters. These neurotransmitters can be affected, often quite dramatically, by a wide variety of everyday behaviors. Our food choices, eating patterns, exercise, creative expression, sleep, intimacy, television, and interaction with others are all examples of ways that we alter our brain chemistry each day, both positively *and* negatively.

One of the neurotransmitters responsible for enhancing your overall feeling of well-being, goodwill, and zest for life is serotonin. This feel-good chemical increases your ability to concentrate on a particular subject or problem for extended periods of time—and to care about the problem. It also provides you with deeper and more restful sleep. When your serotonin is high, you are more relaxed and content. When serotonin is low, energy will also be low and you are apt to be immobilized with bad moods and depression. Concentration becomes difficult and sleep is fitful. Appetite rages out of control—particularly for carbohydrates, which boost serotonin. Many bouts of binges can be traced to a serotonin deficiency.

Dopamine is another vital neurotransmitter, but with the opposite effects of serotonin. A high level of dopamine also brings high levels of energy but in an alert, aroused, "get-things-done" mode. Abnormally high levels of dopamine result in high anxiety, to the point of aggressiveness and paranoia. The resulting message to the brain stimulates production of hormones that contribute to fat cell lock-down.

The stress response causes the production and even flow of dopamine and serotonin to go awry, causing chemical gymnastics. Plummeting energy and brain fatigue result from falling off the chemical high bar. A poorly nourished brain is not able to protect you against the stress response, fatigue, or overeating.

Your Tool Chest for Equalizing Brain Chemistries

We've talked about many of the things you can do to stabilize your appetite and moods and increase your metabolism, but you may not be aware that many of these secrets work because they work in the brain. In order to avoid using food as your chemical boost, use these ten healthy pleasure tools to keep your brain operating optimally.

(1) **EXERCISE!** Nothing will win the brain chemical battle better than a workout. Just a brisk ten-minute walk can produce serotonin that will last for an hour or more. People begin working out for many different reasons—weight control, muscle toning, back pain relief— but equalizing brain chemistries is the number one reason to stay with it. Just the ritual associated with exercise—putting on your shoes, stretching, seeing familiar faces, taking a warm shower afterward—can start the process of making your brain feel great!

(2) **GET OUTSIDE IN THE SUNLIGHT EVERY DAY.** Our brain's neurotransmitters respond well to sunlight. That's why we feel oppressed and trapped in urban centers or enclosed spaces. The more oxygen we get, the more alert we feel. And the more sunlight we get, the more feel-good chemicals the brain produces.

Sunlight, even on cloudy days, helps to set your biological clock, lifts your moods, strengthens your immune system, and even produces vitamin D to keep you healthy. Sunlight is made up of a full spectrum of wavelengths, or colors, each of which affects your body.

The full-spectrum wavelengths produced by the sun create feelings of emotional well-being and physical energy. A few minutes by a sunny window will brighten your day—and a walk outdoors can give you a tremendous boost! Even in the midst of winter, when you can't see the sun, your body responds.

Though not a replacement for natural sunlight, one type of artificial light helps you maintain proper energy levels and good spirits: warm incandescent light. Cool fluorescents have been shown to depress you and deplete your energy reserves. An increase and improvement in office lighting has been found to result in decreased absenteeism and errors—and increased productivity.

(3) CONNECT SPIRITUALLY. Share your thoughts with a trusted friend, pastor, or counselor, and turn to your Creator in prayer. Studies have shown that as little as twenty minutes in reflective prayer a day can prompt an ongoing sense of calm and well-being. The resulting

---

SEASONAL AFFECTIVE DISORDER (SAD) If you are desperately in need of light, suffering from seasonal affective disorder, you may need full-spectrum bulbs that more closely simulate natural sunlight. This form of depression has been linked to inadequate exposure to light, and may be caused by an improper balance of melatonin in the brain. The symptoms of SAD are:

- noticeable lack of energy
- a fairly constant level of sadness
- a desire to sleep as much as possible, but the sleep is fitful
- feeling listless and being less creative than usual
- having less control of your appetite, resulting in significant weight gain.

SAD needs to be treated appropriately. The best treatment has come from bright natural light. Full-spectrum lights are now readily available for both home and commercial use.

change in brain chemistry is believed to be the scientific physiological factor in the proved strengthening of the immunology system that comes through this spiritual endeavor.

(4) SPEND TIME WITH UPBEAT PEOPLE. And participate in upbeat activities with them. Good moods are catching! Look for ways to help someone else: encourage a friend, pray for those in need. Research has shown an increase in serotonin when you refresh someone else.

(5) TAKE CONTROL OF YOUR SPACE. The chronic chaos in your life could be affecting your brain chemistry by keeping your body in a chronic state of stress. Even piles of paperwork can affect your well-being. Researchers have discovered that clutter (paperwork, newspapers, etc.) send impulses to your brain that can cause stress hormones to rise and serotonin levels to drop, affecting your pulse and blood pressure. Just clearing the clutter—even if you hide it in a closet—can bring you a sense of calm and well-being. That is, until you lose something! Like so many other self-care principles, organization takes time and motivation, but it's a tremendous investment.

(6) COLOR YOUR WORLD. Boost the feel-good chemicals in your brain by warming up the colors in your surroundings. Colors actually give off electromagnetic wave bands of energy, which send impulses to the energy control glands in your brain. Just painting a wall or wearing a certain color shirt can energize your day. Fascinating studies have shown that the blind respond to wavelengths of color just as those who see—in both energy levels and moods. That's an amazing thought: color is *felt*, not just seen.

Yellow shades have the most positive effects on brain chemistry, followed by the other warm colors of orange and red. Anything that adds these colors of fire—a flowering plant, a painting or poster, Mexican pottery—will help keep you more alert. Just be careful not to overdo; too much color can be just as damaging as too little.

Extroverts who are easily overstimulated and distracted often respond best to the calming colors of blue or green, but with a warm yellow-tinted shade.

(7) GET SHOWERED IN ENERGY. When you have the time or the place, a brisk shower can truly wash away brain fatigue, giving you just the chemical boost you need! The spray of the water from the shower peps up your body through a powerful energizing reaction that comes through exposure to negative ions (molecules with an extra electron). Although not completely proved, the theory holds that showers, waterfalls, and ocean waves multiply the negative ions in the air, which in turn affects brain chemistry, releasing energy and positive feelings.

You can get a quick, cheap stand-in for a shower with a small atomizer. Fill it with mineral water, hold it six inches from your face or pulse points, and spray. It's amazingly refreshing, like a rain or waterfall mist. It humidifies the air, hydrates your skin, cools you, feels good, and wakes you up.

(8) TURN ON THE TUNES. If you're in a slump, music can lift you up. If you're stressed, music can calm you. Music can open the door to your emotions, stimulate you, restore you, and awaken your creativity. The best brain power response comes from listening to music with a gentle rhythm such as that of the piano or flute—without lyrics or loud drums. It should be music that keeps your mind focused rather than distracted. Rhythmic music affects brain waves in a way similar to color, particularly by inducing alpha waves that have been linked to enhanced concentration.

This impact on the alpha waves of the brain is only one of music's power to relax. Studies show that listening to rhythmic music can reduce blood pressure, heart and breathing rates, and even stress hormone levels—all important in unlocking your fat cells.

(9) **DRINK WATER**—and lots of it! Overcoming dehydration will improve your blood circulation, which in turn will take your brain's feel-good chemicals throughout your body more efficiently.

(10) **FOLLOW THE EAT-RIGHT PRESCRIPTION.** Eat early, eat often, eat balanced, eat lean, and eat bright! Consider taking a multivitamin that contains at least 150 percent of the RDA for B-complex vitamins, which are fuel carriers, to nourish the brain and trigger the release of upbeat serotonin.

Nourish Your Brain

Vital to your brain chemistry is the last tool in the chest—the eat-right prescription: Are you getting enough of the right fuel to nourish your brain and keep essential chemicals stable?

When you eat, your digestive system breaks the food down into individual nutrients, like glucose and amino acids, to be absorbed into your bloodstream. Once absorbed, specific nutrients cross into the brain to speed the production of mood-enhancing neurotransmitters. What we eat—or don't eat—can have a profound effect on our mood, appetite, and fat-burning capacity.

For example, a raging appetite and slowed metabolic rate are clues to a brain fuel deficit, bringing an almost addictive pull toward certain foods. Your brain may need certain nutrients found in everyday foods to bring peace to the warfare within it. Eating, and eating often, is a big part of the solution.

Remember, your brain has only one fuel source: glucose. If deprived of its energy source, the brain functions at a deficit. Fatigue, mood swings, headaches, depression, and poor short-term memory are the early symptoms of insufficient blood glucose levels. By remembering that blood glucose levels normally crest and fall every three to four hours, you can prevent your personal sinking

BRAIN FOOD

Go for the Bs. In addition to fueling the brain with a constant supply of glucose, there are a number of other brainpower boosts that keep your mind sharp, clear, and effective—and your appetite regulated. For example, fuel-carriers are necessary to get the needed glucose supply to the brain. These vehicles are the B-complex vitamins. When the brain sputters along without adequate amounts of B vitamins, disorders like depression—even overeating—may be the result.

Your basic goal is to aim for these daily values: 2 mg of B6, 400 mcg of folic acid, and 6 micrograms of B12. Make foods rich in these brainpower Bs a part of your daily diet.

POWER B FOODS

VITAMIN B6 (needed: 2 mg daily)		FOLIC ACID (needed: 400 mcg daily)		VITAMIN B12 (needed: 6 mcg daily)	
Potato	.91 mg	Chickpeas, cooked (1/2 cup)	140 mcg	Atlantic Mackerel, 3 oz.	16 mcg
Banana	.73 mg	Lima Beans, cooked (1/2 cup)	140 mcg	Beef, 3 oz.	3 mcg
Whole Grain		Spinach, 1/2 cup cooked	140 mcg	Tuna or Salmon, 3 oz.	2 mcg
Cereal (1/2 cup)	.50 mg	Orange Juice, 1 cup	110 mcg	Milk, 8 oz.	1.5 mcg
Lean Beef (3 oz.)	.48 mg	Strawberries. 1/2 cup	110 mcg		
Halibut (3 oz.)	.34 mg				

Go Fish. Ever heard that fish is "brain food"? That's because it's an excellent source of the amino acid tyrosine. This amino acid increases the production of dopamine and norepinephrine, which help the body to buffer the effects of stress. Known as catecholamines, these chemical compounds work to regulate your blood pressure, heart rate, muscle tone, nervous system function, and metabolism. They are "alertness" chemicals of the brain. Studies have shown that people who get an increase in tyrosine foods perform better at mental tasks and show a significant edge in alertness and quick response time. They also experience less anxiety and have more clarity of thought.

Fish is the single best source of tyrosine, and brings it to you in an almost no-fat form. Cold-water fishes like salmon, swordfish, tuna, and mackerel (along with breast milk!) are also the best source of valuable EPA (eicosapentaneoic acid) oils, known to increase the IQ of developing babies. Whether adequate EPA oil intake helps the aging brain has not been established.

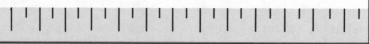

spells by eating smaller amounts of food more evenly throughout the day. Not eating sends you into "brain alert," and the brain sends out the call to eat, eat too much, and eat the wrong things.

You can prevent the alert, by eating the minimeals suggested in *The Smart Weigh* plan. (See specific details in Chapters 6 and 12.) "Power snacking" is also a valuable tool for equalizing brain chemistry because it gives you an immediate supply to meet the demand. (Read about power snacking on page 125.)

SECRET NO. 6:
TAKE CHARGE OF YOUR APPETITE

Many people go wrong not in *what* they eat, but in *how much* they eat. Even if they are eating food that is good for them, they often eat too much of it. Calories *do* count, so learning how to say *enough*—before you've eaten way too much—is vital.

I've got another secret for you: The way to tame your appetite and stop overeating is to *start* eating. You've already gotten a glimpse of this in learning of the power that regulating your blood sugars and equalizing brain chemistries can have over your appetite. It's a fact: wise eating all through the day keeps ravenous appetite away. Enjoying food, not shunning it, is the answer. I know that can strike fear in the heart of any overeater who believes that once he or she begins to eat, there is no stopping. And who has time to eat so often anyway?

American society has become so focused on avoiding and getting rid of fat that we've lost the positive and pleasurable aspects of eating. We've settled for foods that are convenient yet incapable of providing the full sensory experience. And that leads to one thing: overeating. When you've pushed your body through the day on fumes and eat steamed vegetables and plain broiled chicken night

LIQUID SNACKS? Don't make the mistake of slugging down soda to keep from snacking on candy or chips, thinking that *at least it's fat free*. (The average American downs fifty-three gallons of soda a year: 79,146 empty calories!)

In a recent study at Purdue University, subjects were fed extra calories in the form of solid food every day for a month. Their total daily calorie intake—and their weight—remained stable. They made up for the snack calories by cutting back elsewhere in their diets.

During a different month, they were given the same number of extra calories, but this time in a liquid form. Their total calorie intake went up, and they put on pounds. The reason, in theory, is that liquids pass through the digestive tract too quickly to trigger a feeling of satiety, so the "take in more" signal persists.

Other studies have shown that even people who drink diet sodas eat more calories. Of course, diet soda itself has no calories, but the sweet taste can trigger an insulin release that signals you to eat more—which is one of the many reasons that diet sodas have not produced a fit and trim world.

Some solid advice: choose snacks you can chew.

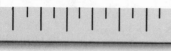

after night, pizza and Haagen-Dazs can sound really good—and a lot of it sounds better! Starvation and sensory deprivation is a sure route to a binge.

Managing Cravings

Sarah has a chocolate fit every month just before she gets her period. After a tough day at the office, Jim covets tortilla chips. Debbie suddenly can't resist pasta with a rich, creamy sauce.

Most of us have experienced a strong, nearly uncontrollable urge for a certain type of food. And while we've struggled to keep away from the refrigerator, we may have wondered why we long so intensely for a particular taste. Why do we have cravings? Are they emotional or physical?

Most people don't sell their soul for a stalk of celery. They are driven toward sugar and salt (inborn preferences for infants to drink breast milk) and fat (inborn preferences for children to sustain growth). The problem is that even though children outgrow their biological needs, their tastes persist because of the foods that are cultural and family favorites. They develop passions for peanut butter and jelly, macaroni and cheese, cheeseburgers, and milkshakes. For the more sophisticated palates of adults, it's

Rocky Road ice cream, fettucine alfredo, creamy chocolate mousse, and nachos.

Diet deficiencies fuel the cravings. As you've read, fluctuating blood sugars—enhanced by unbalanced hormones and stress chemicals—stimulate the driving desire for sweets; fluid imbalances drive the desire for salty foods; a sustained inadequate intake of calories (lack of supply to meet demands) fuels the desire for fats. This is the physical side of the craving, driving us in a general direction.

Our emotions help determine the exact food we arrive at. The body sends out the "I NEED" signal, the emotions send out the "I WANT" signal—and both send us directly the comfort food of choice, particularly when comfort is being called for. Our culture's battlecry is "relief is just a swallow away," and for many of us that spells food. The refrigerator light becomes the light of our life.

Learning Your Hunger Signals

It takes time to recognize the emotional issues behind the "I WANT" signal, but you can take charge of the physical side of your appetite this very day by learning to recognize true hunger. If you've been eating too much, too frequently, or too infrequently, it will take some time and adjustments to learn—and obey—your true hunger signals. Everyone is different; your task is to watch for your own unique hunger and satisfaction clues.

Hunger is not always about stomach sensations; it's more often about energy drops, weakness, fatigue, bad concentration, an empty feeling, crankiness, even cold hands and feet. Satiation has occurred when there is an absence of hunger or a fullness, a level of physical energy, loss of interest in food, and interest in other things. You are more than likely overfull (or as my teenage daughter calls it, "at capacity") when you are feeling bloated, lethargic, and short of breath. Your healthy goal is to eat to your level of satiation. Eat balanced and choose wisely, but *stop* when you are satisfied.

When you're eating right things at the right time, your meals and snacks will satisfy you much more easily. If you find you are feeling hungry between regularly scheduled meals and snacks, wait ten minutes and see if you still are. After ten minutes, ask yourself if there is something going on emotionally—or if you are just bored or stressed. If you're truly hungry, have your power snack at that time, even if you need to add another to that day.

You don't have to rely on iron-will discipline to control your food intake. By following an eating plan that meets the physical needs of your body, you *will* be in control. Follow these ten tips to stay full—and satisfied:

(1) KEEP A LOG ON THE FIRE ALL DAY. Again, the eat-right prescription of eating early and often, balanced and lean, with lots of brightly colored fruits and vegetables will fill you with satisfying protein, appetite-curbing fiber, and energy-boosting carbohydrates. And minimeals or power snacks every couple of hours will keep your metabolism in high gear and your appetite in control. Don't be a rabbit—salad alone won't satisfy you. Eat a well-balanced diet with plenty of fiber.

(2) EAT FRUIT BEFORE EVERY MEAL. These satisfying tidbits can curb your appetite and slow down your eating—*before* you "eat the whole thing!" Listen to your body and focus on fueling it rather than feeding your emotional needs. Remember, it takes most people about twenty minutes to feel full. We often eat too much in three to five minutes, and are left still looking for more. The simple carbohydrates in your fruit appetizer will have reached your bloodstream by then, helping you to reach satisfaction without looking for something sweet.

(3) **PAY ATTENTION TO YOUR FOOD.** Inhaling a sandwich at your desk or in your car can set you up for overeating—it fills you up, but doesn't satisfy you. We often turn to richly flavored candy bars or fat-filled chips to satisfy the flavor needs we didn't get during our meal. Instead, take the time to focus on what you're eating and savor every bite. And make it great! Forego bland and tasteless, albeit quick and easy, meals—go for flavor and pizzazz!

(4) **HAVE A SEAT.** Rushing through a meal can leave you feeling deprived even when your body's signaling that you're full. Savor your food, and avoid distractions like watching TV, which encourages mindless eating. Try to dine at the dinner table only. If you always eat in front of the TV, then every time you nestle in with the remote control, it's a cue to eat. Instead, designate an eating spot for all meals and snacks.

(5) **DRINK WATER, DRINK WATER, DRINK WATER.** And a lot of it! Don't mistake dehydration for hunger. If you yearn for salty foods, a big craving catalyst is probably your lack of proper fluids, which depletes your body's sodium supply. If you're craving chips, try a tall glass of water first! And, have a tall glass of water before and after each meal.

(6) **WAIT OUT CRAVINGS.** Think before you bite. Creating rituals—like the old standby of waiting ten minutes before giving in to a craving—can stop you from eating when you aren't really hungry. Ask before you reach: are you bored, tired, angry, stressed, or lonely? If so, you won't find the answer in food. If you find that your emotions are fueling your cravings, choose a healthier alternative than overeating. Sure, you can eat a bag of Oreos when you're angry or frustrated, but a five-minute walk will work, too. And you'll feel better, not bloated.

If the craving seems stronger than you are, try to make the most of it. If you crave ice cream, choose sorbet and yogurt and top it with fresh fruit. If you crave chips, get the baked version and serve with a fat-free bean dip or top with melted low-fat cheese. Give yourself a treat, not a trick.

(7) TALK TO YOURSELF. At heart, we all crave continuity. So when you try to alter long-standing eating habits, inner voices will pipe up to protest the change. Try to remember specifically why you want to change (e.g., "I'll have more energy when I lose weight").

(8) EXERCISE. Regular exercise keeps you energized and may even suppress your appetite for several hours. Remember, exercise boosts your brain's production of serotonin, which reduces carbohydrate cravings.

(9) PUT A MIRROR ON THE FRIDGE. It may sound strange, but researchers found that people who ate at a table with a large mirror on it were more likely to choose reduced-fat or fat-free products than those higher in fat or calories. That doesn't mean that you need to hang a mirror by the dining room table—a small mirror on your refrigerator or inside the pantry door may get the message across. Keeping a food diary can also serve as a sort of mirror for your eating patterns, helping you to get a grip on reality.

(10) BE PATIENT. Very, very patient! Forget quick diet fixes—it can take three to six months to replace bad habits with healthy ones. Answering the call of an appetite that's run wild is a physical as well as habitual pattern; it takes time to learn how to turn down your personal appetite thermostat, and time to learn how to "just say no" to urges that aren't physical at all. The quickest way to become discouraged is to expect quick success. So give yourself plenty of time to change. This will increase the odds that you'll stay motivated for the long run.

SECRET NO. 7:
STRENGTHEN YOUR IMMUNE SYSTEM

A vital part of the master design plan to keep you living life abundantly is a strong immune system. A good way to picture the immune system is as a disciplined and effective personal "border patrol," with soldiers and scouts on permanent duty throughout your body. These warriors include several different types of white blood cells, each with its own special mission. Together they work to identify a threat to the body, call an alert, and divide into army battalions to attack the enemy and stabilize the body. It all happens so quickly, you often don't even know you were threatened.

Your body's natural ability to lose weight is inherently tied to the energy and healing that is scripted into every cell in your body—and nothing will slow your metabolism and lock down your fat cells into "store" mode like being sick. When battle breaks out in your body, your immune fighting army locks up your fat cells tighter than Fort Knox. This is because your body is on a mission to fight the infection at hand—and signals ring out to produce cortisol from your adrenal glands to steer the immune system's production of white blood cells and steer them to the particular area of your body under attack. As mentioned earlier, heightened cortisol levels slow down the fat-burning capacity—putting your fat cells into a "store" mode to provide an adequate stockpile of fuel for the battle against the offending bug.

Although science has yet to discover a cure for the common cold, there *are* ways to outsmart many bugs. Researchers have begun to unlock some of the secrets of strengthening the immune system. In order to keep your border patrol officers alert and strong, the immune system needs to be kept fit and fueled, mobilized for action. Start eating more of the best and less of the rest. The real world can be a deadly place, so protect yourself with power foods and power living. Outsmart the invisible invaders that get you sick by using these keys to enforce your own personal protective shield—and receive a boosted metabolism as your reward.

(1) EAT POWER FOODS. This is the number-one strengthener of your immunes. Whole-grain carbohydrates not only give you energy, they supply much-needed B6, selenium, and magnesium, which activate your immune troops within. Power proteins provide vitamin D, iron, and zinc. Essential vitamins and minerals keep your immune system humming, so eat lots of brightly colored fruits and vegetables. They are loaded with nutraceuticals like beta-carotene, flavonoids, vitamin A, folic acid, vitamin C, and B vitamins that help to keep natural energy and healing flowing.

(2) TAKE A HIKE. Moderate regular exercise has been shown to boost the immune system significantly. It increases the activity of white blood cells and natural bug-killer cells.

(3) LIFT UP THE STRESS SHIELD. Studies have shown that people who are under chronic stress are more likely to get sick than those under less pressure. This is because during chronic stress situations, hormones (such as cortisol) are constantly circulating in excessive levels— amounts that can suppress the activity of immune system cells and make people more open to attack. It's a different way of responding to stress than the classic "fight-or-flight" response; instead, it's a "play possum" reaction. Just as a possum rolls over and plays dead when threatened, a person may "roll over" in hopelessness, depression, and feelings of being out of control. Physiological reactions include decreased heart rate and muscle tone. When chronic, this kind of "play dead" reaction may actually invite life-threatening illness by deadening the immune system's response, dulling the mind, and causing the organ systems to function less efficiently.

Unprocessed emotions have the same effect on the body, so don't bury them. Instead, deal with problems or get help. As silly as it sounds, even laughing at problems helps. Laughter even helps us fight infection by releasing hormones that can override the immune, dampening effects of stress. You can outsmart the slowdown with a smile.

(4) GET SWEET SLEEP. Studies show that people who are sleep-deprived experience as much as a 50 percent drop in their natural killer cells that fight invaders. The body can bounce back very quickly, though, with a good night's sleep.

(5) BE A GIVING FRIEND. It has been shown that people with a network of friends who give of themselves have four times the immune fighting potential of those who are more isolated and self-absorbed. Showing love can give an amazing boost to the immune system!

WELCOME TO *THE SMART WEIGH*

All of the secrets we've discussed are really process goals: the process of cracking the fat cell code and unleashing your body's natural ability to lose weight becomes your goal and keeps you well and trim for life. These secrets are the foundation upon which *The Smart Weigh* is built. Cracking the fat cell code and living *The Smart Weigh* begins with choosing a way of eating and living that is so comfortable that you can live with it the rest of your life.

The Smart Weigh plan is not a magic formula. It is a nondieting solution to weight management that works to unleash your body's natural healing and weight-loss mechanism. It is based on timeless truths that show you how the body was designed to work and how you can choose food and water, exercise, air, rest, and self-care to work for you, not against you. It enables you to operate from a point of strength physically—and sets the stage for you to meet the deeper needs of your soul.

I won't give you a specific diet to follow because sooner or later you have to go off it—you know that. But I do ask you to do this: throw out your diet books, and just say no to the next "diet answer" that comes to you via your friends, family, or group. Make the decision, today, to turn from the dieting path, and take a small step on the road to looking and feeling better. Refuse to sacrifice your health and your energy at the altar of improper weight loss.

Embrace these simple truths: live *The Smart Weigh*.

THE SMART WEIGH IN ACTION
S: Strategic Eating
M: Movement
A: Air and Water
R: Rest
T: Treat Yourself Well

Is *The Smart Weigh* easy? Quite honestly, because this lifestyle and eating plan represents the ultimate in health and nutrition, you'll probably find *The Smart Weigh* plan a challenge at first, as you adopt some new, powerfully healthy habits. But the results will be worth it. Studies show that each improvement in lifestyle will not only help your weight loss, but also lower your risk of heart attack, high blood pressure, stroke, cancer, diabetes, osteoporosis, cataracts, asthma, diverticulosis, depression, and even PMS.

Many of the steps in the next section will help you change your attitude or lifestyle which in turn will help crack the code of the fat cell. You have to start somewhere—and *The Smart Weigh* is that place. It is not important to enact the lifestyle upgrades in any certain order, or to master one completely before you learn about the others. However, I have put these principles in logical progression, beginning with meeting your body's most pressing physical needs. You will find that fueling your body well will regulate your blood sugars and stabilize your body chemistries to energize you for exercise. Eating well and exercising will promote more restful sleep. You'll start to feel good enough to notice when you feel bad, which will in turn remind you to slow down and take a breather. The stress reduction will lead to greater productivity and the free time to pursue the quality relationships and activities you value.

Can the image of the perfect body. Instead of thinking that you have to reach some unattainable goal, focus on losing just ten pounds over these next six to seven weeks. Keep that off for a while and let your body adjust. Then, if you want to lose more, you can. Or, don't focus on losing weight at all; focus on a new way of living—free of the diet trap. In the meantime, you'll be rewarded with new energy and wellness—not just from weight loss, but from your new marvelous way of eating and caring for yourself. And as you meet your physical need for proper nourishment, you will be better able to work on the deeper needs of your soul.

PART THREE ■ **EMBRACING**
              THE SMART WEIGH

CHAPTER 6 ■ S: Strategic Eating

It is futile to wish for a long life, and then give such little care to living well.

—THOMAS A KEMPIS

What if we stopped trying not to eat, or not to cheat, and started planning how best to charge up our internal motor? Then we'd be eating *The Smart Weigh*—and feel great all day, relax and play all evening, rise to almost any occasion, with activated metabolisms and bodies that are working for us, and with us.

Remember, eating smart isn't about what you *shouldn't* be eating; it's not about how bad potato chips or ice cream or red meat may be

> **SMART WEIGH TIP**
>
> *Stop starving yourself*
> *—eat to lose weight*
> The Smart Weigh.

for you. Instead, it's about the foods and lifestyle choices that power you with high octane energy fuel. The food you eat shapes the optimal performance and effectiveness of all your body mechanisms and allows your metabolism to burn in high gear. Releasing your body's natural ability to lose weight requires a nutrition plan that goes far beyond traditional or fad dieting.

It was only a decade ago that the world of nutrition began to go beyond dieting for weight loss alone and to focus instead on living life well each day while preventing the diseases of tomorrow.

Most of us underestimate the effect of our eating on how we feel. We don't connect morning sluggishness or afternoon sleepiness to when and what we eat. We know that food is our body's fuel, but most of us resist an even flow. As our schedules get full, it's easy for a consistent eating routine to go awry. Eating falls into an erratic, catch-as-catch-can affair that can't supply our body's needs. It seems as if we can't afford the time to eat well—yet the truth is that we can't afford *not* to. Wisely chosen food is a powerful tool to right the wrong of stress, and remove the logjam to your metabolism that it causes. Paying attention to how you eat is a small-time investment with a tremendous return.

Right now, changing your eating patterns may seem like just another duty, another bondage—maybe even another diet. But you will find that choosing to eat the right foods at the right time is choosing freedom. Rather than binding you, wise choices and self-control frees you to be the real you—free from compulsive dieting, overeating, or self-abusive living. Thousands of people have done it—and you can, too!

EDIBLE ENERGY

When it comes to nutrition, calories take a lot of abuse. Most Americans, particularly women, want to cut them, burn them, and otherwise get rid of them. But a certain number of calories are essential. They provide the fuel our bodies need in order to function. The truth about food is simple: food is just tasty units of energy. It takes food to make energy and to activate the metabolism.

As we've already discussed, the food we eat gets converted to glucose, which is the brain and lungs' only energy source and the most efficient and common form for the rest of the body. A single molecule of glucose can trigger the production of nearly thirty-eight

HOW TO REACH YOUR TARGET WEIGHT

To calculate if you are getting enough fuel, use this formula: multiply your current weight by 16 if you're active, by 12 if you exercise by lifting the remote control. This gives you the approximate number of calories you typically burn in a day—and the amount that will give optimal energy and the amount needed to maintain your current weight. An active 125-pound woman burns roughly 2,000 calories, a sedentary one will need only 1,750. An active 175-pound man needs 2,800 calories, a sedentary one will need only 2,100. To gain one pound per week, 500 calories should be added daily; to lose one pound per week, 500 calories should be cut daily—never to less than 1,500 calories for a female or 1,800 calories for a male.

Eating less than 1,500 calories per day can slow down your metabolic rate by 30 percent and leave you without key energy-releasing nutrients. Your memory, concentration, and judgment can all be impaired. Since weight loss means cutting back on those valuable energy-giving calories, it requires upping the ante of quality and timing of eating. To make up the difference, the goal is to become more active and better burn the calories consumed.

To reach your target weight, first figure out how many calories to cut to hit your goal. One pound of fat equals approximately 3,500 calories. Multiply 3,500 by the number of pounds you want to shed. To lose five pounds you'd need to burn about 17,500 calories. If you cut 500 calories daily below what you need for maintenance, you could lose the weight in about five weeks.

An easier approach is to split the equation. By shaving calories from your food intake and simultaneously becoming more active, you can minimize the struggle and maximize the results—reaching your goal sooner. *The Smart Weigh* plan uses the dynamic duo: reducing calories by 250 to 750 per day and burning an additional 250 calories with added exercise.

To Lose	You Need to Use Up	Time to Goal Weight Exercise Alone	Time to Goal Weight Eating well plus exercise
5 pounds	17,500 calories	6 weeks	4 weeks
10 pounds	35,000 calories	12 weeks	8 weeks
20 pounds	70,000 calories	24 weeks	16 weeks

molecules of ATP, the energy molecule that fuels the body's cells. Without ATP, the cells go on a hunger strike and muscles stiffen, refusing to function efficiently. Our moment-by-moment personal energy is, at the most basic level, all about how much ATP our body is producing. Food—and calories—give us the power to breathe, think, move, crack a joke, make love. Taken in appropriate amounts at the proper times, they are a *very* good thing.

Three components in foods provide calories: carbohydrates, proteins, and fats. Per gram (about the weight of a paper clip), each component provides the following number of calories:

Carbohydrates: 4 calories per gram
Protein: 4 calories per gram
Fat: 9 calories per gram

Alcohol also provides calories—7 calories per gram—but no nutritive value. Generally speaking, all calories—whether from carbohydrates, proteins, or fats—supply the same amount of energy. But each provides unique contributions to bodily function and health. Foods high in carbohydrates (including breads and starches) are mostly used for energy. The fiber that is found in many high-carbohydrate foods also helps regulate bowel function and protects against heart disease and certain types of cancer. Carbohydrates should make up about 55 to 60 percent of your total daily calories.

Protein (including meats, legumes, and soybean products) may also be used for energy. But the body uses protein in more vital ways—to make and maintain body tissue such as muscles and organs. In addition, protein is a key component of enzymes, hormones, and many body fluids. When there are enough calories from other sources, the body uses protein for these essential purposes rather than for fuel. Only about 15 to 20 percent of your daily calories should come from protein.

Fat provides the most concentrated source of energy. Even a little fat can provide a lot of calories. In excess, fat can increase the risk of cardiovascular disease and some cancers. Fat comes in two forms: saturated and unsaturated. No more than 30 percent of your daily calories should come from fat, and—ideally—no more than 20 to 25 percent.

Caloric needs vary considerably from one individual to another. A small, elderly, sedentary woman requires fewer calories than a large, young, physically active man. The number of calories you need depends on your age, height, weight, gender, and activity level. But remember, it's not just the energy consumed that counts; it's the energy *burned*. As we've discussed, our stressful, frenzied, and often sedentary lifestyles have slowed our metabolic rate to a snail's pace, resulting in fats being stored rather than burned for energy.

> **THE EAT-RIGHT PRESCRIPTION**
>
> Eat Early and Eat Often
> Eat Balanced and Eat Lean
> Eat Bright and Eat Variety
> Drink Water—and lots of it!

Regardless of the number of calories consumed when we eat, the body can use only a small amount of energy quickly—the rest is thrown off as waste or stored as fat. And most of us eat most of our calories overloaded into just a few concentrated hours in the evening. Because of this our bodies are robbed of precious energy fuel and a metabolism that's burning in high gear for the remaining twenty hours, until the next feeding frenzy. We not only go wrong in how much we eat or what we eat; we also eat entirely too much at the wrong time. Energy after six o'clock in the evening is just *too much too late*.

Instead, we need to activate our metabolism with *The Smart Weigh* eat-right prescription: small meals of high-energy, whole-grain carbohydrates and power-building, low-fat proteins complemented by brightly colored fruits and vegetables, at least every three hours, with LOTS of water.

EAT EARLY

Although it may not seem like news, breakfast is still the most important meal of your day—don't leave home without it! Breakfast begins your day by stabilizing body chemistries and starting your metabolism in high gear. View eating breakfast as a primary metabolic booster.

Breakfast is important to "break the fast" of the body's night rest. Remember the campfire story and your metabolism: think of your body as a campfire that dies down during the night and in the morning needs to be "stoked up" with wood to begin burning vigorously again. Your body is very similar; it awakens in a slowed, resting state, having utilized all the easily available fuel, and it needs breakfast to rev the rate at which you burn calories into high gear. After

CAN'T I JUST EAT A BREAKFAST BAR?

There is a wide variety of bars are available, from grain-and-"fruit" bars to granola or chocolate-covered bars pegged as meal replacements. Although there is certainly nothing "wrong" with these products, we are probably misleading ourselves if we say they are an equal substitute for a balanced breakfast.

Most breakfast bars provide less fiber than you would get from a whole-grain cereal or toast, and most contain substantially more sugar than you might realize. (Check the label for sugar content. Remember that every four grams of sugar equals a teaspoonful.) Even products marketed as containing fruit really contain what is more like sugar-filled jam.

Perhaps heading to bed fifteen minutes earlier would allow you to get up with five minutes to spare for a breakfast that includes a more balanced selection of whole grains, proteins, and fruit without too much of a fat and sugar load. Even if you prefer dinner leftovers to traditional "breakfast foods," the key is the balance—and real foods, not packaged pep.

a night's sleep, it takes 250 to 350 calories to get your metabolism percolating again.

If you choose not to eat breakfast, your body turns to internal sources for energy, burning muscle mass (not fat) for fuel. The metabolism slows down another notch, conserving itself in this disabled, starved state. Continuing to starve your body will leave it dragging through the day, unable to work efficiently and more ready to store whatever food is eaten. When the evening "gorge" begins, much of the nutrients you eat will be wasted and the energy stored as fat. All that food can't possibly be used up because your body isn't burning energy at a fast rate—the fire has already gone out. It's like dumping an armful of firewood on a dead fire.

After a big meal, your body puts out an excess of the fat storage hormone, or insulin. Remember, extra insulin locks down the fat cell, inhibiting it from releasing fatty acids to be burned for energy. Eating smaller meals, more often, is a lot like throwing logs on our slow-burning metabolic fires, getting them to burn better and brighter. It all starts with breakfast.

Don't think for a minute that you are wisely cutting calories or saving time by skipping breakfast. The truth is, those calories would be burned by your body's higher metabolic rate. You are only robbing your body of performance and metabolic fuel. And bypassing this morning metabolic boost doesn't just affect your weight—it can also affect your thinking abilities. Research has shown that missing breakfast can undercut reading skills and the ability to concentrate. A recent breakfast study showed a full letter grade differential in children who had breakfast compared to those who did not. Not only that, the study reported a poorer attitude and behavior problems among the children who missed breakfast. A recent study at the University of Wales found that breakfast-skippers were less able than breakfast-eaters to recall a word list and a story that was read aloud to them.

Because breakfast stabilizes your blood chemistries, you will have more energy and alertness. It allows you to be more productive and effective, allowing you to do what you do quickly and more enjoyably—with fewer mistakes. How's that for a time investment?

But Breakfast Is a Pain!

Actually, people skip breakfast for lots of reasons. Again, some skip it to save calories; others skip it to save time. Some can't face food in the morning, and others just don't like breakfast foods.

If you are not hungry in the morning, it's more than likely because your body has gone through some chemical gymnastics while you've slept, and you may wake up in a state of "morning sickness." It's not that you aren't in need of breakfast—just the opposite. Breakfast will neutralize your blood sugars and stomach acids and make you feel better.

A quite common reason for skipping breakfast is that in some people it seems to start a vicious appetite machine making them hungry every few hours. If this is you, be assured that breakfast is not the problem; you get hungry soon after you've eaten breakfast because you take yourself out of the starved mode and raise your blood sugars. When you starve your body in the morning, the resulting use of your own tissue for energy releases waste products (ketones) into your system that temporarily depress your appetite and give you a feeling of fullness. You can continue to starve for many hours without feeling hunger.

Sadly, this backfires later in the day. As soon as you begin to eat, the appetite really turns on, and you eat too much, too late. In addition, you've let your body go into a slowed metabolic state, and you're setting yourself up for a gorge. Not only will you overeat because your blood sugar level has fallen so low, but, like the campfire, your body will not be able to burn those calories well. Remember, your body just cannot handle such a large intake of food at one time; your needs go on twenty-four hours a day.

In matters of nutrition, I talk a lot about investment and returns. Breakfast calories are a good example of this; the return is greater than the initial deposit—remaining calories eaten during the day burn more efficiently rather than being stored as fat. A Vanderbilt University study showed that overweight breakfast-skippers who started to eat breakfast lost an average of seventeen pounds in twelve weeks. Not only did eating breakfast speed up their metabolisms, but it also caused them to be less hungry the rest of the day. Because they were eating the right foods at the right times, they were less apt to eat the wrong things at the wrong times.

The bottom line: eat breakfast soon after you get up (within the first half-hour of arising), and have three different foods for breakfast—a quick, energy-starting simple carbohydrate (fruit), a long-lasting whole grain complex carbohydrate (grains, cereals, bread, or muffins), and a power-building protein (dairy, egg, soy, or meat). This good-for-you balance will allow a slow and steady release of glucose into your bloodstream to feed your brain and muscles with vital energy. Selecting whole foods, rather than a Danish and fruit punch, also gives your body the vitamins and minerals it needs to transform the energy nutrients into usable fuel.

Go light and easy if time is a push; try some eat-and-go meals like fresh fruit and skim-milk shakes, cheese-toast and fruit, or freshly fruited yogurt with a muffin. And don't be concerned if the meals are not made up of traditional breakfast-food choices. Some nonbreakfast food lovers start their day with a turkey or tuna sandwich or even a cheese quesadilla.

You may want to try the breakfast recipes on page 272—quick meals designed to give you the perfect start to an energy-filled day.

EAT OFTEN

Once you get your day started with breakfast, the goal is to keep your metabolic system and blood chemistries working for you. To prevent your blood sugar level from dropping and to keep your metabolic rate high, you need food distributed evenly throughout the day. Going many hours between meals causes the body to slow metabolically so that the next meal is perceived as an overload. Even if the meal is balanced and healthy, the nutrients cannot be used optimally—again, it's too much too late. And the lowered blood sugar will leave you sleepy and craving sweets. Snacking on the right foods is much more fun—and a lot more healthy.

This is what I call "power snacking"—eating the right amounts of the right foods at regular intervals—and it's an important component of *The Smart Weigh*.

But I Thought Snacks Were Bad

You may be thinking, *But I thought I wasn't supposed to eat between meals.* Wrong! When most people think of snacks, they picture potato chips, candy, and sodas. These types of snacks are "empty calories," providing high amounts of fats, sugars, salt, and calories, but little or no vitamins or minerals. A healthy snack, on the other hand, provides you with real nutrition and will keep your blood sugar levels from dropping too low. It will keep your metabolism burning high, your needs satisfied.

Your daily eating should consist of three meals with at least two healthy snacks. Ideally, eat 25 percent of your day's calories at breakfast, 25 percent at lunch, 25 percent at dinner, and the other 25 percent in healthy snacks, eaten about every two-and-one-half to three hours. This is not mindless grazing, which has been shown *not* to raise your metabolism; instead, it is eating strategically to go for the caloric burn. On average, weight loss winners eat five times a day.

Wise snacking will also invigorate your mind. Tests have shown that a snack eaten fifteen minutes before skill tests of memory, alertness, reading, or problem-solving greatly increased performance in

POWER SNACKS

- Whole grain crackers or Raisin Squares cereal and low-fat cheese (like string cheese, part-skim mozzarella, or Laughing Cow Lite Cheese Wedges)
- Fresh fruit or small box of raisins and low-fat cheese
- Half of a lean turkey or chicken sandwich on whole grain bread
- Plain, nonfat yogurt blended with fruit or all-fruit jam, or Stonyfield Farms yogurt
- Whole grain cereal with skim milk
- Wasa bread with light cream cheese and all-fruit jam
- Baked low-fat tortilla chips with fat-free bean dip and salsa
- Health Valley graham crackers or rice cakes with natural peanut butter
- Popcorn sprinkled with Parmesan cheese
- Homemade low-fat bran muffin with low-fat or skim milk
- Crisp bread with sliced turkey and Dijon mustard
- Small pop-top can of water-packed tuna or chicken with whole grain crackers
- Half of a small, whole wheat bagel or English muffin with 2 tablespoons light cream cheese
- Veggie tortilla rolls: whole wheat tortilla spread with mustard or low-fat mayonnaise, and sprinkled with a variety of shredded vegetables, and 2 ounces low-fat grated cheese
- Fruit shake: skim milk blended with frozen fruit and vanilla
- Trail mix: 1 cup unsalted dry roasted peanuts, 1 cup unsalted dry roasted shelled pumpkin or sunflower seeds, and 2 cups raisins (make it in abundance and bag up into 1/4-cup or 1/2-cup portions for a whole snack)

test subjects, while those individuals who had eaten breakfast and lunch, but no snack, scored lower.

Iron-will discipline has never controlled food intake and never will. No checklist or rigid diet plan will give that control. Wisely chosen foods and well-timed eating is much more powerful and energizing. Strategic eating is essentially a balancing act, achieved by giving your body the right foods at the right time, and put together in effective ways. This means having both carbohydrates and proteins at every meal and snack, and keeping your healthy snack handy. When you don't have good choices available, you're likely to reach for an unhealthy snack or not eat at all, with either alternative setting you up for a later disaster.

Consider the healthy power snack ideas chart on the previous page, and start making them a regular part of your daily diet. Many power snacks do not require refrigeration, so keep them available in your car, in your desk drawer, in your briefcase—wherever you may find yourself at critical times. They can be as simple as fresh or dried fruit with low-fat cheese or yogurt, half a sandwich, or a trail mix of dry roasted peanuts, sunflower seeds, and dried fruit.

EAT BALANCED

Eating evenly throughout the day is not the only important factor in keeping your metabolism burning high and your body working well. Balancing your intake of carbohydrates and proteins is also vital to utilizing nutrients optimally. Every meal (and power snack) should include both whole food carbohydrates and lean proteins.

I know that this notion slaps every pop diet in the face; all quick-weight-loss plans manipulate and throw off this balance to force quick weight loss from dehydration. But the only way to lose body fat without losing your health is to embrace balance. It's this balance

POWER PROTEINS

Anything that comes from an animal (poultry, fish, meat, eggs, cheese, milk, and yogurt) gives you complete protein, supplying all the essential amino acids that your body can't make or store. The only plant source of quality protein, a miraculous one, is the legume family (dried beans and peanuts). Their pods absorb nitrogen from the soil and become an excellent high-fiber, low-fat protein source. Yet, because they lack sufficient amounts of one or more of the essential amino acids, they are considered "incomplete" proteins. They are best eaten with a grain (corn, wheat, rice, or oat product) or a seed (sunflower, sesame, pumpkin) to be complete.

Examples of high-quality dynamic duos are: peanut butter on bread, black beans over rice, beans and tortillas or cornbread, or a peanut and sunflower seed trail mix. Generally a 1/2 cup of cooked beans serves as two ounces of protein when mixed with an appropriate grain or seed, and 3/4 cup equals three ounces of protein.

EACH SERVING EQUALS 1 OUNCE OF PROTEIN (7 GRAMS)

■ nonfat milk or nonfat plain yogurt	6 ounces
■ low-fat cheeses	1 ounce or 1/4 cup grated
■ 1 percent low-fat or nonfat cottage cheese or part-skim or fat-free ricotta	1/4 cup
■ eggs (particularly egg whites)	1
■ fish	1 ounce or 1/4 cup flaked fish, i.e., tuna, salmon
■ seafood (crab, lobster)	1/4 cup
■ seafood (clams, shrimp, oysters, scallops)	5 pieces
■ poultry	1 ounce or 1/4 cup chopped
■ beef, pork, lamb, veal (lean, trimmed)	1 ounce
■ legumes (black beans, garbanzo beans, Great Northern beans, kidney beans, lentils, navy beans, peanuts, red beans, split peas)	1/4 cup
■ Soybeans and soy products (such as tofu and soy milk)	8 ounces
■ natural peanut butter	2 tablespoons

ENERGY-BOOSTING CARBOHYDRATES

Carbohydrates are found in plant foods (wheat, corn, oats, rice, barley, fruits, and vegetables), and are nutrition heavyweights themselves. When chosen in their whole food forms, they are packed with fiber, vitamins, and minerals that allow your body to stay operative from a point of strength. Contrary to what you may have heard, carbohydrates are low in calories. It's what we cook them in or top them with (butter, mayonnaise, heavy oils, and dressing) that moves us into weight-gaining territory.

Some carbohydrates are digested and absorbed quite easily, allowing them to be quick-burning forms of energy. These are the simple carbohydrates, found in fruits, unsweetened juices, and crunchy vegetables. The closer the food is to how it is grown, the slower will be the release of its sugars into the bloodstream. Complex carbohydrates, found in root vegetables, legumes, and grains that have been processed and refined, require more time to convert into a usable form of energy; they are digested more slowly and absorbed more evenly into the system as fuel. An eating plan high in whole-food forms of carbohydrates is your best bet for living long and well.

SIMPLE CARBOHYDRATES

FRUITS

All fruits and fruit juices like apples, apricots, bananas, berries, cherries, dates, grapefruit, grapes, kiwis, lemons, limes, melons, nectarines, oranges, peaches, pears, pineapples, plums, raisins (Generally one serving of simple carbohydrates is obtained from 1/2 cup fruit, 1/2 cup fruit juice, or 1/8 cup dried fruit. This gives 10 grams of carbohydrates)

NONSTARCHY VEGETABLES

asparagus, beets, broccoli, brussels sprouts, cabbage, carrots, cauliflower, celery, green beans, green leafy vegetables, kale, mushrooms, okra, onions, snow peas, sugar snaps, summer squash, tomatoes, zucchini (Generally one serving of simple carbohydrates is obtained from 1/2 cup cooked vegetables or 1 cup raw vegetables or juice—this gives 10 grams of simple carbohydrates)

COMPLEX CARBOHYDRATES

GRAINS

The following amounts provide one serving of complex carbohydrates, giving 15 grams:

barley, bulgur, couscous, grits, kasha, millet, or polenta, cooked... 1/2 cup
bread... 1 slice
cereals... 1 ounce (1/4 cup of concentrated cereal such as Grape Nuts or granola, 1/2 to 3/4 cup flaked cereals, 1 cup puffed cereal)
1 cup crackers or mini-rice cakes... 5
crispbread or rice cakes... 2
oats, uncooked... 1/3 cup
pasta or rice, cooked... 1/2 cup
fat-free tortillas... 1
wheat germ... 1/4 cup

STARCHY VEGETABLES

black-eyed peas, corn, green peas, lima beans, rutabagas, turnips, potatoes (white and sweet), winter squash (Generally one serving of complex carbohydrates is obtained from 1/2 cup cooked starchy vegetables, giving 15 grams)

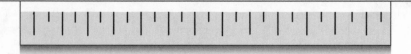

that produces the metabolic burn we are seeking the most. In a study published in 1999, researchers found that healthy young women burned almost 50 percent more of their daily caloric intake when they ate meals that were low in fat and high in carbohydrates (with proper protein balance) than they did when eating meals that were lower in carbs but higher in fat.

Remember, carbohydrates and protein have very different functions in your body. Proteins are the vital building blocks for the body. Carbohydrates are 100 percent pure energy—your body's fuel, designed to burn fast, clean, and pure. When carbohydrates are eaten alone, the body uses them like kindling on a fire. It burns brightly and quickly, but the body-building functions of protein do not take place. While protein can be used as an energy source, it has another much more vital function—which is why carbohydrates should be eaten *with* a protein to protect this building nutrient from being wasted as a less efficient source of energy. This allows protein to be used for building new cells, boosting your metabolism, building body muscle, keeping body fluids in balance, healing and fighting infections, and making skin, hair, and nails beautiful.

Women generally need at least 50 to 55 grams of protein per day; men generally need 65 to 70 grams (these estimates are based on percentage of lean body mass). More protein is needed in times of stress, or when actively working to build muscle or to maintain muscle mass while losing fat weight. Generally, one ounce of meat contains about 7 grams of protein, meaning women need a minimum of 7 to 8 ounces per day and men need a minimum of 9 to 10 ounces per day. Generally, your power snacks should include at least 1 to 2 ounces protein, and your meals should provide 2 to 3 ounces (after cooking). If possible, get a food scale and periodically weigh your protein portion to be sure you are getting enough.

But the *amount* of protein eaten is not the only secret to abundant energy and wellness; equally important is the need to take in protein in smaller, evenly distributed amounts throughout the day. Because protein is not stored, it must be replenished frequently throughout the day, each and every day. And this is where people go wrong. Never, never believe anybody who tells you that you don't need protein, or to eat it only once a day. You will be robbing your body of protein's healing and building power all day long.

The bottom line: be sure to eat proteins and carbs together. At every meal and power snack have a balance of high-quality, whole-food carbohydrate and lean proteins. Always remember: carbohydrates *burn* and proteins *build*. You need them both.

Best-Choice Carbohydrates

When choosing carbohydrates, go for the most whole form possible and thus benefit from all the fiber, nutrients, and natural chemicals they were created with. This means eating fruits and vegetables with well-washed skins on, and choosing fruit rather than fruit juice. Choose whole grains when you can, such as brown rice and stone ground 100 percent whole grain breads, crackers, pastas, and cereals. Look for the word WHOLE as the first ingredient on the label. These foods supply much-needed vitamin B6, chromium, selenium, and magnesium, all nutrients that are critical for activating energy production and release. They also have a lower glycemic response.

Whole-grain carbohydrates are particularly valuable because they have not had the outer layers of grain removed; they contain many more vitamins, minerals, and fiber than the refined, white products. Don't be fooled by manufacturers and advertisements. White, refined carbohydrates, even when enriched, are never as good nutritionally as whole grains. In fact, to your body, refined white flour is the same as sugar, making a diet high in white-flour foods the same as a high-sugar diet. Start reading the ingredients lists of all your grain products and remember to choose the ones made with 100 percent whole grain. Many manufacturers call products whole grain even if they contain only minimal amounts of bran. Brown dye does wonders in making food look healthy.

Whole grains satisfy and keep you full, so you may eat less in general. The fiber they contain slows the rate of nutrient absorption following a meal, reducing the rise of blood sugar levels and secretion of insulin that causes the fat cells to lock down. Fiber serves as a "time-release capsule," releasing sugars from digested carbohydrates slowly and evenly into the bloodstream. This helps keep your energy levels up and even.

EAT LEAN

One of the drawbacks to eating more protein, more often, is that many popular choices are also high in fat. But does fat make you fat? It's not quite that simple, but fat *is* more than just a disease culprit; excess intake is also a culprit in fat storage and metabolic lock-down. It's theorized that overeating fat sends fat molecules into your bloodstream, increasing the thickness, or viscosity, of the blood, and reducing its oxygen-delivery capacity. And it's the oxygen that's needed for energy to be metabolized rather than stored. In addition, the excess calories we consume as fat are converted and stored as fat more readily than those from other sources. One reason for this is that fat is a more concentrated source of calories (all fats contain twice as many calories as equal amounts of carbohydrate or proteins, about 9 calories per gram, or 120 calories per tablespoon). Also, the body is more efficient in storing fat as fat. This is why the weight control experts of today consider "trimming the fat" from our diets to be much more important in weight loss than just watching our calories.

FIBER: A POWERFUL WEIGHT-LOSS BOOSTER

Dietary fiber (the part of plants not digested by the body) promotes weight loss by helping to block the body's digestion of fat. A recent study of 3,700 men and women ages 18 to 30 showed that those who had the highest intakes of fiber-rich whole grains also tended to have lower body fat. The study showed that at all levels of fat intake, individuals eating the most fiber gained less weight than those eating the least fiber.

HIGH-FIBER FOODS

Peanuts and peanut butter
Cooked dried beans
Sunflower and sesame seeds
Apples, apricots, peaches, pears, bananas, pineapple, plums, prunes
Broccoli, carrots, corn, lettuce, peas, potatoes (including skins), spinach
Bran (unprocessed wheat and oat)
Bread (whole wheat)
Brown rice
Cereals: whole grain, bran type, oatmeal, Wheatena
Whole wheat pasta

In another study, people absorbed fewer calories when the fiber content of their meals was increased. Individuals who upped their daily fiber intake from 18 grams to 36 grams (a bowl of high-fiber cereal can contain 25 grams) absorbed 130 fewer calories per day. Over the course of a year, that reduction in calorie uptake would bring a loss of roughly ten pounds.

There are two types of fiber: the water-soluble fibers found in oats, barley, apples, dried beans, and nuts, which have been found to lower serum cholesterol and triglyceride levels and to help control blood sugar levels; and the water-insoluble fibers found in wheat bran, whole grains, and fresh vegetables, which are excellent means of controlling chronic GI problems.

Think of fiber as a sponge that absorbs excess water in the GI tract to curtail diarrhea but provides a bulky mass which will pass more quickly and easily to relieve constipation and diverticulosis and possibly prevent hemorrhoids. Fiber needs water to make it work the way it should, ideally 8 to 10 glasses a day. The best way to drink water is to have a glass before and after every meal and snack rather than with a meal when it dilutes digestive functions. Try filling a two-quart container with water each morning and make sure you have drunk it all before bedtime.

To increase the amount of fiber you get in your diet easily, choose more raw and lightly cooked vegetables but in as nonprocessed form as possible. As a food becomes processed, ground, mashed, puréed, or juiced, the fiber effectiveness is decreased. Add unprocessed raw bran to your cereals. Raw oat bran (from oatmeal) is particularly useful in stabilizing blood sugar and cholesterol levels; raw wheat bran is useful for a healthy gastrointestinal tract. Be careful to add bran gradually. Begin with 1 teaspoon wheat bran and 1 teaspoon oat bran and increase slowly as your body adjusts to more fiber.

Of course, fatness or thinness is not the only issue involved in our food choices. Even if you have been blessed with a metabolism that burns ever brightly, allowing you to maintain your weight easily, excess fat intake can bring problems. You may not be seeing the problem, on the scale or on your waistline, but it's an energy drain and a disease flag just the same.

Intriguing research on fat's effect on our metabolism has come out of Duke University, showing that Type II diabetic mice put on a radically reduced fat intake (10 percent of total calories consumed) were cured of their diabetes. This reflects the impact that an excess fat intake can have on blood sugar levels—of both mice and men. It also makes a statement about the risk of diets that push fat and radically cut valuable carbohydrates as a diabetes cure. The truth is that excess fat fed to animals with a genetic susceptibility to diabetes made them far more likely to develop the disease.

And there's more. Look at these vital facts about fat:

Daily Calories	Grams of Fat Suggested
1,500 calories	42 grams of fat a day
1,800 calories	50 grams of fat
2,000 calories	55 grams of fat
2,500 calories	67 grams of fat

- Excess fat intake increases your cholesterol level and your risk of heart disease and stroke.
- Excess fat intake increases your risk of cancer.
- Excess fat intake, particularly saturated fat, has been shown to elevate blood pressure, regardless of your weight or sodium intake.

The bottom line: choose your proteins wisely by making them low-fat. You certainly do need fat; it is an essential nutrient needed

ALL ABOUT OIL

We eat five kinds of oil: saturated, hydrogenated, polyunsaturated, monounsaturated, and omega-3 fatty acids. Each has the same fat content and number of calories that contribute to the fat budget: 5 grams of fat and 45 calories per teaspoon.

But these oils vary greatly in the effects they have on our bodies—good and bad. Some are damaging to the arteries and heart.

Artery-clogging fats that increase blood cholesterol include:

SATURATED FAT: Found in dairy and meat products, including milk, cheese, ice cream, beef, and pork. It also can be found in coconut and palm oils, nondairy creamers, and toppings.

HYDROGENATED FAT: Also called trans fat, hydrogenated fat is formed when vegetable oils are hardened into solids, usually to protect against spoiling and to maintain flavor. Examples include stick margarine and shortening, deep-fried foods such as French fries and fried chicken, and pastries, cookies, doughnuts, and crackers. Read the ingredient list of any processed foods you buy. If you see the words "partially hydrogenated," look for a different product—especially if it is one of the first three ingredients. Hydrogenation is a manufacturing process that converts a polyunsaturated or monounsaturated oil into a saturated fat.

Fats that do not clog arteries include:

MONOUNSATURATED FAT: Found in olive, canola, and peanut oils. These fats increase good HDL cholesterol and decrease bad LDL cholesterol, and thus the risk of disease.

OMEGA-3 FATTY ACIDS (EPA AND DHA OILS): Found in all fish and seafood, particularly cold-water fish such as salmon, albacore tuna, swordfish, sardines, mackerel, and hard shellfish. The only plant source is flaxseed. Omega-3 fatty acids decrease triglycerides and total and bad LDL cholesterol. They reduce the tendency of the blood to form clots, stabilize blood sugars, improve brain function, and reduce inflammation.

POLYUNSATURATED FATS decrease both bad LDL *and* good HDL cholesterol, so they aren't the desired choice. These fats are those in corn oil, cottonseed oil, safflower oil, sesame oil, sunflower oil, as well as avocado, sunflower seed kernels, sesame seeds, almonds, walnuts, and pecans.

Try to get most of your fat from monounsaturated olive and canola oil (or salad dressings made from them), nuts, and the Omega-3s found in fish and flaxseed. And spread your fat throughout the day—a little fat helps you absorb fat-soluble nutrients from vegetables and fruit.

in limited amounts to lubricate your body, transport fat-soluble vitamins, produce hormones, and fill you after eating. But it needs to come from the healthiest sources, not from bacon fat and butter.

Cutting calories is easier if you focus on limiting fat to less than 30 percent of daily calories. Cutting back on calories from fat allows you to eat more nutrient-rich foods like whole grains, fruits, and vegetables. You can also eat more food for fewer calories.

Determining Your Personal Fat Budget

As much as we need a balancing act of carbohydrates and proteins at each meal, we don't need fat in the quantities we consume. On the average, too much of our calorie intake is from fat—35 to 40 percent rather than the recommended 25 to 30 percent. The typical adult eats the fat equivalent of one stick of butter a day. Even if *you* don't eat that much fat, chances are you are eating a lot more than you realize.

To really understand your fat limit, you need to know your calorie limit. Remember, to lose weight, a moderately active woman will probably need to keep her daily caloric intake to around 1,500 calories. A moderately active man shouldn't exceed around 1,800 calories. To determine your 25 percent fat allowance, use this formula:

25 percent of 1,500 calories = 375 calories
375 calories divided by 9 calories per gram of fat = 42 grams of total fat suggested each day.

Once you know your fat budget, see whether you are staying within the bounds by adding up the grams of fat for all the food that you eat in a day. This is both the fat hidden in foods you eat—what is in chicken, fish, and cheese—as well as the added fat you cook with or add to your food, like oils or butter. Almost all food labels will tell you the grams of total fat in a serving.

Like any worthy goal, reducing your personal fat intake requires some effort and commitment—to learn new ways to season foods without fat, to order more healthfully at restaurants, to discover the right snack foods. Be assured that the benefits far exceed the effort. Smart eating does not doom you to nutrition martyrdom—eating flavorless foods that taste like cardboard. Nor do you have to become a chemical analyst to stay within these guidelines while dining out, grocery shopping, or cooking. Use the Practical Strategies For Living in Part 4 to help you trim the fat without cutting flavor.

> **SMART WEIGH TIP**
>
> *Get back to basics—
> limit your portions.*

Think of a move toward nutritious, low-fat eating as a permanent change instead of a dieting regime that you go on, and off. Don't keep a calculator at your bedside, and don't get stuck in a deprivation mode. Be easy on yourself, and go slowly, taking practical, feasible steps one at a time. Focus on good foods, well prepared, and your desires will begin to shift. Give your taste buds time to return to how they were created; high-fat foods will have less and less appeal as you begin to eat foods that kick up your metabolism and give you energy, better digestion, and a sense of well-being.

If motivation to cut back on the fat in your diet comes hard, consider this mental picture: imagine hamburger grease after it cools and hardens. Then imagine that grease trying to circulate through your bloodstream.

EAT BRIGHT

Brightly colored fruits and vegetables are loaded with antioxidants like beta-carotene and vitamin A, folic acid, and other B vitamins, along with vitamin C. These nutrients are vital to wellness since they neutralize chemicals believed to damage body processes and serve to boost metabolism by boosting the immune system.

Generally, the more vivid the color of the fruit or veggie, the higher in nutrients it will be. The bright color signals that these are treasure chests of protection, and triggers for releasing energy and raising immunities. That deep orange-red color of carrots, sweet potatoes, apricots, cantaloupe, and strawberries is a sign of their vitamin A content. Dark green leafy vegetables like greens, spinach, romaine lettuce, broccoli, and brussels sprouts, also have the extra bonus of being *the* source of folic acid (folate), a must-have for health and wellness. The presence of folate in the blood seems to lower the level of homocysteine, an amino acid that may be a cause of stroke and heart disease. A variety of foods contain folate, including breakfast cereals as well as beans and green vegetables. Since January 1998 the federal government has insisted that folate be added to all flour. So it's in your bread, whether you eat it sliced, wrapped, or by the baguette.

Without trying to calculate every milligram of this vitamin and that mineral in the foods you eat, the best way to assure that your vitamin intake is optimal is to go for whole-grain carbohydrates whenever possible, and choose meals full of a variety of brightly colored fruits and vegetables.

The ideal is nine servings of vegetables and fruits every day. Veggies and fruit are the foundation of *The Smart Weigh* plan, as opposed to grains, the foundation of the traditional food pyramid. You should be eating nine 1/2-cup servings (about 4 1/2 cups) of a variety of brightly colored fruits and veggies every day.

Sound like overkill? In reality, it could spell extra life. Study after study links diets highest in fruit and vegetables with less cancer,

> **TIPS TO RETAIN NUTRIENTS**
> - Buy vegetables that are as fresh as possible. When not possible, frozen is the next best choice. Avoid those frozen with butter or sauces.
> - Use well-washed peelings and outer leaves of vegetables whenever possible because of the high concentration of nutrients found within them.
> - Store vegetables in airtight containers in the refrigerator.
> - Do not store vegetables in water. Too many vitamins are lost.
> - Cook vegetables on the highest heat possible, in the least amount of water possible, and for the shortest time possible. Steaming, microwaving, and stir-frying are the best cooking methods.
> - Cook vegetables until tender crisp, not mushy. Overcooked vegetables lose their flavor along with their vitamins.

heart disease, diabetes, even osteoporosis. The landmark DASH (Dietary Approaches to Stop Hypertension) diet study found that nine servings a day lowered high blood pressure as much as some prescription drugs. More and more research suggests that nine a day—five vegetables and four fruits—is the optimum. Yet most Americans get only four servings a day.

Antioxidant Power

For fifty years or so, a leading hypothesis has been that aging and disease are promoted by highly reactive molecules called free radicals. The older we get, the more free radicals are released into our systems, where they destroy tissue. The villain is oxygen. In effect, we rust as we get older! But the body also has a network of defenses against free radicals, called antioxidants. Some are produced internally; others are derived from what we eat.

Vitamin E is one such antioxidant. Many other antioxidants also promise protection against diseases. One is lutein, found in leafy green vegetables, which may help protect against degeneration of the macula in the eye, the leading cause of blindness in those sixty-five or older. Another is lycopene, contained in tomatoes, apricots, guava, pink grapefruit, and watermelon, which may help prevent prostate cancer. And exciting beneficial effects are being shown through the antioxidants contained in red wine, blueberries, and strawberries as well.

As the research continues to pour in, this is the best health insurance policy: five servings a day of brightly colored fruits and vegetables will help to keep the doctor away... and ten servings will allow you to thrive, especially if complemented with other antioxidant-rich foods such as garlic, hot peppers, green tea, and soy.

FOOD HEALS

A discussion about strategic eating wouldn't be complete without some comments on the pharmacological wonders of food. If you have been eating foods just to lose weight, or gain weight, or just because it's dinner time, you are missing an important and exciting truth: food is filled with healing agents, like the antioxidants mentioned above, that energize and power you. Food is *medicine* for your body.

If you desire to get well, stay well, and live a life filled with energy, you must expose your body to food because of what's *in* food: natural healing agents, mood enhancers, and energy boosters. There

EAT LIKE THE GREEKS!

A Mediterranean diet may help protect people against rheumatoid arthritis, Greek investigators report. Study findings published in the *American Journal of Clinical Nutrition* from the University of Athens Medical School show that a high intake of cooked vegetables and olive oil may reduce the risk of developing the disease. The research team compared the diets of 145 rheumatoid arthritis patients with the diets of 188 people who did not have the disease. All of the study participants lived in southern Greece, where the average diet consists of less meat and more cooked and raw vegetables, fish, and olive oil than most diets in Westernized countries. Participants who ate the greatest number of servings of cooked vegetables were about 75 percent less likely to develop rheumatoid arthritis than those who reported eating the fewest servings. People with the lowest intake of cooked vegetables ate 0.85 servings of cooked vegetables a day, on average, and people with the highest intakes ate an average of 2.9 half-cup servings a day.

THE NUTRITIONAL TOP TEN

(1) **OATS:** The b-glucan in whole oats reduces the risk of coronary heart disease. The soluble fiber is instrumental in lowering cholesterol and stabilizing blood sugars.

(2) **SOYBEANS:** The bioactive ingredients in soy products suppress formation of blood vessels that feed cancer cells. Soy helps stabilize hormone levels in women, as well as decrease the risk of heart disease, osteoporosis, ovarian, breast, and prostate cancer.

(3) **TOMATOES:** Lycopene, a potent antioxidant, is a carotenoid that fights the uncontrolled growth of cells into tumors. It fights cancer of the colon, bladder, pancreas, and prostate. Men who eat ten servings of tomatoes per week have been shown to decrease their prostate cancer risk by 66 percent.

(4) **COLD-WATER SEAFOOD:** Healthy EPA/omega-3 oils are shown to turn on fat oxidation, decrease risk of coronary artery disease, stabilize blood sugars, increase brain power, and reduce the inflammatory response. Seafood reduces LDL cholesterol and triglycerides, while raising levels of HDL cholesterol.

(5) **FLAXSEED:** A unique source of lignans, powerful antioxidants that are believed to stop cells from turning cancerous. Flaxseed also contains alpha-linolenic acid, the plant version of the omega-3s found in fish oils; it makes a great healthy option for people who won't eat fish.

(6) **GARLIC:** Rich in allicin, which boosts immune function and reduces cancer risk. Garlic also has strong antiviral effects and has been shown to lower blood pressure and cholesterol levels.

(7) **HOT PEPPERS:** A source of capsaicin, a vital immune, mood, and metabolic booster with powerful antiviral effects. Capsaicin is linked to decreased risk of stomach cancer due to its ability to neutralize nitrosamines, a cancer-causing compound formed in the body when cured or charred meats are consumed. Capsaicin also kills bacteria believed to cause stomach ulcers, and appears to turn on the fat-burning capacity.

(8) **SWEET POTATOES:** A rival of carrots as a potent source of beta-carotene and other carotenoids, which help prevent cataracts and protect the body from free radicals and cancer—particularly cancer of the larynx, esophagus, and lungs.

(9) **GRAPES:** Grape skins contain a high concentration of resveratrol, which appears to block the formation of coronary artery plaque, as well as tumor formation and growth. Red grape juice or red wine is considered a better source of resveratrol than white, which is made without the grape skins.

(10) **CRUCIFEROUS VEGETABLES:** Broccoli, cabbage, cauliflower, and brussels sprouts contain indoles, sulforaphane, and isothiocyanates which protect cells from damage by carcinogens, block tumor formation, and help the liver to inactivate hormone-like compounds that may promote cancer.

are certain foods that pack a powerful punch when it comes to wellness. In addition to their wealth of vitamins and minerals, these foods contain nutraceuticals, the food pharmacy for the new millennium.

This may be a new thought for you. Most of us are much more aware of the food/*disease* connection: if a person has diabetes, refined sugar is a bad thing; if he's allergic to shellfish, eating lobster is a bad thing; if she has high cholesterol, saturated fat is a *very* bad thing. Yet most people are just becoming aware of the food/*wellness* connection. And it's the most exciting part of health research today—a focus on the essential building blocks in food that make us well and keep us well.

This new perspective takes us beyond Mom's chiding to "eat your vegetables" because they're good for us. Instead, it's an understanding of what, in broccoli, makes it exciting to eat—indoles and sulforaphanes that protect against cancer and aging, folic acid that protects against heart disease, and vitamin C that boosts immunes.

These truths are why I'm a "food pusher." This perspective builds appreciation and awe for lycopene in tomatoes—the antioxidant mentioned above that strongly protects against prostate and cervical cancer. Or for the b-glucan in whole oats that does medical magic by reducing cholesterol levels, increasing protection from cancer, regulating blood sugars, and serving as a gastrointestinal stabilizer.

These are just a few of the foods in my "Nutritional Top Ten" that can make all the difference. Review this list, and then review your food choices over the past week. How are you measuring up? It may be time to go to the grocery store and to start saying *yes*, not yuck, to power foods for your body.

There are *so* many other foods that could be placed on this Nutritional Top Ten list, some that may surprise you—like blueberries as a potent anti-ager and green tea as a brew for a slimmer you.

That's right, energy expenditure scientists in Switzerland have found that the flavonoid in green tea—epigallocatechin galate (EGCG)— has been found to "turn up the burn" in fat oxidation, helping the body to better burn body fat rather than store it. If you must turn to caffeine for an energy hit, turn to green tea instead of espresso.

WHAT ABOUT VITAMINS AND MINERALS?

Vitamins and essential minerals are required in tiny amounts to promote essential biochemical reactions in your cells. Together, vitamins and minerals are called micronutrients. Lack of a particular

YOUR SUPPLEMENT GUIDE

Supplements are not substitutes. They can't replace the hundreds of nutrients in whole foods needed for a balanced diet. But if you do decide to take a vitamin supplement, here are things to consider:

STICK TO THE DAILY VALUE — Choose a vitamin-mineral combination limited to 150 percent DV or less. Take no more than the recommended dose. The higher the dose, the more likely you are to have side effects.

DON'T WASTE DOLLARS — Generic brands and synthetic vitamins are generally less expensive and equally effective. Don't be tempted by added herbs, enzymes, or amino acids — they add nothing but cost. If you are going to use an herbal remedy, do that separately.

READ THE LABEL — Supplements can lose potency over time, so check the expiration date on the label. Also look for the initials USP (for the testing organization U.S. Pharmacopeia) or words such as "release assured" or "proven release," indicating that the supplement is easily dissolved and absorbed by your body.

STORE THEM IN A SAFE PLACE — Iron supplements are the most common cause of poisoning deaths among children. Keep them out of little hand's reach— and in a cool place.

DON'T SELF-PRESCRIBE — See your doctor if you have a health problem. Tell him or her about any supplement you're taking. Some supplements may interfere with medications.

micronutrient for a prolonged period can cause a specific disease or condition, which can usually be reversed when the micronutrient is resupplied.

A vitamin deficiency takes you down over time. It may take months, but it's a slow decline into fatigue and weakness. As your body becomes depleted of certain vitamins, various biochemical changes take place that result in a general lack of well-being. This occurs long before any symptoms of a specific vitamin deficiency can be noted. For example, a thiamine deficiency can ultimately exhibit itself as nerve damage, but appetite loss, weakness, and lethargy will proceed it.

Your body can't make most vitamins and minerals. They must come from food or supplements. Vitamins are organic minerals that the body does not produce on its own but cannot do without. As chemical catalysts for the body, they make things happen. Though vitamins do not themselves give energy, they help the body convert carbohydrates to energy and then help the body to metabolize it.

There are thirteen vitamins. Four—vitamins A, D, E, and K— are stored in your body's fat (they're called fat-soluble vitamins). Nine are water-soluble and are not stored in your body in appreciable amounts. They are vitamin C and the eight B vitamins: thiamine (B1), riboflavin (B2), niacin, vitamin B6, pantothenic acid, vitamin B12, biotin, and folic acid (folate).

In addition to their impact on your metabolism, vitamins in the right amounts are needed for normal growth, digestion, mental alertness, and resistance to infection. They enable your body to use carbohydrates, fats, and proteins. They also act as catalysts in your body, initiating or speeding up a chemical reaction. But you don't "burn" vitamins, so you can't get energy (calories) directly from them.

Your body strives to maintain an optimal level of each vitamin and keep a constant amount circulating in your bloodstream. Surplus water-soluble vitamins are excreted in urine. Surplus fat-soluble vitamins are stored in body tissue. Because they're stored, excess fat-soluble vitamins can accumulate in your body and become toxic. Your body is especially sensitive to too much vitamin A and vitamin D. For example, taking large amounts of vitamin D can indirectly cause kidney damage, while large amounts of vitamin A can cause liver damage. Even modest increases in some minerals can lead to imbalances that limit your body's ability to use other minerals. And supplements of iron, zinc, chromium, and selenium can be toxic at just five times the RDA. Megadose formulas can also cause stomach pains, diarrhea, and kidney stones. Virtually all nutrient toxicities stem from high-dose supplements—more is not necessarily better, and can even be harmful.

Minerals, unlike vitamins, are inorganic compounds. Some minerals are building blocks for the body structures such as bones and teeth. Others work with the fluids in the body, giving them certain characteristics. Some thirty minerals are important in nutrition, though most are needed in small, yet vital amounts.

Like an insufficient intake of vitamins, mineral deficiencies also zap your metabolism, particularly when there is a lack of the high-energy nutrients iron, magnesium, and zinc. Your body also needs fifteen minerals that help regulate cell function and provide structure for cells. Major minerals include calcium, phosphorus, and magnesium. In addition, your body needs smaller amounts of chromium, copper, fluoride, iodine, iron, manganese, molybdenum, selenium, zinc, chloride, potassium, and sodium.

Vitamin hucksters spend millions planting the fear: "Are you getting enough vitamins?" They recommend vitamin, mineral, and nutritional supplements as "vitamin insurance." But there's no need for most people to bank on vitamin insurance. The American Dietetic Association, the National Academy of Sciences, the National Research Council, and other major medical societies all agree that as your first choice you should get the vitamins and minerals you need through a well-balanced diet. Although certain high-risk groups may benefit from a vitamin-mineral supplement, healthy adults can get all necessary nutrients from food. But most people don't.

And they don't due to a different reason from what you might think—it's not a nutrient deficiency of our food supply, it's that most people don't eat properly. Only one person in ten, for example, regularly consumes the recommended five to nine servings a day of fruits and vegetables. Skipping meals, dieting, and eating meals high in sugar and fat all contribute to poor nutrition. For these people, taking supplemental vitamins would be reasonable and wise, although the best course would be to adopt better eating habits.

Food is better than supplements because food contains hundreds of additional nutrients, including phytochemicals. As already discussed, phytochemicals are compounds that occur naturally in foods containing important health benefits. Scientists have yet to learn all the roles phytochemicals play in nutrition, and there's no RDA yet established for them. But this is known: If you depend on supplements rather than trying to eat a variety of whole foods, you miss out on possible health benefits from these natural protectors. In addition, only long-term, well-designed studies can sort out which nutrients in food are beneficial and whether taking them in pill form provides the same benefit. In the meantime, it's best to concentrate on getting your nutrients from food.

Having said which, it is admittedly difficult to get enough of some vitamins from the most conscientious diet. Vitamin E, for example, in high dosages may help prevent some cancers and cardiovascular disease. To get that much from your diet, you'd have to consume 1 1/2 quarts of olive oil a day! Overall, however, it is better if your vitamin sources come from natural food rather than supplementation. But a cautionary note: the full benefits of a high dosage of vitamin E are not yet proved. In fact, still troublesome research reports are cropping up showing that antioxidant supplementation can actually trigger cancer cell growth and depress immunities.

The most intelligent course is to get the maximum vitamin and mineral intake you can from food—then use supplements. If you choose to take a multivitamin mineral supplement, look for one that has no more than 150 percent of the RDA. Name-brand multivitamins sold at pharmacies are fine.

And be aware that a multivitamin mineral supplement will not fully meet your needs for certain nutrients like calcium and it will never be a substitute for food. The additional supplements I most commonly recommend are: 100 to 400 international units (IU) of vitamin E and 100 to 500 milligrams (mg) of vitamin C. On days when you may eat only two calcium-rich foods, take 500 mg of calcium if you're under fifty; take 1,000 mg of calcium (divided into

MINERAL TONICS: DO THEY HELP?

So-called tonics of "colloidal" minerals (tiny particles of minerals suspended in liquid), which are touted to increase energy, are brisk sellers in multilevel marketing organizations and health stores alike. But there's no evidence that these drinks do any good, and because they contain potentially toxic heavy metals, they may do a great deal of harm. Many contain arsenic and dolamite, which can build up to toxic levels in the body.

two separate doses of 500 mg each) if you're fifty or older. Calcium citrate has been found to be the most absorbable supplement form.

The bottom line: If you want to improve your nutritional health, look first to a well-balanced diet. In most cases, making changes in your diet has a far greater chance of promoting health than taking supplements. However, even if you don't have a documented deficiency, your doctor or dietitian may recommend a vitamin-mineral supplement if:

YOU'RE OLDER — Lack of appetite, loss of taste and smell, and denture problems can all contribute to a poor diet. If you eat alone or are depressed, you also may not eat enough to get all the nutrients you need from food. Evidence, moveover, shows that, if you're older, a multivitamin may improve your immune function and decrease your risk for some infections.

In addition, if you're age sixty-five or older, you may need to increase your intake of vitamins B6, B12, and D because your body may not be able to absorb these as well. And women, especially those not taking estrogen, may need to increase their intake of calcium and vitamin D to protect against osteoporosis.

YOU'RE ON A RESTRICTIVE DIET — Although certainly not advised, if you are eating fewer than 1,000 calories a day, or your diet has limited variety due to intolerance or allergy, you may benefit from a vitamin-mineral supplement.

YOU HAVE A DISEASE OF YOUR DIGESTIVE TRACT — Diseases of your liver, gallbladder, intestine, or pancreas, or previous surgery on your digestive tract may interfere with your normal digestion and absorption of nutrients. If you have one of these conditions, your doctor may advise you to supplement your diet with vitamins and minerals.

YOU SMOKE — Smoking reduces vitamin C levels and causes production of harmful free radicals. The RDA for vitamin C for smokers is higher—100 milligrams (mg) compared to 60 mg for nonsmokers. Still, you can easily get this much by eating foods rich in vitamin C. If you smoke, try to stop. And don't depend on high-potency supplements to provide necessary nutrients. Two studies of beta carotene have shown an increased risk of lung cancer in smokers who take these supplements.

YOU DRINK ALCOHOLIC BEVERAGES TO EXCESS — If you regularly consume alcohol to excess, you may not get enough vitamins due to poor nutrition and alcohol's effect on the absorption, metabolism, and excretion of vitamins through the urine.

YOU'RE PREGNANT OR BREAST-FEEDING — If you're pregnant or breast-feeding, you need more of certain nutrients, especially folic acid, iron, and calcium. Your doctor can recommend a supplement.

YOU'RE IN ANOTHER HIGH-RISK GROUP — Vegetarians who eliminate all animal products from their diets may need additional vitamin B12. And if you have limited milk intake and limited exposure to the sun, you may need to supplement your diet with calcium and vitamin D.

The beautiful thing about good, balanced nutrition is this: everything fits together in such a perfect way that just eating a wide variety of different foods in their whole form will more than likely give you an adequate intake of essential nutrients. Eating well is the time-tested answer to the vitamin–mineral question, so don't let a junk diet vandalize your metabolism and energy stores any longer. Determine to make changes for the long haul. Learn how to eat and live with it for the rest of your life.

Eating to boost your metabolism and wellness has another payoff: it energizes you to exercise! Eating smart is only half the battle in your quest for an active metabolism—regular exercise is also a key to keeping your body burning calories at a high rate.

CHAPTER 7 ■ M: Movement

You cannot get fit in one workout, just as you cannot live your life in one day.

—**JOHNNY G.,** creator of spinning cycling classes

Exercise is critical to weight management success. In fact, it's the single best predictor of whether you'll keep off excess weight once you've lost it. A study done in Boston over a decade ago showed that weight loss people who dieted but did not exercise gained back nearly all their weight, while those who exercised along with dieting, and continued to do so, didn't regain any.

This is primarily because of the impact exercise has on muscle mass. When you start using muscle during exercise rather than losing it to dieting, you release your fat-burning

> **SMART WEIGH TIP**
>
> *Set small goals—just ten minutes of exercise will do your body good!*

potential. Strong muscles are a lot like the Energizer Bunny: they just keep going and going, activating your metabolism and boosting your calorie burn even while you sleep. New research shows that by building muscle, you can further boost the calorie burn you get out of any kind of exercise.

You probably know that the amount of calories that you burn during exercise depends on what type of exercise you do, your level of effort, and how much you weigh. Yet when researchers at the

Human Performance and Fitness Department at the University of Massachusetts compared bodybuilders with lots of muscle and little fat to men of the same weight who had less muscle and more fat, they found that the bodybuilders burned about 100 calories more during the same thirty-minute walk. They theorize that the good news will hold true for anyone building muscle, in any amount. Strong muscles rev up the body's calorie-burning ability. That is why exercise, particularly strength training, is the anti-aging solution. Lifting weights curbs muscle loss—along with shaping a sleeker, firmer body.

Aerobic exercise (meaning, "with oxygen") is a powerful metabolic enhancer because it boosts the oxygen-carrying capacity of the bloodstream. During aerobic exercise, your heart pumps more blood, your lungs take in more oxygen, and your blood carries more oxygen and fuel to your muscles. The glucose from your food combines with oxygen in your cells, producing and releasing the energy molecules you need for a fast-burning metabolism. This means exercise gives you more metabolic-boosting oxygen where you need it, faster, and more efficiently. And by making your heart more efficient in its function, aerobic exercise improves brain circulation and function as well.

In addition to increasing your caloric burn while you're running the track or pedaling the stationary bike, exercise is a gift that keeps on giving. The "after-burn" of exercise boosts your metabolism so you use up more calories for hours *after* you finish your workout. This is the real impact of exercise and is especially beneficial if you exercise at higher rather than lower intensities—walking, running, or riding just a little faster, or adding some hills or incline to crank up the calorie burn and keep it up, even after your workout.

Exercise also decreases your appetite and gives you a healthy outlet for stress—it douses the emotional fires behind overeating. Endorphins—the powerful morphine-like chemicals that promote a sense of well-being—are also released in your brain during exercise. And moderate regular exercise can create a change in biochemistry that launches you into a state of confidence and exhilaration. Studies have proved that just thirty minutes of aerobic activity—all at once or in three, ten-minute spurts throughout the day—will boost your energy, moods, and alertness. The overall effect of consistent exercise is to provide you better fuel to work with and a better engine to put it in.

Yet most people don't exercise at all. Surveys show that only 40 percent of Americans are involved in any kind of focused exercise on even a weekly basis—which adds up to from 40 to 50 million people.

"JUST DO IT!"

Why *don't* people exercise? I believe the answer is simple: too many of us are stuck in a viscious cycle of exhaustion. We know we need to exercise, but we are simply too done in to get it done. That's why I usually develop a phased *Smart Weigh* plan for my clients, first getting them to eat well and to start easy walking. After two to three weeks, a more focused exercise plan will emerge as a result of the overflow of energy. With this dynamic duo, the exercise adds significantly to their energy level and a positive cycle replaces the negative, downward energy cycle.

When you feel too tired to "just do it," keep reminding yourself of this: *the fastest way to feel energized is to exercise*. That "I'm too tired to work out" feeling will get out of your head once you start moving. You just have to override the message of your stressed-out brain and do something—anything—physical when you're in an energy slump. When you get home feeling totally beat, push yourself a bit:

change into sneakers and go out for a brisk walk. You'll feel a burst of energy afterward. Then the next time you're feeling too pooped to exercise, you'll remember that "buzz" and be quicker to get off the couch. You may even be inclined to expand your workout into a more ambitious run or bike ride, or even a visit to the gym. Soon you'll be healthfully hooked on the buzz of working out and won't even hear those "I'm just too tired" messages from your brain.

Not exercising is associated with an increased rate of illness and disease of nearly every type, from the common cold and flu to heart disease and stroke. People who don't exercise are more apt to die from cardiovascular incidents than to survive them. And because of the interconnected nature of the muscular system, brain, and other processes of the body, being sedentary also depresses your mood, your thinking, and your ability to work productively.

Here are fourteen motivators to get you going and keep you going:

(1) YOU'LL LIVE LONGER. An apple a day may keep the doctor away, but a two-mile walk may keep the coroner at bay. Researchers at the Honolulu Heart Program found that adults who walked an average of two miles a day reduced their risk of premature death by half. For the subjects who walked even more, the risk of death fell even further.

(2) YOU'LL BURN CALORIES. Particularly when you walk. Researchers at the Medical College of Wisconsin and Veterans Affairs Medical Center in Milwaukee tested the calorie burn of six indoor exercise machines and found the treadmill burned the most. When study participants exercised "somewhat hard," they burned a full 40 percent more calories walking on the treadmill than when on the stationary bike.

(3) YOU'LL GIVE YOUR BACK A BREAK. The best thing you can do for a painful lower back is to perform moderate, low-impact exercise, like

walking thirty to forty minutes, three to five days a week. Just avoid hills (which stress your back) and use good technique. Stand up straight, and don't let your stomach stick out or your head droop down.

(4) YOU'LL BUILD BONE MASS AND SLIM YOUR MIDDLE. Weight-bearing exercise like walking or weight-lifting promotes bone growth—a big plus in the battle against osteoporosis. And if you walk at a brisk clip (four mph), you may encourage your body to secrete more growth hormone, which strengthens bones and increases lean body mass.

(5) YOU'LL FEEL LESS PAIN. Researchers at the University of Florida in Gainesville corralled sixteen brave volunteers willing to have their index fingers pinched for two minutes before and after thirty minutes of exercise, then again after thirty minutes of quiet time. Once they recovered the power of speech, all the volunteers reported that the pain was most bearable right after exercise.

(6) YOU'LL NEUTRALIZE PMS SYMPTOMS. Regular aerobic exercise like walking can tame even the worst case of premenstrual syndrome (PMS) by raising the level of endorphins in the brain and by increasing your circulation, which helps minimize bloating.

(7) YOU'LL GET A GOOD NIGHT'S SLEEP. A Stanford University study of forty-three men and women with mild insomnia revealed that those who walked briskly for thirty to forty minutes four times a week for four months slept almost an hour longer per night and fell asleep faster.

(8) YOU'LL LOOK BETTER. Regular exercise gets your blood as well as your body moving. This increased circulation transports nutrients to your skin and quickly flushes out waste products. This leaves your skin glowing with enhanced health.

(9) YOU'LL OUTSMART MIDDLE-AGE SPREAD. You know it's true: metabolism slows naturally with age—but not necessarily because of aging. The decline in metabolic rate over time has less to do with advancing age than with declining activity. A University of Colorado study revealed that middle-aged and older women who exercised regularly didn't experience the age-related decline in their resting metabolic rate as did their sedentary counterparts. As a result, they stayed thinner and healthier—despite their advancing age.

(10) YOU'LL TAKE STRESS IN STRIDE. When you're confronted with a stressful situation, your body prepares to fight or take flight, in part by secreting catecholamines, chemicals that raise your heart rate and blood pressure and pump blood to large muscles in your legs and arms. Your fight-and-flight response then "burns off" those calories. The problem is this: Most often you don't have the option to fight or flee, yet your body is still releasing catecholamines that it doesn't use up. And your heart rate and blood pressure, as well as your stress level, remain elevated. The best way to get rid of those chemicals? Simulate the fight or flight: walk or run.

(11) YOU'LL HAVE A HEALTHIER HEART. Exercise helps to clear the fats that contribute to disease by stimulating fat-clearing enzymes. Fats are either broken down and excreted, or taken up by muscle and fat tissue. Either way, they're out of the bloodstream and less able to increase LDL cholesterol and heart disease risks. This also raises levels of HDL, which protects against heart disease. When a heart is well conditioned, it is like any other muscle: it becomes stronger and more efficient. A normal heart beats at a rate of approximately seventy beats per minute at rest or about 100,000 beats a day. The well-conditioned heart can actually beat as few as forty times a minute at rest or approximately 50,000 beats per day. A well-conditioned heart conserves energy and can supply oxygen-rich blood to the rest of the body with half the effort.

(12) YOU'LL BE A MORE CREATIVE THINKER. According to many recent studies, regular aerobic exercise can improve your memory, enhance your imagination, and make you more creative. The right side of your brain—the area that specializes in creative thought and solving problems—becomes more active when you exercise. It ignites your ability to solve problems, thrive under pressure, and perform at peak levels of effectiveness. As you dramatically increase your oxygen uptake, as well as the production of the red corpuscles that carry oxygen to your brain, the influx enhances the functioning of every organ in your body. Your thinking power receives a forceful boost because 25 percent of your blood is in your brain at any time during exercise.

(13) YOU'LL PROTECT AGAINST SERIOUS DISEASE. A Harvard University study found that women who run regularly produce a less potent form of estrogen than women who don't, resulting in half the risk of developing breast cancer. Researchers at the Harvard School of Public Health found that a thirty minute brisk walk or jog cut the risk of colon cancer in half. And physicians at Case Western Reserve University and University Hospitals of Cleveland report that regular exercise seems to reduce the risk of developing Alzheimer's. Exercise enhances your immune system, and generally improves the function of almost every organ and system in your body. One study found that people who walked briskly for forty-five minutes a day, five times a week, had half as many colds and flus as nonexercisers.

(14) YOU'LL HANDLE STRESS BETTER. Regular exercise can also help protect against the physical effects of daily stress, according to a report in the November 1999 issue of the *Annals of Behavioral Medicine*. In the study, college students who exercised on a regular basis were more likely to take life's daily stresses in stride, compared with their less physically active counterparts. Previous studies have shown that mental stress takes a toll on physical health, causing such problems as increases in blood sugar levels among diabetics, worsening of joint pain in people with arthritis, and symptoms of psychological distress such as anxiety and depression. Minor, everyday stress contributes to the development and exacerbation of physical and mental health problems. However, people experiencing minor stress develop different degrees of symptoms, depending on their level of physical activity. During periods of high stress, those who reported exercising less frequently had 37 percent more physical symptoms than their counterparts who exercised more often. In addition, highly stressed students who did less exercise reported 21 percent more anxiety than those who exercised more frequently. Exercise helps people get their mind off stressors. This temporary escape from the pressure of stressors acts as a kind of rejuvenation process.

GET F.I.T.T.

You don't have to take up the latest exercise craze in order to become fit. Instead you can forge your own path, at your own pace, and in your own direction. The frequency, intensity, and duration of your workouts will influence the extent of the health benefits you reap. The type and time of exercise you choose will determine whether you stick with it.

Consider this exercise guide to be F.I.T.T.:

FREQUENCY—Four to six days a week. Exercising *less* will produce some benefit, but not enough. Exercising *more* may be useful for athletic training, but can lead to injury.

INTENSITY—At a level where you feel slightly out of breath, *without gasping.* Exercise should not hurt. If something hurts, stop and rest. If the pain persists, check with your doctor.

TIME—Thirty to sixty minutes, at a time of day when you feel good and your schedule allows you to build a routine.

TYPE—Whatever type of aerobic exercise you enjoy (or could enjoy) and can do regularly.

Choose a time of day that best suits your schedule. Is it early morning? This is a great choice to beat schedule surprises later in the day. Research has shown that those who begin exercising in the morning are more likely to be at it a year later. Another reason to set the alarm for morning exercise: after a night's fast, two-thirds of the calories you burn come from stored fat rather than stored glycogen.

If you do exercise first thing, grab a glass of energy-boosting juice first (4 to 6 ounces of apple, white grape, or unsweetened cranberry juice is great), then eat breakfast right after your workout. If you exercise outside, pay attention to the weather. If you live in a hot climate, be sure you are drinking lots and lots of water to replenish the fluids you are losing to perspiration. And don't forget your water needs even when it's very cold outside. You can still exercise in winter, but be sure to bundle up in layered clothing that can "wick" the perspiration away from your skin. And cover your head and hands.

If you choose midday as your exercise time, don't let it interfere with your lunchtime fueling or let the exercise break turn your lunch break into a frenzied spin. If you don't have at least an hour, exercise will best wait for another time of day.

If you combine lunch and a workout, be sure you have your midmorning power snack about two hours before your midday workout, then have a piece of fruit (a quick-release carbohydrate) and a twelve-ounce glass of water right before you warm up. Exercise for thirty minutes, freshen up, and then have at least a fifteen-minute lunch.

Is early evening best for you? Although this is a difficult time to stay consistent (easy to "just say no" after a hectic day), it's a tremendous time to take advantage of the stress-busting, energizing power of exercise. By diverting yourself from your day's activities, you can downshift from stress to relaxation. It's a good time also to review the day's events—the good, the bad, and the ugly—and get a pulse on how you feel about them.

If you exercise after dinner, make it a half-hour afterward so you won't be doing battle with your natural digestion process. And don't exercise within half an hour of bedtime; your geared-up metabolism can interfere with restful sleep.

Aerobic workouts are best for morning and midday, serving to maximize energy, reduce tension, and enhance physical and mental performance. Cross training and interval training (more about these later) can energize your performance even more. Anaerobic work, such as conditioning and strength training, may tire you out and is best saved for later in the day.

JUST GET MOVING

No time to get to the gym because of all those household chores? Just get busy and get them done—and you'll get a fitness reward in the process. Studies have shown that you can ward off weight gain, lower blood pressure, and improve your cholesterol levels just by adding even a *little* extra activity to your day, instead of a full-fledged workout. Research done at the Cooper Center for Aerobics Research in Dallas shows that to improve your fitness you have to get your heart rate up, but that can be done if you just *get moving.*

The ways to increase your level of activity without having to adopt a program or invest chunks of time—or money—are endless. And, over time, being more active during the day can have a significant effect on weight loss and maintenance. Each activity below will burn off about 250 calories. And bear in mind that the harder you work, the more calories you'll burn. By pushing yourself to walk faster, scrub harder, or dance more vigorously, you can burn as much as 40 percent more calories in the same amount of time.

I recognize that these kinds of guidelines can sound like heresy for the avid fitness buff—or simply a nod of the head to our sedentary society. But just look below at the metabolic burn that can come from even moderate daily activities, and what it adds up to for a 130-pound woman by week's end.

The point is that *any* amount of physical activity can improve your level of fitness. Fitness is not thinness or being bulked up—it is being able to perform demanding activities without getting out of breath or becoming unduly fatigued.

Monday total: 525 Walk (30 min) 141 Cook dinner (1 hr) 162 Do light housecleaning (1 hr) 222	Tuesday total: 342 Take dancing lesson (1 hr) 180 Cook dinner (1 hr) 162	Wednesday total: 537 Walk (30 min) 141 Mow the lawn (1 hr) 396	Thursday total: 462 Weed the garden (1 hr) 228 Do laundry (1 hr) 234
Friday total: 342 Cook dinner (1 hr) 162 Take dancing lesson (1 hr) 180	Saturday total: 726 Walk the dog (1 hr) 282 Baby-sit nephew (2 hrs) 444	Sunday total: 618 Cook dinner (1 hr) 162 Do laundry (1 hr) 234 Do light housecleaning (1 hr) 222	Grand total: 3,552

NO PAIN, NO GAIN?

If you don't like exercising for the sake of exercise, just do fun things to make you active: take the dog out for a walk, chase a football with the neighborhood kids, get your toddler out for a power stroll, jog, swim, bike, dance. Even gardening and mowing the lawn counts. Or find a passion: ballroom dancing, tennis, volleyball, hiking. If you love it, you'll do it.

A NEAT WAY TO TURN UP THE BURN

In one study, researchers correlated the calorie burn from daily activities to why some people can seemingly eat whatever they want and not gain weight. They burn off the extra calories they consume through everyday activities such as walking, climbing stairs, doing household chores, even fidgeting and maintaining posture—a process researchers call NEAT (nonexercise activity therogenesis).

When researchers fed sixteen normal weight people an extra 1,000 calories a day for eight weeks, the amount of weight they gained varied from 3 to 16 pounds. The reason for the difference: some burned fewer calories (just 98) per day through NEAT than they did before the study, while others burned more (up to 692 calories). As reported in the January 8, 1999, issue of *Science*, it appears that when some people overeat, their NEAT switches on to burn this excess energy. Conversely, the failure to switch this on allows the calories to be stored as fat.

Better news: it appears that you can train yourself to increase NEAT. Here are five ways to do it:

1. Every time the phone rings, stand up before you answer it.

2. Whenever a commercial comes on TV, take out the garbage, put in a load of laundry, pick up the newspaper—anything to get moving.

3. Put on music when you're doing dishes or ironing and folding clothes and bop to the beat.

4. A bit obsessive, but helpful: Set your watch timer to beep every thirty minutes or so. When it goes off, tap each foot ten times.

5. Even more obsessive, but effective: Pick a cue word when you're at the movies or in a meeting, and whenever the speaker says the word rotate each ankle five times or shift the way you're sitting. Remember, you're in training!

The goal is simply to stand instead of sit, sit instead of lie, and walk instead of standing still.

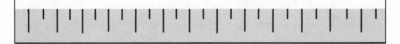

The notion of "no pain, no gain" is an exercise lie. If you are in pain, you'll stop exercising or get hurt, and the benefits of activity will come screeching to a halt. The key with exercise is not to let it *become* a stress. Too much, too hard—two to three hours of hammering the body—zaps energy. Moderation in all things, even exercise, is the age-old word of wisdom.

Before beginning or increasing physical activity, you should take some precautions to ensure a healthy start. To avoid soreness and injury, start out slowly and gradually build up to the desired amount to give your body time to adjust. Most healthy individuals can do this safely.

But if you have chronic health problems such as heart disease, diabetes, asthma, or obesity, you should consult your doctor before you increase your level of physical activity. Also, the American College of Sports Medicine recommends that healthy women over fifty and men over forty who wish to start a vigorous exercise program should check with their doctor to make sure they do not have

LOSE TWICE AS MANY POUNDS

Researchers at the University of Pittsburgh School of Medicine found that women who exercised for at least 150 minutes a week (that's 30 minutes, five times a week) lost nearly twice as many pounds—25 versus 14—as women who exercised less. Losing weight and keeping it off may require more exercise than previously thought—maybe as much as an hour each day, according to this new research.

In another study from Brown University, researchers found that 2,500 people who lost an average of 60 pounds and kept it off for a year exercised about an hour a day. Most of the people in this study walked about 10 miles a week, then did aerobics, weight lifting, or other activities.

A key to remember is that the more fit you are, the more efficiently you'll burn the calories you eat. If three people of similar weight exercise for 50 minutes at a moderately high intensity, the least fit person would burn about 250 calories, the moderately fit person about 400 calories, and the very fit person about 600 calories.

TWENTY-FIVE WAYS TO BURN 250 CALORIES	
Activity	Minutes to burn 250 calories
Cleaning the House	68
Cooking	93
Dancing	58
Doing Laundry	64
Frisbee Playing	43
Gardening	56
Golfing	50
Hiking	52
Ironing	132
In-Line Skating	36
Jumping Rope	26
Making Love	36
Mowing the Lawn	38
Playing the Piano	104
Playing Racquetball	24
Playing Tag with Kids	29
Playing Tennis	39
Playing Volleyball	83
Scrubbing Floors	39
Shopping	81
Surfing the Net	148
Swimming	27
Vacuuming	66
Walking the Dog	54
Walking Fast	44

risk factors for heart disease or any other health problem. Women under fifty and men under forty should also see a physician if they have two or more risk factors for heart disease, such as elevated blood pressure or cholesterol levels, smoking, diabetes, or obesity. And at any age, you should check with your physician first if you have cardiovascular, lung, or joint-muscular disorders (or symptoms that suggest such disorders).

At the very least, you may want to begin your exercise program with a fitness physical, which can be performed by your doctor or wellness professional. An ideal fitness physical is an "all points check" testing the following: cholesterol, EKG stress test, VO2 max, fat/lean body composition, blood pressure, and resting heart rate. This battery of tests helps you to discover if there are any potential risk factors in your planned exercise program, and to set realistic goals. It's a terrific benchmark, and can be highly motivating.

A WELL-ROUNDED WORKOUT

Fitness is most easily understood by examining its components. Basically, four types of exercise are needed to provide the best workout and to work all the muscles of your body: warm-up/cool down, aerobic exercise, conditioning/strength exercise, and stretching for flexibility.

Warming Up/Cooling Down

Use warm-up exercises, such as light side-to-side movements, to limber up your muscles and prevent injuries from the other types of exercise. Never skip the warm-up—it prepares your muscles for the workout (muscles work best when they're warmer than normal body temperature). A warm-up also allows your oxygen supply to get ready for what is to come, alerting your body to oncoming shock or stress.

You can warm up with stretching, jumping jacks, skipping rope, or jogging in place. You can also warm up with stretching and then beginning a less intense version of your exercise activity—for example, walking before jogging. An adequate warm-up time is three to five minutes.

Then, at the end of your exercise time, spend three to five minutes cooling down. This allows your body's cardiovascular system to return to normal gradually, preferably over a ten- to fifteen-minute

EXERCISE BEFORE YOU INDULGE

Take a long, brisk walk before your friend's wedding, and the hors d'oeuvres and cake may not be a heart attack on your plate. In addition to its benefits to your waistline, exercise can help override some of the nasty effects of fat in your blood.

High-fat meals cause spikes in the amount of triglycerides in the bloodstream, which wreak havoc on cholesterol by decreasing good HDL and increasing bad LDL. Over time, these contribute to atherosclerosis and heart disease. But researchers recently found that the timing of exercise can affect these fat levels significantly.

When a group of twenty-one men exercised twelve hours before a high-fat meal, they cut the mount of fat in their blood by half. (Exercising one hour before the meal lowered fat by nearly 40 percent.) Working out *after* a high-fat meal reduced it by only 5 percent.

EXERCISE ON TARGET

When doing aerobic exercise, it's a good idea to keep track of your heart rate. This is especially important when you are building up to a pace and distance that's ideal for you.

Your maximum heart rate is the fastest your heart can beat. The best activity level is 60 to 75 percent of this maximum rate. The 60 to 75 percent range is called your heart rate target zone. In this zone, your muscles are moving, you're breathing deeply, your blood is delivering ample amounts of oxygen to your body systems, and you're burning fat as your major fuel source. At this level, you should be breathing deeply but comfortably enough that you can hold a conversation or sing to yourself.

To find your heart rate target zone, subtract your age from 220. Your exercise zone will be 60 to 75 percent of that number. So, a forty-five-year-old would subtract forty-five from 220, getting an average maximum heart rate (100 percent) of 175. Sixty to 75 percent of this number would be 105 to 131 beats per minute.

When you begin your exercise program, aim for the lower part of your heart rate target zone (60 percent) during the first few months. As you get into better shape, gradually build up to the higher part of your target zone (75 percent).

To see if you are within your exercise heart rate zone, take your pulse periodically throughout your exercise time. Place the first two fingers of your hand at either side of your neck just under your jaw. You should feel your pulse easily at your carotid artery. If not, try the underside of your left wrist. Using your watch or the clock, count for six seconds, then multiply by ten. This is your heart rate per minute.

A fun way to determine whether you are exercising within your ideal zone is to buy a pulse meter, a gadget worn on the wrist or chest that monitors heart rate. It works great for those who have a difficult time mastering the art of checking their heart rate while continuing to exercise.

If you don't exercise hard enough to get your heart rate up into your target zone, you won't produce the changes in your body and brain that boost your metabolism, energy level, and mood. But exercising harder than your target heart rate is self-defeating; it can diminish the effectiveness of your workout. Working to such elevated levels causes you to burn more glucose as an energy source, detracting from fat loss and conditioning of your body. It can also leave you feeling exhausted rather than exhilarated.

period. This can be considered a "warm-up-in-reverse" because it consists of the same types of exercises as your warm-up.

Warm-up and cool down are just as important as the main event. Both can prevent many of the common injuries that take you out of the race.

Aerobic Exercise

Aerobic exercise is any large-muscle activity that gets your heart pumping and that you can sustain for twenty to sixty minutes. Jumping rope, jogging, cycling, stepping, and other cardiovascular activities are aerobic exercises that leave you energized.

> **SMART WEIGH TIP**
>
> *Up the ante. If you walk, try walking faster or running.*

Your heart and lungs work together to supply oxygen to tissues in your body. Aerobic exercise forces the lungs and heart to work harder and, in so doing, strengthens and conditions them. It is crucial for overall body wellness and for fanning the flame of the metabolic fire that burns fat. *Continuous* activity most activates the metabolism, not the stop-stand-start type that you do in softball, volleyball, or golf. And the routine of exercise is what builds a conditioned body—one that adapts much more resiliently to stress.

The minute you start to exercise, your metabolic rate (the amount of energy you expend) immediately increases to somewhere between five and twenty times what you expend sitting down. This change is very healthy when done on a regular basis. The goal is to try for some kind of activity every day. Even if it's not a hard workout at the gym, just a walk after dinner can do miraculous things for your body.

Vary your routine to rev up the calorie burn—different forms of exercise build and strengthen muscles in more parts of the body. Cross training is a technique you can employ that drives up the effectiveness of your aerobic workouts. Quite simply, it is alternating the aerobic activities you do. Instead of using a treadmill four days a week, alternate it with two days of biking. Instead of running every day, run three times a week, swim for two, and cycle for another. Your body perceives the different forms of exercise as more demanding (even though they may seem less demanding), and will trigger greater internal exertion. As a result, you will burn more fat for fuel and become a more efficient energy producer.

Interval training is a technique in which you vary the intensity at which you exercise. If you normally jog at a slow pace, periodically pick up the pace to a run, maybe for a minute, and then return to a slow jog. Alternate this during your entire exercise time. It can give a significant boost to your fitness gains and energy levels.

If your main concern is shedding some body fat, the key is to do longer, more frequent aerobic sessions at an easier pace. This approach burns more calories. Even though vigorous exercise burns more calories per minute than an easy effort, an extra fifteen or thirty minutes of easy exercise will more than make up the difference.

Longer bouts of exercise also burn proportionally more fat. Harder, but shorter exercise draws more on carbohydrates. If you walk or do some other activity for more than an hour, your body will start to burn significantly more fat for the rest of the workout. Why? Because the carbohydrate stores in your muscles begin running low after an hour.

Once you've settled into a routine of exercise:

- Do five to seven aerobic workouts a week.
- Make your effort as easy as possible so that you're able to exer-

cise continuously for forty-five to sixty minutes without strain.

- Try to do one or more "long" workouts (over sixty minutes) per week.
- Ignore any pounds lost in the first week (which are mostly water) and concentrate on a steady, consistent weight reduction of about a half-pound to one pound per week.

Conditioning/Strength Exercises

Conditioning or strength exercises are those that tone, shape, and define various muscles through repetitive movements against resistance. Conditioning exercises activate the metabolism by making demands on the muscles that change their chemistry, making them more energy efficient. Conditioning increases muscle strength and mass by putting more than the usual amount of strain on a muscle that stimulates the growth of small force-generating proteins inside each muscle cell. These proteins feed the "fibers" that grow during exercise. When you make muscles work harder, you actually tear these fibers. As they rebuild, they get stronger and bigger, resulting in harder, tighter, and more defined muscles.

WEIGHT TRAINING INCREASES:
Muscle strength
Muscle mass
The body's average calorie-burning rate
Tendon and ligament strength
Bone density

WEIGHT TRAINING REDUCES:
Body fat
Risk of diabetes
Risk of osteoporosis
Risk of heart disease
Risk of colon cancer
Lower back pain
Arthritis pain
Blood pressure
Cholesterol

WEIGHT TRAINING IMPROVES:
Balance
Digestion
Mood
Sleep

Resistance training can also have a beneficial effect on your body composition. As sedentary people age, from about age twenty or so, they lose 1 percent of their muscle mass each year. By age forty, it has amounted to 20 percent. Between the ages of twenty and sixty, inactive people can lose up to 40 percent of their muscle mass. And the flabbier muscles are, the less muscle fuel (energy) they can store. That means less strength and stamina for you. By the age of forty, up to one-half pound of muscle—and the energy stocked inside—is generally replaced with a half-pound of fat.

By reversing this process, weight training can see you into middle age with the energy, strength, and metabolism you had at twenty. As your muscles grow and become more active, the level of energy within the muscles increases, making you more vital. In addition, stronger muscles offer more support to your joints, pump up your sports performance, improve your balance, and help prevent injuries. And regular weight training exercises can boost your cardiovascular health by improving your levels of good cholesterol (HDL). Resistance training also strengthens your bones and helps increase bone mineral mass to help prevent osteoporosis, a disease that afflicts twenty million women in the United States.

A conditioning or resistance workout usually involves various exercises that focus on different muscle groups. This is the essence of circuit training on machines like Nautilus, which were built for this purpose. Normally the exerciser does one to three "sets" of each exercise (a set can be anywhere from eight to fifteen repetitions, and takes about one minute to complete). A typical session lasts about thirty minutes. But any kind of repetitive resistance training is effective, whether it's circuit training on weight machines; an arm workout with barbells or full soup cans; calisthenics such as chin-ups, push-ups, and sit-ups; or arm and leg extensions with exercise bands.

Just doing a few simple ten- to fifteen-minute strength-training routines at home or at the gym, two times a week, can turn the tide on muscle loss and activate your metabolism. You may notice an increase in the strength and the size of the exercised muscles in just a few weeks.

The good news is that strength and conditioning exercises are easy! You don't even need to change your clothes to get all the benefits with little or no sweat. A few years ago, I made a $20 investment in a pair of three to five pound dumbbells and a rubber exercise band, which is about four inches wide and three feet long and comes in different resistance levels. My best way to build strength has been to lift weight in three sets of eight to twelve repetitions. Lifting a lighter weight for more repetitions is the technique I use to build endurance and tone.

Here are some other tips to keep in mind as you build conditioning into your workout:

■ If you have access to a gym or health club that has Nautilus machines or other weight-lifting machines, sign up for an orientation to learn the proper use of each machine. You may consider a session with a certified personal trainer to get an individualized program worked out for you to reach your goals.

■ If you plan to work out at home, purchase a pair of three to five pound hand-held weights or adjustable-weight dumbbells (with metal plates that can be added or taken off).

■ Before trying any strength exercise, practice it several times with a very light weight, to learn the movement correctly.

■ Start with weights that feel comfortable for you and that allow you to do eight to twelve repetitions without pain. If you can't make eight repetitions of a given exercise, switch to a lower weight. Each lifting motion should take two seconds (counting "one-1,000, two-1,000"), while the recovery motion (returning to starting position) should take four seconds. If you're using a weight machine, one set per exercise is enough.

If you're using dumbbells, two sets (with a couple of minutes of rest in between) are recommended.

■ As you work out for several weeks or months, your muscles will get noticeably stronger, to the point where you'll need to increase the amount of weight you're lifting to continue improving. Whenever the twelfth repetition becomes easy on a given exercise, add three to five pounds to each dumbbell, or ten pounds to the load on the weight machine for that exercise.

■ Each strength workout should include a variety of exercises that work both the pushing and pulling muscles of the upper body (arms, shoulders, abdomen, and back) and lower body (legs, hips, and buttocks).

■ Always allow at least forty-eight hours of recovery time between strength workouts, to give your muscle tissue time to rebuild.

■ Choose your equipment wisely. For example, vinyl-coated dumbbells are comfortable to lift, and the bright colors lift your spirits, too. These are great weights for beginners because they come in one-pound increments (up to eight pounds), with a ten-pound option as you progress. (Beyond ten pounds, you'll have to opt for the more traditional chrome or cast-iron types.) Hand weights are also a good option for beginners, especially for people who have arthritis in their hands. Designed with either a strap or handle, you don't have to use a tight grip to hold onto them. Strapping weights to your ankles or wrists instead of carrying them in the hands is another great choice for people with arthritis, high blood pressure, or any other condition in which you should avoid tight grips. And whether you exercise at home or travel a lot, elastic exercise bands are a great way to enhance your workout.

These bands are lightweight, easy to use, and allow you to do exercises that normally require expensive machines.

THE EXERCISES

These are some exercises that can form the core of a regular strength-training program. You may want to begin with the first four exercises below and supplement them with the next four exercises if and when you want to expand your strength training program.

DUMBBELL SQUAT (LOWER BODY) OR LEG EXTENSION MACHINE

Stand holding a dumbbell in each hand with your feet flat on the floor, shoulder-width apart, and your arms down at your sides. Keeping your head up and your back straight, slowly lower your hips until your thighs are parallel with the floor. Then return slowly to starting position, still keeping head up and back straight. Repeat eight to twelve times.

DUMBBELL LUNGE (LOWER BODY) OR LEG CURL MACHINE

Stand holding a dumbbell in each hand, with your arms down at your sides and your feet slightly less than shoulder-width apart. Looking directly ahead and keeping your left leg straight, take a long step forward with your right leg, bending your right knee so that the knee is lined up directly above your right ankle. Distributing your weight equally on both legs, bend your back leg until your knee is almost touching the ground. Then push slowly off your right foot, stepping back into your starting position. Repeat eight to twelve times, then switch legs and repeat.

DUMBBELL CHEST PRESS (UPPER BODY) OR CHEST PRESS MACHINE

Lie face up on a flat bench or on the floor, with your feet flat on the floor, and hold a dumbbell in each hand. Extend your arms and then lower them to starting position against your chest (your elbows should point out to either side). Slowly push the dumbbells upward together until your arms are fully extended and the dumbbells are directly above your chest. Repeat eight to twelve times.

DUMBBELL ROW (UPPER BODY) OR LATERAL PULL-DOWN MACHINE

Holding a dumbbell in your right hand, rest your left knee on a low bench or step, and place your left (free) hand down flat in front of your knee on the same bench. You should be leaning forward so that your back is horizontal, and your right foot should be flat on the floor, with the right knee slightly bent. Lower the dumbbell so that your right arm is fully extended and slowly pull it to your chest, then return slowly to starting position. Do eight to twelve repetitions, then switch sides and repeat.

DUMBBELL CURL (UPPER BODY) OR BICEPS MACHINE

Holding a dumbbell in each hand, stand comfortably with your arms down at your sides. Slowly bend your arms, curling both dumbbells up to your shoulders, then slowly return to starting position. Keep your head up and your eyes looking straight ahead at all times.

DUMBBELL TRICEPS EXTENSION (UPPER BODY) OR TRICEPS MACHINE

Holding a dumbbell in your right hand, place your left knee on a low bench or chair, and place your left hand in front of it, flat on the bench. Hold the dumbbell with your palm facing inward, and your right elbow slightly bent so the weight is at hip level. Keeping your right shoulder still, slowly straighten your right arm, then slowly return to starting position. Repeat eight to twelve times, then switch arms and repeat.

DUMBBELL SHOULDER PRESS (UPPER BODY) OR OVERHEAD PRESS MACHINE
Holding a dumbbell in each hand, sit on a bench or a chair with your feet flat on the floor. Position both dumbbells at shoulder level, with your elbows pointing downward. Then slowly press both dumbbells upward, until your arms are straight but not locked (think of squeezing your shoulder blades together as you lift). Then return slowly to starting position. Repeat eight to twelve times.

DUMBBELL DELTOID RAISE (UPPER BODY) OR LATERAL RAISE MACHINE
Standing comfortably and with a dumbbell in each hand, hold your arms at your sides so that your elbows are bent at right angles, with your palms facing downward. Slowly raise both dumbbells until your upper arms are parallel to the ground. Then slowly lower your arms to starting position. Repeat eight to twelve times.

Here are three sample exercises you can do with exercise bands:

- Keeping your arms parallel to the floor, hold the band in front of your chest (at armpit level) with your hands about six inches apart. Slowly bring your elbows toward your back, as if you were squeezing a pencil with your shoulder blades. Hold for two seconds, then bring your elbows forward again. (If this is too difficult for you, use a band with less resistance; if it's too easy, switch to a band with more resistance.)
- Stand on one end of the band and hold the other in one hand. With your palm facing upward, slowly bring the band up to your shoulder, using only the lower part of your arm. It's important to keep the elbow close to the body and the upper arm straight. Repeat with the other arm.
- To target the large latissimus dorsi muscle of your back, a

muscle particularly difficult to get at using dumbbells, attach a band to the top of a door using a specially designed door anchor. (If you don't secure the band, it may slide off the door and smack you in the face!) Then sit or kneel on the floor, facing the door and holding the band so that it and your arms are fully extended. Your hands should be about shoulder-width apart. Squeezing your shoulder blades, pull your hands down toward your chest. Elbows should be pointing behind you and down. Hold, and then release.

CALISTHENICS TO REDUCE BELLY BULGE

No matter what the cause of extra abdominal fat—a recent baby, too many brews, or too much time on the sofa—this program will work for you. Do these six exercises three or four times a week to tone and tighten your abs.

Get started today! But go slowly for best results. Forget doing hundreds of crunches. You'll get a flatter tummy quicker if you slow down. Each repetition of an exercise should take about six to eight seconds to complete. For example, slowly count one, two, three, four as you lift during a crunch, and then five, six, seven, eight as you lower. If you experience back pain with any of these exercises, stop the exercise and check with your doctor before continuing. Do each exercise three or four times a week.

CRUNCH

Lying on a mat or carpeted floor, place your hands lightly behind your head, bend your knees, and put your feet flat on the floor. Using your abs, slowly lift your head, shoulders, and upper back off the mat. Keep your abs tight and exhale on the way up. Hold, and then lower. Do ten to fifteen repetitions.

TWISTING CRUNCH

Start in the crunch position. As you lift, twist your torso, bringing your left shoulder toward your right knee at the top of the crunch. Hold, and then lower. Repeat on the other side. Do ten to fifteen repetitions on each side.

ROLLDOWN

Sit on the floor with your knees bent, feet flat. Keeping your arms out in front of you, slowly roll down—one vertebrae at a time—until you're lying on the floor. Then roll to your side and sit up. Do four to six repetitions.

LEG DROP

Lying on your back, bend at your knees and hips so your legs form a right angle. Keeping your back pressed to the mat, slowly lower your right leg until your toe touches the mat. Then slowly return it to the starting position. If your back starts to arch, stop at that point. As your abs get stronger, you'll be able to go farther. Do four to six repetitions with each leg and then do both legs together.

SITTING KNEE LIFT

Sit up straight in a firm, armless chair. Place your hands on the sides of the chair in front of your hips. Tightening your abs and supporting yourself with your hands, slowly pull your knees up toward your chest. Hold and then slowly lower. Keep your lower back against the chair back. This is an advanced exercise, so you may want to start by alternating your legs, lifting one at a time. Do four to six repetitions.

As with any other exercise program, before starting a strength-training regimen, you need to get a medical exam to rule out any possible underlying health problems or any existing conditions that could be aggravated.

EXERCISING FOR FLEXIBILITY

Flexibility is the ability of joints and muscles to achieve a full range of motion. Exercising for flexibility helps prevent injuries, improves your posture, provides for better breathing, and even lowers blood pressure. Despite popular opinion, there's no evidence that you should lose flexibility as you build muscle.

Flexibility exercises use gentle, stretching movements to increase the length of your muscles and the effective range of motion in your joints, allowing you to perform better at daily tasks—from bending over to tie your shoe to lifting a baby out of a car seat to carrying a heavy computer bag. They may consist of a series of specific stretching exercises or be part of a larger exercise program such as aerobics or dance classes.

Since one of the main goals of stretching is to lengthen the connective tissue surrounding your muscle fibers, flexibility exercises should be done after you've already warmed up your muscles with a few minutes of aerobic activity. A typical session involves a minute or two on each stretching exercise. As with aerobics, you can break up your stretching routine into shorter sessions before and after your other workouts.

All stretching movements should be done slowly, to the point where you feel a gentle pleasant tension—not pain—in the muscle being stretched. For an effective stretch, you need to hold the position for fifteen to thirty seconds, then work toward holding all stretches for a full minute. Breathe deeply through your nostrils, concentrating on the muscles you're stretching. Never "bounce" as you hold a stretch, because this will activate your stretch reflex (an automatic, protective contraction). If you feel any pain, stop immediately.

If you regularly stretch your muscles after they're fully warmed up—at the end of an aerobic workout, for example—you can gradually increase their resting length by lengthening the connective tissue that surrounds your muscle fibers. Improving flexibility in this way will make movement easier and more fluid. The more often you stretch, the longer your muscles. For maximum benefits, do a stretching routine several times each week.

THE STRETCHES

Here are some flexibility exercises to add in to your exercise routine. The ideal is to do two thirty-minute flexibility workouts each week, or ten minutes each day incorporated into your aerobic workout.

HAMSTRING STRETCH

Sit with your right leg extended in front of you, your left leg bent with your left sole resting against your right thigh. Place your right hand on the floor slightly behind you as you slowly reach forward with your left hand. Grasp and flex the toes of your right foot, if you can. Repeat four times, then switch legs.

THE BIG V

Lie on your back with legs straight and stretched out to the sides so that they form a V in the air. Your feet should be flexed. Place your hands on the inside of each thigh just above the knee and slowly press until you feel a gentle tension in your inner thighs. Repeat four times.

TOWEL STRETCH

Stand with your feet together, knees soft. With your arms overhead, hold a towel taut (if you feel too much tension, get a longer towel so that your hands are positioned farther apart). Take the towel a few inches behind your head, then slowly lower it. Keep your elbows soft. When you feel the stretch across your chest, take a few deep breaths and hold it. As your flexibility improves, slide your hands closer together.

CALF STRETCH

Stand comfortably with your hands on your hips, or place both hands on a wall (shoulder's width apart), and step forward with your right foot (about a half-shoulder's width). Bend both knees, keeping your feet flat on the floor, and shift your weight to your forward foot. Slowly lower your hips, until you feel a gentle stretching sensation in the calf muscle and Achilles tendon of your left (rear) leg. Hold for fifteen to thirty seconds, then switch legs and repeat.

TRICEPS STRETCH

Stand tall, with your feet shoulder width apart. Reach down the middle of your back with your right hand, pointing your elbow toward the ceiling. Keeping your shoulders down, use your left hand to pull your right elbow gently toward the center of your body. Imagine that you're trying to align your forearm with your spine to form a continuous straight line. Repeat four times. Switch arms.

CROSS-LEGGED PULL

Lie on your back with your right leg bent, foot planted on the floor. Cross your left ankle over your right thigh. Clasp your hands behind your right thigh and gently coax the leg toward your chest. Feel the deep stretch in your left hip. Repeat four times, then switch sides.

WALK FOR LIFE

Want to drop a size, stabilize hormones, sleep better, and live longer? I can't say it enough: putting one foot in front of the other does your body, mind, and spirit a world of good!

There are many unquestionably good exercises, but all are not everyone's cup of tea. For those that cringe at the thought of jogging, can't easily get to a pool for swimming, and don't have the time, place, or desire for aerobic dancing, fitness walking is a tremendous alternative.

Walking is structured, simple, easy, quick, and cheap—and is guaranteed to make you feel better and look better in just a couple of weeks. It's also a social contribution: researchers have concluded that you help the national economy just by taking a walk. Two doctors at Brown University have calculated the amount spent nationally each year on heart-disease treatment and the added amount wasted as a result of lost employee productivity. They estimated that $5.6 billion in health care costs would be saved if only one out of ten nonexercising adults started a regular walking program.

Even if you haven't exercised in a long time, remember that walking is natural and easy. You need not "gear up" mentally, so walking is easy to build into your life's routine. Even if you don't walk far, just get out and move.

SIX REASONS WHY WALKING RULES

YOU CAN DO IT FOR LIFE. Forty years from now, you may not be rollerblading every morning. But you could still be walking—around your neighborhood, to the park, maybe in the mall. With little risk of injury and great opportunity to see gains in fitness, walking is a sport you can keep for life.

YOU CAN RUN OR WALK NO MATTER WHAT YOUR BODY TYPE. You may not ever have the muscular makeup to do marathons, but as long as you start slowly to prevent injuries, anyone—short, tall, big, or small—can walk or run.

YOU CAN WALK NO MATTER WHAT YOUR CONDITION. Whether you're pregnant, elderly, or obese; with arthritis, diabetes or osteoporosis; even recovering from heart surgery or chronic fatigue—you can walk safely.
YOU CAN LOSE WEIGHT WALKING. The faster you walk (and the more you weigh), the more calories you use.
YOU CAN GET WELL WALKING. Walking's health benefits include an increase in HDL levels, a reduced risk of bone loss and resulting fractures, a decrease in blood pressure, a stabilization of blood sugar levels in diabetics, and an increase in mobility for people with arthritis.
YOU CAN FEEL WELL BY WALKING. Walking has immense emotional benefits: it counters depression, relieves stress, and refreshes your spirit. You can talk to God, yourself, or a walking companion.

TURNING A WALK INTO A WORKOUT

Find a block of time in the morning (before breakfast) or after work (ideally, before dinner) to go for a brisk walk around your neighborhood. If you are traveling, or don't feel comfortable walking in your own neighborhood, stop off on the way home at an area where you feel safe. Just remember to pack your walking shoes!

Look for a shoe that offers stability, good arch support, and durability, with a half-inch maximum heel height. The heel should be rolled and tapered, and the heel cushion should be about one-half to three-quarters of an inch thick. Combine good shoes with good-quality athletic socks that fit smoothly and evenly on your feet. Don't wear running shoes for walking; walking shoes help your feet roll along in a heel-toe motion and have more flexible soles for faster walking.

Before and after each walk, gently stretch to keep muscle soreness and tightness to a minimum. Do gentle, nonbouncing stretches for your shin muscles, calf muscles and tendons, hamstrings and front thighs with a slow, steady pull until you feel the muscles ache slightly. Trunk rotations (turning the upper body while feet remain planted) and side bends are helpful as well. Hold each stretch for fifteen seconds. Do these stretches even on days you don't exercise, to keep your muscles from tightening.

Walk fast enough to work up a light sweat (swing your arms, take long, but comfortable strides), but not so fast that you become breathless. This is your ideal "aerobic" pace. You should always be able to talk to a companion (or hum to yourself) during exercise. If you can't do this, slow your pace. When you feel like extending yourself a bit more, research indicates that you will benefit as much from extending time as from increasing pace and stepping more frequently rather than trying to stretch your stride, which can injure your knees.

Proper posture is very important to protect against fatigue and injuries. Stand up straight and walk with your ears, shoulders, hips, knees, and ankles in a vertical line. Keep your head erect, chin pulled in toward your neck, back straight, and buttocks and stomach tucked in. Avoid leaning forward when walking to prevent back strain.

Walking will satisfy all your body's needs for aerobic exercise if you do it in such a way to raise your heart rate to its training zone. If your heart rate is not elevated at the end of a forty-five minute walk, try walking faster, at least part of the time, or look for some long, gradual hills to climb. You may also try walking with weights.

Plan to get some walking in every day, or at least four to five days a week. In a few weeks, your exercise program will be a habit and you'll feel uncomfortable if you have to miss a day. I've done a lot of different forms of exercise at different times in my life, but I always come back to walking. It's simply the best exercise for me to rely on to keep my body operating at its metabolic best.

STICKING WITH IT

Just knowing the benefits of exercise isn't enough; more people *don't* exercise than do. What's the problem? For a lot of us, it's just that exercise is no fun—and it's hard to stick with something every day that's not. To "Just Do It," and keep on doing it, we have to find an exercise that matches our lifestyle, our fitness needs, and our own definition of enjoyment. Follow these guidelines to increase your enjoyment of an exercise routine.

KNOW YOURSELF. The exercises you'll find most enjoyable will probably be those you feel you can best handle. If you have difficulty with eye-hand coordination, you may be frustrated by a sport like tennis but would do well with walking or swimming. If you are not naturally flexible, you may be happier with bicycling than ballet. And you may just want to choose aerobic gardening! Exercise doesn't have to be running a marathon—you just need to get moving, get your heart rate up to your target zone, and keep it there for at least twelve minutes. Playing with your kids or grandchildren may work just fine!

CONSIDER YOUR CURRENT CONDITION. If you are overweight, beginning with an activity that involves pounding on your feet, such as running or aerobic dance, may stress your joints by placing too much weight on them. Try riding a stationary bike or swimming instead. And remember, if you're over thirty-five, see a health professional for an "all-points" check before beginning an exercise program.

USE THE BUDDY SYSTEM. Exercising with a friend will not only give you an opportunity to socialize, but you'll also be more motivated to show up and keep your commitment. Other people's enthusiasm and energy may be just the inspiration you need.

DISTRACT YOURSELF. If your exercise of choice isn't particularly interesting, combine it with something that is. Do the Stairmaster while listening to books on tape, or sing along to uplifting music while walking on the treadmill.

HAVE FUN. Take up a sport that allows you to get exercise while working on skills and having fun. Volleyball, racquetball, in-line skating, even badminton, are activities that provide terrific fitness benefits but don't feel like exercise. Pick activities that reduce stress, not those that add to it. If risk-taking isn't your idea of fun, leave sky-diving to someone else!

REMEMBER THE PAYOFF. Keep your focus on how good you'll feel after you exercise. Keep envisioning exercise as a sword that cuts away at the stress response. Remind yourself of the long-term benefits you're getting: better energy, a better body, and better health. Choosing to exercise daily is giving yourself a precious gift. And your body was created to reward you by strengthening your "armor": building up protective barriers against heart disease, diabetes, bone loss, arthritis, even cancer.

FINE-TUNE YOUR WORKOUT. You're thinking of chucking it all because you're not seeing the payoff? You're still carrying around an extra fifteen pounds? Or maybe you're not getting stronger, faster, or any more energized? Before you give up, use these five steps to fine-tune your workouts for maximum results:

(1) **BE A LITTLE PUSHY.** If you've been doing the same type of exercise for more than three months, you may be stuck. It's easy to amble on walks or coast along on your bike. But for meaningful results, you've got to challenge yourself. Push to go just a little faster, a little longer (even an extra five minutes can do the trick), or to do it more often. (To avoid injury, increase only one aspect of your workout at a time.)

(2) **EXPERIMENT.** The more proficient your muscles become at a

particular activity, the fewer calories you burn. Add a new activity such as biking, swimming, jumproping, even kickboxing or volleyball to your usual exercise routine. You'll burn more calories as you master a new skill—and you'll have fun! Cross training is also a great way to prevent injuries and boredom.

(3) BE ACTIVE ALL DAY. Don't think that you can veg out the rest of the day just because you took a low-impact aerobics class or a brisk hour-long walk. The 300 to 400 calories that you likely burned won't make up for all the calories you're not burning throughout the day thanks to the TV remote, automatic garage-door opener, e-mail, and more. It's estimated that in the past twenty-five years, labor-saving devices have decreased the number of calories we burn daily by 800 or more.

(4) CHECK YOUR FRIDGE. Exercise is key to losing weight and keeping it off, but you can't ignore what you eat. An extra slice of pizza, for example, can put right back the 240 calories you burned jogging for half an hour. And even if you're choosing low-fat, nutritious foods, eating too much of them can have the same effect. Be aware of what and how much you're eating so that you don't negate the calorie-burning benefits of exercise.

(5) TAKE A BREAK. Doing too much, particularly vigorous, high-intensity exercise, can actually hinder your progress. Your body needs time to recover from intense workouts in order to get stronger. Take at least two or three days off between these high-intensity workouts to let your muscles recover, or mix in some lower-intensity walking, swimming, or stretching.

If you are ready to move beyond the reasons why *not* to exercise and join the ranks of those who successfully develop a regular exercise routine and enjoy its benefits, take note: initiating a well-designed exercise plan will create a wave of positive changes in your life. You'll work with a higher level of energy, think with greater mental clarity and concentration, build confidence, quell negative anxiety, and cut away at the stress response—and all the while lose body fat; build and tone firm, lean muscle; stabilize blood chemistry; and increase your strength. It's an incredible package that shouldn't be hard to sell, even to ourselves!

Exercise is a powerful tool in your stress-fighting and pound-shedding tool chest. Another is healthy, full breaths of air—and lots and lots of water.

CHAPTER 8 ■ A: Air and Water

One reason for doing the right thing today—is tomorrow.

—ANONYMOUS

E ver breathe a sigh of relief? Gasp in shock or pain? Feel the need to vent at someone? These all express the close connection between the way we breathe and how we feel.

The pressure of a deadline can leave us wiped out for the afternoon. Fear makes us tense our muscles, which leads to fatigue, just as if we were working out. Fear can also make us hold our breath, depriving us of oxygen. This not only can lead to fatigue, but it can kick up the stress response and slam shut the fat cell door.

> **SMART WEIGH TIP**
>
> *Just breathe.*

Breathing isn't something we normally have to think about—we inhale and exhale at a fairly steady pace, without much thought or worry over how we're doing. We take on average 28,000 breaths each day. But how we take those breaths contributes to our body's metabolic response—it revs it up or locks it down. While losing weight, we have much to gain from learning how to breathe *correctly*.

In addition, deep and slow oxygenating breaths are one of the simplest things you can do to relieve stress, energize yourself, and keep control of yourself in any situation. Healthy breathing can help you to overcome the low energy and high stress levels that result from rapid, shallow, or deep, heaving breaths.

Again, because breathing seems so simple, so automatic, it's difficult to think that our metabolism and energy can be boosted just from taking a breath of air. And it certainly is automatic, but so is eating. And how many people do that right?

BACK TO BASICS

Getting the right amount of oxygen into the bloodstream depends on a balance of carbon dioxide and oxygen in the blood. When you breathe in a panicked way, each breath throws that balance off. But you can actually train yourself to breathe in a way that energizes you.

When you're relaxed, you breathe slowly and deeply, inhaling vital, energy-producing oxygen. When you're tense or just not breathing correctly, you tend to breathe lightly and rapidly from your chest, which delivers less oxygen to your body's cells. As professional singers will tell you, only 30 percent of your full oxygen capacity is available when you're not breathing in a deep, diaphragmatic way—it suffocates your blood cells.

To test your breathing, place one hand on your upper chest and one hand on your abdomen. If the hand on your chest rises when you inhale and contracts when you exhale, you're chest breathing. This type of breathing brings in large amounts of air at one time and activates the fight-or-flight alarm reaction. This is good in a life-threatening emergency, but not in daily living.

Chest breathing keeps your body in a state of chronic stress. It also impairs circulation, depletes energy, and slows the metabolism because, without adequate oxygen, the body cells cannot burn fat effectively nor produce a full measure of energy. The brain reads this as stress, and produces stress hormones. Yet the shallow breathing that accompanies stress decreases the oxygen intake and transfer—and we become even more stressed. Another vicious cycle.

Studies suggest that 80 percent of us don't know how to breathe in a metabolically activating and energizing way; we put our emphasis on inhalation, but the energy and stress release is in exhalation.

Freeze for a moment, holding your body in its exact position. Notice that your shoulders may be shrugged or tense. Correct your posture; imagine being suspended from above with your head erect, light and alert. Next, exhale slowly, draining your lungs—concentrating on the stress being blown out of your body, out through the mouth. Now, slowly fill your chest with air, taking the air in through your nostrils. Expand your diaphragm (the cone-shaped muscle that forms the floor of your chest cavity) by pushing your stomach down and out. Then breathe again... in and out... fully. In and out... in and out.

A RELEASING BREATH WORKOUT

Breathing in this way—from your diaphragm—tells your body: "Everything is okay... you are in control." So, before the pressures of life attack again, take two minutes to practice this type of breath work.

The best way to get started in a focused releasing/relaxing breath pattern is to place one hand on your upper stomach, just below your chest. Inhale while you imagine you're filling a small balloon inside. Fill it in all directions—top, bottom, forward, backward. Breathe in until you feel comfortably full, but not too full. Your stomach should gently rise and then fall as you exhale. Make the exhalation a little bit longer than you think you should. Hold it for a half-second before you inhale again. Your upper chest should stay flat throughout. Once you're breathing from the right spot, focus on making your breath as even and steady as possible. You'll find that your tension dissipates.

Ready to blow a gasket because your computer just froze *again?* Put your hands flat on your desk and take about fifteen slow, deep breaths. Breathe in, breathe out. You'll feel calmer, and you'll unwind all the energy-depleting tension before it has a chance to overtake you. Practice this energizing and relaxing deep breathing so that you can do it automatically when under stress. Try it whenever the tension builds—in meetings, during a crisis, when you feel tired, unfocused, confused, mad, scared, anxious, or bored.

Repeat breathing "in and out" fully, at least ten times, whenever you feel tired or stressed. Your body and mind will soon feel the release and refreshment.

HYPERVENTILATION

Many people are being robbed of energy and metabolic power because they breathe shallowly and rapidly (more than eighteen times per minute), leading to an excessive loss of carbon dioxide. The loss of carbon dioxide due to chronic hyperventilation syndrome (HVS) affects the blood's hemoglobin, making it less able to carry oxygen throughout the body. So even though you are breathing quickly, you are getting less air. Among the symptoms are fatigue, anxiety, frequent sighing or yawning, and a tingling, coldness, or numbness in the fingers. Many of these symptoms are due to holding your breath to make up for the carbon dioxide lost in hyperventilating. In addition, you have to work harder to breathe, which in and of itself is tiring.

How to overcome hyperventilation problems? First, sit or stand up straight—correct your posture. Keeping your tummy firmly tucked in when you stand or sit up straight will relax your diaphragm muscles and improve their movement during breathing. Second, if you breathe from your nose, keep your mouth closed. Your nasal passages are too narrow to allow for hyperventilation. Third, practice breathing into a closed paper bag held tightly against your face. With this bag-breathing, carbon dioxide is trapped into the bag where it is recirculated, preventing carbon dioxide levels from falling. Finally, learn the art of breathing to release stress—getting your breath working for you, not against you.

TWO/ONE BREATHING

You can further expand your stress-busting expertise by learning how to manipulate the way you exhale. Since exhaling slows the pulse, a technique called two/one breathing—in which you exhale for twice as long as you inhale makes diaphragmatic breathing even more effective.

To practice the two/one breathing technique, follow these steps:

(1) Sit quietly and do diaphragmatic breathing.

(2) When your breathing becomes balanced and even (it will take a few minutes), gently slow your rate of exhalation until you are breathing out for about twice as long as you breathe in. The easiest technique: count six when you exhale, three when you inhale—or eight and four. You shouldn't end up doing deep breathing; you want to alter the rhythmic motion of your lungs, not fill or empty them completely.

(3) Once you've established your rhythm of breathing, stop the mental counting and focus on the smoothness and evenness of your breath flow.

You receive more than air through proper breathing—you invite regeneration into your body. Breathing for energy gives you a recharge, along with a sense of rest and relaxation. So take a nice, long, slow breath. Now, take another one. Feel better?

SCENT THE AIR

Now, consider the air you are breathing in—is it pure and clear? Toxic air depresses your immune system—and slows your body. Even the scent in the air can lessen your body's ability to lose weight because of the air quality's affect on your brain chemistry.

Pleasant scents stimulate a nerve in the body that triggers wakefulness and alertness. They also can impact the nerve response that triggers appetite—and satiety.

You don't need fancy fragrances or potpourris—they sometimes overwhelm the olfactory sensors, particularly when synthetic. Go the most natural way you can: keep a basket of oranges or lemons on your desk, and slice one when you're feeling fatigued. The sniff will trigger alertness. A mint plant on your desk will provide the same boost when you break off a leaf to breathe in its aroma. Because of intriguing research, many Japanese corporations pipe the scent of peppermint through their air-conditioning systems in midafternoon to perk up energy and boost concentration and productivity.

Another energizing scent is jasmine, which actually alters brain waves and energy levels. It increases the beta waves in the frontal lobe of the brain, stimulating alertness. Jasmine plants or essential oils will supply the refreshment.

A splitting headache, and still more to do on the report? Well, a green apple a day may keep your migraine away—smelling it, that is! Research by Dr. Alan Hirsch of the Smell and Taste Treatment and Research Foundation in Chicago found that for those who like the smell of green apples, the scent produces a marked reduction in the severity of their headaches. This may also be related to the alteration of brain waves.

Feeling overwhelmed by the stress of the day? The scent of lavender has been found to induce alpha waves in the back of the brain which relax and calm. Certain scents, such as those from strawberries and popcorn, can even distract you from the stress you are feeling.

The easiest way to provide the specific scent you need is to purchase a small vial of an essential oil, a concentrated mixture extracted from a plant. (Be sure to get pure, natural scents only, available from natural foods stores, bath and body shops, and certain drug stores.) An effective way to put the scent where it counts is with a small atomizer (less than a dollar) filled with water and just a few drops of the essential oil. Shake before using, then lightly spray on the pulse points of your wrists, or into the air as a freshener.

Some of the more stimulating scents are lemon, peppermint or spearmint, pine, rosemary, eucalyptus, jasmine, and basil. Among the known relaxing scents are lavender, chamomile, orange blossom, rose, marjoram, sage, and patchouli.

PURIFY THE AIR WITH PLANTS

Plants give off low levels of hundreds of different chemicals that purify the air. Although the chemicals are designed to protect the plant against insects, they also help and energize *us* by protecting against "sick-building syndrome." In addition, plants absorb many toxins like formaldehyde and benzene; the root systems of plants actually feed off pollutants and toxins in the air. After absorbing the contaminants, the plants "breathe back" clean air.

The build-up of air contaminants in many buildings and homes can cause flu-like symptoms and fatigue, even cancer. Plants are a friendly, "green" way to clear the air. Just seeing the plants may stimulate a sense of well-being. One study of surgery patients showed quicker recovery rates when their hospital rooms gave a view of a garden or an area with trees.

It is suggested that maximum air purification comes when you have a minimum of one plant for every 100 square feet of living space. Don't worry about overestimating—the more the better, especially if you have central heat and air. The plants will help control the humidity of your living space, absorbing the humidity when it's thick in the air, releasing it when it's dry. That adds up to you being more comfortable—and energized.

To get the best humidity control from your plants, keep them well watered but not drowned. Water them the way you need to be watered—when needed. This will keep your plants thriving and more healthy than a massive watering once a week. They also need more water in the winter when the humidity is low, just as you do. A good watering can do you both a world of good.

DRINK PLENTY OF WATER

Too tired for that walk? It may be hard to believe, but the number-one factor in fatigue is dehydration. If you do nothing else in your quest for weight loss but begin to drink water each day—and drink a lot of it—you will experience a phenomenal boost in your energy and sense of well-being. Few of my clients think of water as their most important energy enhancer, yet many of the symptoms of fatigue that we blame on too much stress and too little sleep are simply the result of thirst.

At the end of a long workday, when you feel rotten and headachy and unwilling to exercise—in a strange zone between sore and numb—your body is crying out to be hydrated. Chances are you've only drunk enough water to wash down a few aspirin and have had little else since that coffee or diet soda this morning. You've been breathing dry, air-conditioned or heated air at the office, and the chronic stress in your routine has caused some moments of intense perspiration. And of course, you've been losing fluids through the day through normal body functions—fluids that haven't been replaced. You're parched!

Water is important for your energy metabolism for several vital reasons. Consider that your body is comprised primarily of water (it's

> **SMART WEIGH TIP**
> *Drink water—and drink a lot of it!*

92 percent of your blood plasma, 80 percent of your muscle mass, 60 percent of your red blood cells, and 50 percent of everything else in your body). Every cell in your body relies on water to dilute biochemicals, vitamins, and minerals to just the right concentrations. Your body also depends on the bloodstream to transport nutrients and other substances from one part to another, and this too depends on optimal fluid concentration. Blood volume actually decreases and "thickens" when you are dehydrated, meaning that the heart has to work harder to supply your body with needed oxygen. And remember, oxygenated blood is the key for effective energy metabolism.

Water is also vital for maintaining proper muscle tone, allowing muscles to contract naturally and increase in mass. When dehydrated, the muscles are more injury-prone and will not work to optimal performance. In fact, dehydrated muscles will only work to 30 or 35 percent of their capacity. This spells mediocre performance for athletes, tiredness, achiness, and headaches for you—and an inability to build body muscle while losing body fat. Without oxygen getting to the cells, fat cannot be burned for energy.

DRINK YOURSELF WELL

Drinking more water is a challenge for most of us. Most Americans have grown up drinking just about anything but water. We list our favorite beverages as soda, coffee, tea, juice—with water only for washing down pills, washing away dirt, and brushing teeth.

Water is an essential nutrient. Without food, a person can survive (although not well) for days, even months. But without water, the human body can survive only three to five days.

Again, water is a metabolic booster because it is a critical component of basic functions to your body's health. First, along with proper protein and salt intake, water works to release excess stores of fluid, much like priming a pump. It is *the* natural diuretic. No other beverage works like water to prevent the body from holding excess fluids. Second, water transports the energy nutrients throughout your body and is essential for maintaining your body temperature. Third, water helps you digest food and maintains proper bowel function and waste elimination. Being a mild laxative, water actually activates the fiber you eat, allowing it to form a bulky mass that passes through the gastrointestinal tract easily and quickly. Without proper water, fiber becomes a difficult-to-pass "glue" in your colon. Big water drinkers get less colon and bladder cancer.

Water is the only liquid we consume that doesn't require the body to work to metabolize or excrete it. Even fresh juices do not provide the solid benefits of pure, wonderful water, since your body must process the substances they contain. With soft drinks, your body has to work overtime to process and excrete the chemicals and colorings. Although based on water, sodas are "polluted" water.

Many other beverages, particularly those with caffeine, actually remove more water than contained in the beverage itself. Coffee, tea, and some sodas contain tannic acid, a product that interferes with iron and calcium absorption and competes for excretion with other bodily waste products such as uric acid. When not properly excreted, this uric acid can build up in the body and crystallize around the joints. This build-up leads to joint pain in elbows, shoulders, knees, and feet, especially former injury spots, and is a type of gouty arthritis. Men are particularly prone to uric acid excesses. This is one reason why a cup of tea or coffee, although fluid based, just doesn't do the job. Furthermore, water works to lubricate joints.

If you're still not convinced about the wonders of water, consider this: Water also works to keep the skin healthy, resilient, and wrinkle-resistant. It could honestly be labeled an "anti-aging" ingredient!

HOW MUCH DO I NEED?

Eight to ten eight-ounce glasses each day—more when you exercise, travel by plane, or live at high altitudes. Sound overwhelming? Never thirsty? You're not alone. The water prescription brings out cries of anguish from many people.

But you really do need that much because you lose that much every day. Your body continually loses water as it performs necessary functions. Even breathing uses up your fluid stores; every time you exhale you blow off water—a total of about two cups per day. Water evaporates from your skin to cool your body, even when you aren't aware of sweating. These losses, along with what is lost in regular urination and bowel movements, total up to ten cups per day. When perspiring heavily, the amount lost can double or triple.

Take heart! As you begin to meet your body's needs by drinking more water, your natural thirst will increase. You may find water drinking habit-forming; the more you drink, the more you want.

Start increasing your intake any way you can: through a straw, in a sports sipper, from a silver pitcher. Add fresh lemon or lime, drink sparkling water, buy bottled water—just drink it! Try filling a two-quart container with water each morning, and then make sure it's all gone before you go to bed. I also encourage drinking a twelve- to sixteen-ounce glass of water right after each meal and snack throughout the day. If you are eating as often as you should, every three hours or so, this will provide a large proportion of the fluid you need.

TIPS FOR STAYING HYDRATED

START YOUR DAY WITH EIGHT TO SIXTEEN OUNCES OF WATER. While the coffee or tea is brewing, drink a cup or two of water. You wake up with a water deficit, so drinking water soon after waking will gently restore hydration. Many of my clients swear by a cup of warm water with a squeeze of lemon first thing in the morning to jumpstart their digestive system gently. They declare it's the answer to their "regularity" problems.

GET YOUR EIGHT-A-DAY. This isn't a diet principle; it's just how your body is wired. Take water breaks routinely, at least every thirty-five to forty-five minutes, even more frequently when the air is dry or hot. Try to drink little or nothing with your meals (sip water if you must), because washing food down with water dilutes the digestive function.

GET MORE WHEN YOU NEED IT. You may not automatically know when you need more, but look for the subtle signs of dehydration—dry eyes, nose or mouth, impatience, slight nausea, flushed skin, dizziness, headaches, weakness, and mild fatigue. Also, drink when you're more stressed than normal. Not to make you obsessive, but it's a good idea to glance at your urine occasionally. Other than first thing in the morning, a dark yellow color is a sign your kidneys are having to concentrate the waste in too-small a volume of liquid. Pale-colored urine indicates good hydration.

DON'T WAIT UNTIL YOU'RE THIRSTY TO DRINK. It's already too late. Once you feel thirsty, you've already lost a significant amount of fluid. So don't rely on your thirst mechanism. It will prompt you to replace only thirty-five to forty percent of your body's hydration needs. And if you don't take in adequate water, your body fluids will be thrown out of balance and you may experience fluid retention, constipation, unexplained weight gain, and a greater malfunction in your natural thirst mechanism.

KEEP WATER WHERE YOU ARE. You're more apt to keep up with water needs if you keep drinking water close at hand. Freeze large bottles of water overnight and pull them out in the morning. The water thaws through the day, but is still chilled. Keep a glass or a pitcher of water at your desk, and refill it often. At home, keep a pitcher or large bottle of water in the refrigerator, with a glass on the counter as a reminder.

AVOID DEHYDRATING FOOD AND DRINKS. Caffeine-containing and alcoholic beverages act as dehydrators, further increasing, and never replacing, your fluid needs. In fact, each cup of coffee or tea adds an extra cup of water to the eight- to ten-a-day basic requirement. Who has the room—or time?

FILL UP BEFORE YOU WORKOUT. Drink sixteen ounces of water fifteen to thirty minutes before your workout. Avoid starting to exercise when you're already thirsty; you're guaranteed a substandard performance.

CONTINUE TO FILL UP WHILE YOU'RE WORKING OUT. Drink six to eight ounces of water every twenty minutes during your workout or training. This may seem like a lot, but even this doesn't begin to keep up with typical sweat losses. When possible, drink cool water—it is absorbed into the system more quickly. No need for a sports drink to replenish electrolytes unless you're exercising longer than ninety minutes.

PRACTICE AIR TRAVEL SMARTS. Drink as if you're going into an exercise workout: sixteen ounces before your flight, then at least eight more every hour aloft. Stick with water or juices.

IF YOU START CRAVING SALT, GO FOR WATER. Once your fluid stores drop below a certain level, your thirst mechanism cuts off altogether. (Possibly to preserve your sanity if you're lost in the desert?) What turns on is a desire for salt—or salty foods. It's one of those magnificent things the body does: because extra sodium holds more fluids in the body, the salt craving is a survival mechanism to slow life-threatening dehydration. Notice a craving for hot dogs and nachos at the beach? Look for a water bottle instead.

IS TAP WATER OKAY?

Be sure not to let the bottled versus tap versus treated water controversy get in the way of your health. Many people do; they don't trust their tap water, so they drink no water at all.

Public water systems today are well monitored for safety, and bottled water companies are now beginning to fall under similar standards. You can assure yourself of the purity and safety of your local drinking water by checking with your local EPA or health department, or by contacting EPA's Safe Drinking Water Hotline at 800-426-4791. If you lack confidence in the answers you receive, you can have your water tested privately. The agencies listed above can give you the names of testing laboratories.

If you drink bottled water, choose brands that bottle their water in glass or clear plastic containers and are able and willing to provide an analysis or certification of purity. And buy only spring or purified water—a bottle labeled "drinking water" may just come from your municipal water system. You would do just as well turning on your faucet.

The biggest concern with tap water is that it is treated with chlorine to remove contaminants. As important as chlorine is for purifying our water, questions have been raised about its contribution to heart disease risk, to miscarriage, and to long-term effects on the immune system. I encourage my clients to avoid, when possible, water that has an obvious taste or smell of chlorine. When you travel, consider ordering bottled water.

You may want to get information on a water purifying system for your home. Steam distillation is the most reliable, and most expensive, form of filtration. The next best is reverse osmosis, which forces the water through a cellophane-like, semipermeable membrane that acts as a barrier to contaminants like asbestos, copper, lead, mercury, and even some microorganisms. Reverse osmosis systems require a good bit of water pressure to function and are often difficult to access for necessary filter changes. And the replacement filters can be quite expensive.

Activated carbon filters use granules, precoat (a fine powder), or a solid block to remove unpleasant odors, colors, and bad tastes from drinking water, and do a very good job in removing chlorine and some contaminants. If all you're after is good taste and less chlorine odor and aren't concerned about microorganisms or other contaminants, a simple table-top pitcher with a carbon filter (such as Brita) will suffice. If you drink tap water, the taste may improve after refrigerating it for twenty-four hours (the chlorine will dissipate). This can be a low-cost way to get the more refreshing taste of bottled water without the cost. Your choice of which water to drink comes down to taste, cost, and availability.

Regardless, the bottom line is this: drink eight to ten glasses of water every day, and more if you exercise heavily. Don't allow anything to become a substitute for the beverage your body likes best: water, the beverage of champions!

CHAPTER 9 ■ R: Rest

The best bridge between hope and despair is often a good night's sleep.

—ANONYMOUS

R est is something we read about, talk about, and long for, but don't often get. How many of us fall into bed at night, literally "dead to the world" (or is it dead from the world?), seeking a few hours of relief from our lives? Too many days of doing whatever it takes have taken their toll. Too many hours of just getting through have gotten to us. Bedtime comes, but refreshing sleep may not.

For some, it's as difficult to turn off the day as it is to turn off the TV. There is simply too much to do and not enough time to do it, and robbing from sleep seems an easy way to make up the difference. Ask ten people how disciplined they are with a sleep schedule and you'll

> **SMART WEIGH TIP**
>
> *How well you live your day affects how well you rest at night.*

be likely to hear variations on a single theme: "I go to bed when I finish doing what I have to do." Bombarded by increasing demands on their time from work, travel, play, family, and social obligations, most people steal time from sleep. In fact, some are downright proud of under-sleeping. Getting by on four hours has a superhuman sound.

A National Sleep Foundation survey found nearly two out of three people do not get the recommended eight hours of sleep each night. A third of those get less than six hours of sleep. Other surveys have shown that in the past year, one-third of American adults have had trouble falling asleep or staying asleep and two-thirds complained of sleep-related problems such as insomnia, snoring, or restless legs. The late hours designated for rest mirror our days: we fight through them.

LACK OF SLEEP

Sleep is a little known and often missed component in the weight-management game: a bad night's sleep might do more than give you the early-morning blues; it can actually play a central role in locking down your fat cells. Results from studies of the impact of sleep deprivation on the body indicate that a chronic lack of sleep may affect metabolic function as much as living a sedentary lifestyle. Being consistently deprived of sleep can also increase the severity of age-related chronic disorders, including diabetes, obesity, and hypertension.

Sleep is the repair shop of the body and brain, the process that most thoroughly restores our psychological and physiological vitality after the strain and exertion of life. Along with building and repairing our muscle tissue, bones, cells, and immune system, restful sleep allows the release of important hormones such as the human growth hormone, which is critical for vitality and metabolic burn.

Sleep researchers have shown that cheating on sleep for only one night increases evening cortisol to levels that can adversely impact health by lowering immunes and slowing the body's fat-burning potential. Because cortisol helps to regulate blood sugar concentrations, the sleep-deprived body metabolizes glucose less effectively.

Increased levels of cortisol can also damage brain cells, causing shrinkage in the hippocampus, the critical region of the brain that regulates learning.

Small sleep losses can be cumulative. Research has revealed that after even one week's lack of sleep, there are striking alterations in metabolic and endocrine function and a rapid deterioration of the body's functions. The good news is that these studies also show that the negative effects of sleep deprivation can be corrected by normal sleep. Just as a lack of sleep can harm the body, getting sleep can help it.

HOW MUCH IS ENOUGH?

Believe it or not, research still shows that the average adult needs seven-and-a-half to eight hours of deep, restful sleep a night to stay healthy and alert. There are exceptions: one in ten needs ten hours of sleep each night, one in one hundred can be refreshed with five. Again, new studies show that cutting back on sleep to below the seven-and-a-half hours most of us need can be as dangerous to health as a poor diet and no exercise.

> **SMART WEIGH TIP**
>
> *Sleep is the repair shop of the body—aim for 7 1/2 to 8 hours a night.*

There appears to be a biological feedback loop between the body's use of energy, its need to resupply it, and the brain's mechanism for maintaining the proper energy balance. This need of the brain for energy helps to explain why lack of sleep dulls the brain, saps energy, increases irritability and depression, and turns up the appetite thermostat. We think we can lose sleep and be a little tired, but otherwise we'll just be fine. The truth is we won't—we ultimately have to pay the piper. We may be living life in the modern age, but we still have the same bodies, living by the same principles, that we were created with.

If you desire more sleep, but your body simply won't cooperate, check this list for sleep robbers that may be stealing your much-needed rest.

SLEEP ROBBERS

BLOOD SUGAR FLUCTUATIONS. Sleep deprivation and the resulting cortisol production causes impaired blood sugar regulation. In turn, blood sugar fluctuations are a prime culprit in restless sleep. A sudden drop in your blood sugar level, characteristically occurring at 2:30 to 3:00 AM, causes a surge in adrenaline. This can bring on a panic response, which is why you often wake with a start, with your heart and mind racing. Once awakened, it's difficult to get back to restful sleep.

HOT FLASHES AND NIGHT SWEATS. The results of blood sugar crashes, menopause, and panic attacks last only a few minutes but are notorious for disrupting sleep. If they are hormone related and you're a female approaching menopause, please don't ignore the hormone issue. Let troublesome hot flashes and night sweats motivate you to consider hormone replacement therapy or healing soy foods.

GETTING OLDER. It's a myth that you need less sleep as you age. But, your sleep patterns will likely change. You may sleep less in one stretch. You also get less of the deeper, most restorative sleep. Consequently, you awaken more often and are more easily aroused by a snoring spouse or a call to the bathroom.

STRESS. It's the top cause of short-term sleep problems due to the chemical gymnastics it causes in your body. Even worrying about your insomnia can worsen the problem.

MEDICATIONS. Steroids and some drugs can disrupt sleep. The most common troublemakers are some blood pressure medications, diet pills, diuretics, antidepressants, cold and allergy remedies, and asthma medications. Check with your physician and pharmacist.

(6) CAFFEINE. Americans drink 400 million cups of coffee each day, and get extra doses of caffeine in tea or cola-type sodas, cocoa, and chocolate. Caffeine's stimulants are still at work five to seven hours after you've ingested it, preventing your body from falling into deep sleep and often awakening you prematurely by disrupting sleep patterns.

A NIGHTCAP OR NIGHT SMOKE. Alcohol in the bloodstream makes staying asleep more difficult. In addition, it suppresses dreams, depriving your body of its normal, refreshing sleep cycle. Nicotine is also a stimulant that keeps your body from easily falling asleep. One more reason to kick the habit!

ILLNESS. Arthritis, asthma, and sleep apnea (breathing cessation characterized by loud snoring and gasping) can interfere with sleep.

DEPRESSION can also cause insomnia, just as insomnia can bring on depression.

ABCS OF GOOD ZZZS

If it's a little harder for you to shut off the business of your mind than it is to shut off the light, you may need some tips for sweet sleep. Rather than endure one more sleepless night or another morning dragging out of bed, use these tips to keep your body programmed for restful sleep.

BE CLOCK-DRIVEN. When it comes to catching up on lost sleep, timing is everything. Block in sleep as a priority part of your schedule. By doing this you are making an advance decision that sleep is important because being your very best is important.

Your body's internal time clock is daily reset by getting up at the same time each day. "Sleeping in," even for an hour, can disrupt your biological clock and end up making you feel even more fatigued. This is why getting to bed earlier in the evening is better than sleeping late the next morning—it gives you the extra rest without upsetting your rhythm. Stick with it. People who are just starting to make up lost sleep can take six weeks to recover fully.

I know this is hard, but try to get up at the same time every day, regardless of when you fall asleep. Set your alarm clock—then put it out of sight. You want to be clock-driven, not clock-obsessed.

CHOOSE NIGHTTIME SNACKS WISELY. Overeating, or high-fat, high-sugar snacks after dinner can so overload your body that it will resist getting to sleep or staying asleep. The classic pattern is being awakened around 3:00 AM, eyes open, heart racing, unable to get back to sleep. Eating too much too late has put your body into chemical gymnastics. Going to bed hungry can be a sleep-robbing culprit as well. When you're hungry your brain will try to keep you alert until you eat.

A great bedtime snack is a small bowl of whole grain cereal with low-fat milk or half a turkey sandwich or a banana with skim milk. All keep the body chemistries undergirded through the night, allowing you to waken rested and refreshed.

WORK YOUR BODY DURING THE DAY. Exercise, with its ability to physically process the stressors of our day physically, gives sweeter sleep; it's nature's best tranquilizer! People who work out for thirty to forty minutes, four times a week, fall asleep faster and sleep longer than nonexercisers. Just don't exercise less than an hour before bedtime—the rise in your body temperature can keep you awake.

KEEP IT COOL, DARK, AND QUIET. People sleep best in rooms that are between 60 and 65 degrees, pitch-black, and silent. If that's a far cry from your bedroom, put up heavy drapes or a light-blocking shade. To drown out traffic noises or a snoring spouse, try wearing ear plugs or adding "white noise" like a fan or air-conditioner.

CHECK YOUR NIGHTTIME POSTURE. One of the often overlooked causes of daytime fatigue is nighttime posture. Sleeping on your stomach can cause a strain on your back that might be just painful enough to keep you from getting a good night's sleep. For the most restful repose night after night, sleep on your side. This promotes easier breathing and reduces snoring, which can wake you up. Consider keeping a pillow under your knees; this comfortably flexes your lower spine, making it say Ahhhh.... To avoid neck and shoulder aches, use a pillow that's low enough to support your head without flexing your neck. Down pillows work best; foam ones are often too springy. Also be sure you're warm enough. If you have to stay curled up all night to keep warm, your back is likely to get sore.

DEVELOP A SLEEP RITUAL. Remember the bedtime story that helped to calm you down as a child? An adult bedtime routine gives your brain strong cues that it's time to slow down and prepare for sleep. It can be as simple or as elaborate as you like—a warm bath, lighting a candle (particularly a calming lavender one), putting a "brow pillow" on your forehead, snuggling up with your loved one, or listening to classical music. (Just ten minutes of Mozart has been shown to rein in the racing mind—both for sleep and performance.)

Some people are avid writers before bed, particularly when their mind is racing. Writing down what you're thinking and feeling helps to "drain the brain" for restful sleep. I have more than a few clients who lie down for five minutes, then get up and make a to-do list, writing down everything that needs to be attended to the next day. Then they set it aside, and set aside time the next day to deal with their list.

LET BED BE BED. Don't let it be an office, a place to pay bills, or a home theater. Make your bed restful by using it only for sleeping and romance.

Don't force the sleep issue. If you're still awake thirty minutes after going to bed, get up and do something calming, such as reading, until you're groggy enough to fall asleep. Try to stay awake until your eyes close involuntarily. This works best if you don't keep track of time.

OTHER BRIGHT IDEAS—LIGHT

Sunlight is the "spark of life," without which there would be no plant growth, no photosynthesis, no oxygen. On a more personal level, light causes normal physiological fluctuations that can affect the way we feel, think, and sleep. Depending on personal sensitivity and the extent of light changes in your environment, the effects can range from mild fatigue to severe depression.

What keeps us tied to light is a cleverly balanced internal clock, known as circadian rhythm, which synchronizes a wide variety of physiological systems including heart rate, body temperature, and sleep cycles. This internal clock is set by light; it can be reset by changes in the timing or duration of light exposure.

Most of us don't think twice about our circadian rhythms. We take for granted that we become tired and sleepy at night, awake and alert during the day. We notice the effects only if our internal clock is "out of sync." Most people notice the effects of circadian rhythms when they gain or lose time such as in traveling, or during seasonal changes in light. Even small changes can cause dramatic symptoms in some people.

To help smooth out your sleep-wake cycle, try these simple measures to manipulate your exposure to light:

- If you get up in the middle of the night, avoid turning on bright lights. Light suppresses melatonin production and may make it more difficult to fall back to sleep. Put dimmer switches or nightlights in bathrooms and hallways.

- If you have trouble rising in the morning, maximize the amount of light in your bedroom as soon as you wake up.
- If you wake up too early in the morning, minimize the amount of dawn light. Wear a sleep mask or put blackout shades on your windows. When you wake, keep lights dim to help gradually shift your usual pattern.

In all of creation, the principle of rest is modeled for us. The soil of the earth needs a rest from time to time, allowing it to become more productive. Bears hibernate, fish sleep with their eyes open, the most beautiful plants have a period of dormancy. Our needs are no different: we need rest in order to heal and rejuvenate. So treat yourself well: give yourself time to recharge and replenish so you can keep your metabolism burning brightly.

CHAPTER 10 ■ T: Treating Yourself Well

Climb the mountains and get their good tidings.
Nature's peace will flow into you as sunshine flows into trees.
The winds will blow their own freshness into you, and the storms their energy,
while cares will drop away from you like leaves of autumn.

—JOHN MUIR, Naturalist who helped establish Yosemite National Park

T he lives of so many of us are two-dimensional—work and food. Doing and eating. It's hard to find a place for relaxation and replenishment—sometimes even relationships. You know you should spend more quality time on yourself but just thinking about how to fit it in gives you a migraine. It's easier just to hit the sofa— take in some food and tune out with TV.

Many of us push ourselves into prolonged periods of exertion without adequate periods of rest and relaxation. Some of us push ourselves through long days with barely time for a bathroom break, and definitely no time for lunch.

> **SMART WEIGH TIP**
>
> *Indulge yourself in healthy pleasures that replenish, refresh, and relax you.*

Some go months, even years, without a vacation, or a relaxing weekend. No wonder we get run out and run down, and robbed of the joy and peace we so desire.

This breakneck pace not only inflates your stress level, but takes a hefty toll on your metabolism and your quality of life. It signals the body to eat, and overeat, in order to provide the energy to keep up with the demands of your daily grind, yet slows you down to conserve what energy you do have. When life borders on depletion, food (and storing that food) takes center stage. Losing weight becomes impossible.

If you are approaching meltdown, the best thing to do, ironically, is nothing at all. You were created with a need to rest, to recreate, to reflect, and to be regenerated. Treating yourself well is really a lifestyle—it makes a statement that "you deserve a break today."

Here are some ways to achieve a wiser, saner, and metabolically boosted you.

CHILL OUT!

Countless studies have documented the benefits of chilling out. Anything that relieves stress also boosts physical, spiritual, and emotional energy and becomes a metabolic booster. Fatigue disappears; backaches vanish; colds and flu are kept at bay; blood pressure drops; and chronic conditions—such as migraine, irritable bowel syndrome, insomnia, even acne—improve.

Sure, it used to be a little easier to get a break. Ten years ago, most stores were not open on Sundays. Now, Sunday is a day for shopping. The notion of the Sabbath being a day of rest has disappeared. You can go to the all-night supermarket and get your entire week's food at 3:00 AM. And holidays—even those like Labor Day and New Year—are a merchant's delight: a time for some of the biggest clearance sales of the year.

To really enjoy life physically, emotionally, relationally, and spiritually, we must have a way, and take the time, to recharge our physical batteries and renew our spirits. Here's how.

TRIM YOUR CALENDAR

Just because you *can* do everything doesn't mean that you *must* do everything. Ruthlessly cross out unnecessary events in your calendar. Time pressure is a huge metabolism zapper. Research tells us that although we feel more rushed and harried than we did twenty or thirty years ago, we actually have more free time than we used to. We just feel pressured to do more because of our super-speedy culture. E-mail, laptops, and cell phones create the illusion that we can, and should, be busy and productive every minute of the day.

While you can't always stop responsibilities from piling up, you can pick what requires immediate attention and what can be put on the back burner. So go ahead, cancel some social events and not-so-vital work commitments and do *exactly* what you want. It will energize you beyond words and remove a major logjam to your metabolic burn.

MAKE A DATE WITH YOURSELF

At least once a week, carve out one hour (or longer) for your own— an hour in which you have nothing to do. Plan ahead on when the hour will be, but don't plan what you'll do—otherwise it will become one more thing on your "to-do" list.

I actually try to spend one day a week in time-out rest, whether it's Sunday or another day, I need a consistent weekly withdrawal to do replenishing activities. A day of rest for me means a day of activities that personally revitalize me. It may mean reading novels, taking leisurely walks, napping, enjoying friends, window shopping, or just sitting, daydreaming, and writing.

For some people, this kind of activity would *provoke* anxiety. To relax and be replenished, they need to be skydiving, or driving a race car! And that's fine—"relaxing" means different things to different people. But just switching to a *different* activity, even if it's physically strenuous, can revive you. Studies have shown that curiosity increases our performance capability. When devoid of stimulation, people become disorganized, lose their intellectual ability to concentrate, and decline in coordination. So read a new book, paint your masterpiece, and seek out new situations, work opportunities, and challenges. We are stimulus-hungry beings, and denying our nature can lead to inertia and listlessness.

Does all this sound more like the ideal than reality? It needn't be. This is a great time to carve out our personal hours of renewal, because living in contemporary society has made our need desperate. With determination and a little creativity, anyone can make the time for time-out.

Something happens to me when I choose to relax and be replenished. I return to what I was created to be: a *human being.* With time invested in recharge I can review how I'm normally spending my time and reevaluate according to the purposes that have been placed in my heart. Otherwise, I stay too busy for issues of the soul.

START YOUR DAY WITH A TIME-OUT

Many of us have learned the power of starting the morning with a quiet time of reflection and spiritual connection. This is a daily part of my life because I know that I could be doing nothing more important, and that it is the only way to start my day with strength. It is a time-out in the midst of my busyness to reflect on what my source of strength really is, who I really am, and that nothing, NOTHING, is worth being robbed of the joy of life. Starting my day with quiet reflection is like the warm-up for my exercise—a time to stretch spiritually and get my soul circulating.

I get up and eat breakfast (body fuel) while reading inspirational words (soul fuel). Then, I walk. While walking, I'm also reflecting—not just going through a mental checklist and to-do list, but taking a step beyond to look at the "why" of my life: What's the passion, what's the purpose, why am I doing all these things, and why am I spinning all these plates? Sometimes I need to focus more on what I need to say no to, more than on what to say yes to. After this time of listening and reflecting, writing is my way to get my thoughts and feelings into a place where I can take action. Writing down what's inside is a ten-minute investment that yields huge dividends for me.

TAKE POWER BREAKS—EVEN POWER NAPS

Research shows that no matter how busy people are, they would work better, faster, and more productively if they took a break. True, withdrawing from your endeavors for a few moments temporarily halts your output, but research shows that doing so can erase tension, enhance optimistic attitudes, focus the mind, jump-start creativity—and give a significant energy and metabolic boost. Why work hours on end at a slightly unfocused 75 percent performance, when a fifteen-minute power break can help you work at an efficient 100 percent for the next few hours?

And that's exactly what happens. Research shows that after every few hours of focused activity, your brain and body take a downturn. Blood sugars begin to drop, energy levels fade, alertness dims, and metabolism slows. You need to get up, get a snack, get water, get moving, and get your mind off the work. If you ignore this need, or try to shake it off, you'll only achieve a lower level of productivity.

You may need to write breaks into your schedule as a priority appointment—as important as any other. It *is* that important. Even the busiest people—a surgeon doing open-heart surgeries, a judge hearing back-to-back cases—can manipulate their difficult schedules to allow for break time. If you realize how important it is, you can make it happen. Remember this: *More breaks, more breakthroughs!*

Using your break for a power nap can also be very refreshing—relaxing your body, clearing your mind, improving your mood, and boosting your energy levels. Studies show that you don't really have to sleep to get the rejuvenation you need—just shut the door, unplug the phone, turn off the lights, and close your eyes. Rest and be replenished. Then get up and have a power snack. Stretch or take a quick walk at the end of your break to rejuvenate yourself for the work at hand.

If you choose to nap, make it short and sweet. Don't tell toddlers this, but a fifteen- to twenty-minute nap seems to be ideal for the maximum energy boost. You can stretch it a few extra minutes, but don't go over an hour. Napping too long can be counterproductive; long naps can allow you to enter into the deeper delta-type sleep, causing a groggy, disoriented state when you wake that takes a long time to snap out of. If you seem to need more than an hour's nap in the afternoon, you're probably not getting enough sleep at night.

END YOUR DAY WITH A TIME-OUT

I have recently begun to end my day with a time-out. This is very difficult for me; I have to tell myself more than once that *there is nothing more I should be doing.* I then enjoy some of my favorite things that don't seem very productive in the scheme of life, yet I know are vital to recharge my energy: reading travel magazines, listening to favorite music, whatever.

Again, it doesn't come naturally for me; I'm a "doer" by nature. The first one up in our household, I go nonstop till the sun goes down and beyond. Even my "breaks" have often been purposeful: planning, researching, meeting with a small group. I have laughed for many years about being a "human doing" rather than a "human being," but only in recent years have I realized it's not something to laugh about. Ending my day with a time just to "be" reaffirms in my own mind that I am only human—and that's more than enough!

EXTEND TIME-OUTS TWICE A YEAR

I try to begin each year with a personal retreat, a time to write and reflect on where I've been and where I'm going. Is it the direction I want, propelling me toward my dreams?

I try to take another time to pull away midyear to do a midpoint check. What have the past six months done to me and for me? Am I on track with the goals and priorities I established six months earlier? Am I treating myself well—and honoring my body, soul, and beliefs?

At least twice a year, schedule time to pull away and completely change your scenery. Even if it's only for a weekend, physically separating yourself from your daily obligations can do a world of good for your energy level. Leaving your familiar environment is a surefire way to

> **SMART WEIGH TIP**
>
> *Divert Daily,*
> *Withdraw Weekly,*
> *Abandon Annually.*

recharge and refresh your batteries. Viewing life in a new context is itself invigorating. When you return, you'll have a new perspective.

Let your time away build your motivation for making your day-to-day world more beautiful, more relaxing—and definitely more energizing. Treating yourself well is more than just taking action—it is a state of mind, a state of soul. You can enter into rest anytime you choose to let go of all the stuff you don't want, won't use, and don't need. You feel uplifted and drawn to the new because you aren't struggling to carry the old.

SHAKE THINGS UP!

Embracing *The Smart Weigh* will work wonders with your metabolism and well-being—and it will bring something else into life: *change.* We humans are prone to fall into ruts in life—in the way we eat, the way we live, the way we interact with others. These ruts may provide safety, but they also bring boredom and weariness. So shake things up! Taking different actions will give you a different point of view, and that will remind you that you're in control of your choices and can change things for the better.

You probably have a suitcase full of habits and ruts that you aren't even aware of. By becoming conscious of them and then breaking or altering them, you can stir up your old thought patterns and emerge from your slump. Consider moving the furniture; mix up your schedule of doing things in the morning; do your work in a different location; eat a different breakfast; listen to some new music; cross train in exercise; take a new route to the office or school; change the lighting; paint a room; try some unfamiliar fruits and vegetables.

The power of rearranging one's external environment has been well documented in studies since the 1960s when it was first reported. For years, Weight Watchers and other eating modification groups have used this strategy to help countless people to lose weight by modifying their behavior and "stimulus environment." For example, external changes like eating from smaller plates or eating only at the table with a place mat—even just rearranging the refrigerator—can have a huge impact on the inside of you.

You will see how all these truths operate as you learn to implement them through the seven-week plan in the next chapter. Let it become the beginning of a new way of living!

CHAPTER 11 ▪ Your Seven-Week Plan to Lose Weight and Feel Great

The task ahead of you is never as great as the power behind you. You have been created with a genetic heritage for wellness—claim that power.

—ANONYMOUS

There's a good reason why most people fail at sustaining a new way of living: they don't plan to fail, but fail to plan. The best way to reach long-term goals is with short-term steps. But most people try to make changes without understanding that changing behavior is a process, not a once-a-year New Year's resolution.

The reality is that change is difficult—especially if you haven't figured out the steps. You must know where you are beginning, you need to know where you are going, and you have to figure out how to get there. By implementing certain behavioral steps, you can increase the likelihood of achieving your goal.

> **SMART WEIGH TIP**
>
> *Don't focus on perfection, rather focus on progress. Look at how far you've come!*

For instance, when the goal is weight loss, the first step is to set a realistic weight-loss goal within an appropriate amount of time—about one pound per week. Accept that the healthful weight loss is slow and steady. If you want to keep it off, you have to change your behavior and eating habits permanently. But you don't have to do it all at once. Make small changes, like walking two or three days a week, cutting out frequent desserts—things you can achieve without much trouble. If you set goals you can achieve, it reinforces a positive feeling that helps you go on. And success breeds success.

PLAN FOR SUCCESS

Many people have had excellent long-lasting results in making change with the SUCCESS plan, a series of steps to help them reach their goals developed by Harold Shinitzky, Psy. D. Consider these elements in your own plan for SUCCESS.

Set Your Goals

Decide what changes you want to make, keeping in mind that you should be specific and realistic. "Lose weight" is a broadly defined goal. A more specific and realistic goal would be, "Lose ten pounds within two months." The key word here is *realistic*—try achieving a comfortable weight you maintained easily as a young adult. If you've always been overweight, reaching a weight at which levels of triglycerides, blood sugar, blood pressure, and energy improve may be a realistic goal for you.

"My first goal was to lose only ten pounds," says Rebecca. "I had very high blood pressure, and my doctor said if I would just lose ten pounds, he believed that I could get off the pills. Every other doctor before said I had to lose 100 pounds, and I thought, 'I can't do that.' But ten pounds—I thought, 'Maybe I can do that.' Doing it one bite at a time made it more achievable for me."

Write down your goals and then let others know about them. That will increase the likelihood that you'll follow through and get support when you need it.

Understand Your Passions

Lose weight because you want to, not to please someone else. You must want to lose weight because it's what *you* want to do. Know what really makes you feel good, what you like to do, and use that to help guide you to your long-term goals. If you want to be fit, or to become a better athlete, focus on what it will take, such as increasing your cardiovascular workouts or weight training. This step requires you to narrow your focus to one or two specific goals. Which goals do you value most? These will become your priorities.

Critically Plan Your Steps

Determine small steps that will lead to the larger one. If your goal is to become more fit, you can join a gym and/or schedule a workout three times a week. If you want to drop ten pounds, follow the guides for weight loss that will bring your calories down and your nutrition up. Exercise appropriately to come up with a 500-calorie-a-day deficit. This will allow you to lose the weight in one- or two-pound increments per week.

Challenge Yourself

That means be willing to work hard, push yourself, and feel a little discomfort (not pain) if it means helping you to reach your goals. Realize that if you want to lose weight, you might feel discontented sometimes, or feel a little out of breath while working out. Acknowledge that change is not easy. If it were, you would have already accomplished your goal.

When things get difficult, we tend to revert to previous comfortable behaviors. But now is the time to develop *new* lifestyle behaviors. To do that, you have to change the behaviors that resulted in weight gain in the first place. Lifestyle changes involve taking a realistic, sometimes painfully honest look at your eating habits and daily routine. Were you taught as a child to clean your plate? If so, do you still feel compelled to eat everything, even when you're full? Examine your eating style. Do you eat fast? Do you take big bites? When do you eat? While watching TV? All the time? Examine your shopping and cooking techniques.

Evaluate Your Progress

Are you making headway? If not, why not? Adjust your plan to meet your long-term goal. Are you meeting your weekly or monthly weight-loss goals? If not, determine what the problem might be. Do you need more consistency with exercise? Do you need to be eating more often—or become more careful with portion sizes?

Stay Focused

That means not being deterred by obstacles that threaten to obscure your goal. Are you invited to a great party where there's lots of food? Look past the buffet table and envision yourself as the fit and trim person you want to be. That should help you control yourself. Remember, "if it's meant to be, it's up to me."

Savor Your Accomplishments

Reward yourself for reaching small goals along the way. As you lose weight and become more fit, buy yourself some new clothes. Have you developed a pleasant routine of walking? Treat yourself to a walk on the beach or around a lake.

BUILDING A HEALTHY FOUNDATION

I have taken the principles from the previous chapters and arranged them in the form of week-by-week suggestions to help you change your lifestyle in a way that releases your body's natural ability to lose weight. Each week's suggestions build on what you have done in the previous week; after seven weeks, you will have created the foundation of a healthy lifestyle—one that is free of the diet trap. This exclusive plan combines the best of the best: it combines every top strategy shown by research to increase your chances of reaping the joys of fitness and good health.

There is no need to do this plan in just seven weeks. You may want to slow the pace and incorporate the principles over the next seven months, or even over the next year. Remember, it has taken you a lifetime to accumulate your current habits and attitudes; it will take longer than a few weeks to weed out the negative ones, plant new ones, and allow them to grow into a new you. Of course, I have many clients who are the all-or-nothing type people, and they make a total about-face and dive into the whole seven-week plan the very first day. But, as I've said before, these truths are simple, but they are not easy. Give yourself time to succeed.

Read over the plan below, then try to set a date to begin. You may not be ready now to invest yourself fully in these changes. You may already be on a diet and thrilled with it—for now—and not too thrilled with my opinions about it. If that is the case, I'd love to see you make an appointment with yourself and this book to reexamine your feelings about that diet in two months, or next year. Ask a friend or family member to check in with you at that time, and see if you are then ready to embrace a new way of living—for life.

YOUR SEVEN-WEEK PLAN

WEEK ONE:
STOKE YOUR METABOLIC FIRE

Begin to eat early, often, and balanced; drink water,
get moving, and get some sleep.

ACTION STEPS

- For the first three days, keep a diary of everything you eat and drink, the time that you eat, how you are feeling, and any exercise you may do (see sample and blank diary pages on page 389). As you keep track of how you are living each day, look for the areas that may be contributing to your metabolism slow-down and fat cell lock-down. What patterns do you see with your eating, your exercise, your moods, and your feelings?

- Next, begin a new food diary for the remainder of the week using the "Eat Right Prescription" to activate your metabolism (eat early, often, balanced, lean, and bright). This is a time to focus on what to eat rather than what to avoid. Have a balanced breakfast every day, and power snacks or meals every two-and-a-half to three hours (see page 125 for power snack ideas or creatively put together your own). Also keep track of the eight to ten glasses of water you drink each day.

- Try to walk at least ten minutes a day for five days of this week. If you are already exercising aerobically at least four times a week, keep it up—and do the walk in addition.

- Look at your sleep patterns and the hours you invest in this vital key to wellness. If you aren't getting at least seven to eight hours of sleep each night, try to get to bed a bit earlier two nights this week.

WEEK TWO:
EQUIP YOUR BODY FOR STRESS RELEASE

Be sure to eat early, often, and balanced—with special attention to eating lean and bright. Choose whole-grain foods, low-fat proteins, and a variety of brightly colored fruits and vegetables. Increase your exercise time, using it as a time to reflect and be refreshed. Breathe *deeply and fully.*

ACTION STEPS

- Compare your last week's food diary to the guidelines of *The Smart Weigh* eating in the next chapter, and note adjustments you might want to make in timing or balance of eating. After you've evaluated your present-day eating habits and have found your weak spots, you can get on your way toward eating *The Smart Weigh*. Begin to eat in a focused way, using a goal-appropriate meal plan in Chapter 12 as your guide.

- This week, choose foods and portions for your meals and snacks based on your new plan. Keep in mind that these are guides for minimum portions and proper balance to achieve your desired goals for healthy living, putting you on the road to losing weight and feeling great. Get started with these amounts for the next two weeks to allow your body to stabilize before making adjustments, and keep a diary of what, when, and how much you eat and drink as well as exercise times and types, and how you feel. The sample diary on page 389 provides space for you to list your protein choice, carbohydrates, and added fats.

- Increase walking to twenty minutes a day, either at one time or in two, ten-minute sessions. If you are already exercising aerobically four times a week, do the twenty-minute walk on the other days.

- Begin to do the releasing/relaxing breathing described on page 189. Choose a time every day to practice your new focused breathing to release stress and breathe in life. Start with fifteen deep breaths at a time.

WEEK THREE:
CULTIVATE A POSITIVE PERSPECTIVE

Treat yourself well by eating well, exercising, resting, and making time for time-outs to reflect on your attitude and life purpose.

ACTION STEPS

- Review your day. Is there adequate time for time-outs? Carving out even ten minutes to reflect and be redirected is an excellent beginning. You may focus on writing this week as a way to study your thoughts. What negative thoughts about your progress seem to be recurring? What positive thoughts can you replace them with?

- Continue the breathing exercises. Practice the relaxing breath exercise whenever you feel anxious or upset, as well as at the beginning of your quiet time and exercise time. Try to have two focused breathing sessions each day.

- Treat yourself well by doing something nice for yourself: Go to a park or art museum, get a massage or pedicure. Or maybe just take a long, warm bath.

- Go through your pantry and refrigerator and aggressively remove the foods that no longer fit into your healthy lifestyle. Why keep them? Box up unopened cans and cake mixes and donate to a local shelter for the disadvantaged. After planning your meals and snacks for the coming week, use *The Smart Weigh* grocery list on pages 263-266 to shop smart. Pick up some fresh flowers to enjoy.

- Increase your walking to thirty minutes, at least five days this week. If you are doing another form of aerobic exercise, continue to walk on the other days.

WEEK FOUR:
REGULATE YOUR BLOOD SUGARS

Use the dynamic duo of healthy eating and exercise to stabilize the rise and fall of your blood sugars and body chemistry.

ACTION STEPS

■ Continue to choose foods and portions for your meals and snacks based on the meal plan that is appropriate for you. Review your food diary—are there times of the day when you are hungry, or crave certain foods? How about your moods and energy? Are there times of the day when you are particularly high, or low? Adjust the timing of your eating to best under-gird your blood sugars. Also review your diaries for food choices that may contribute to better stabilization. For example, you may need to choose more of the best-choice whole grains and legumes on page 92.

■ Check the mileage you are walking in your thirty minutes. If you are walking less than two miles, pick up your pace a bit. Continue exercising at least five days a week, and add in the conditioning exercises on page 171-173 on two of the days.

■ Choose four nights this week that you will go to bed early enough to get seven to eight hours of sleep. If you are waking up in the middle of the night, unable to get back to restful sleep, try a bowl of whole-grain cereal as your bedtime snack to stabilize your blood sugars through the night. Also review your day to be sure you are eating in even ways. Remember: how well you live your days affects how well you rest at night.

WEEK FIVE:
EQUALIZE YOUR BRAIN CHEMISTRY

Change your body physically by changing your environment and habits.

ACTION STEPS

- Look around your world. Is there something that may be preventing a positive balance of the chemicals in your brain? Use the tools on pages 95-99 as a guide to look for ways to brighten up your world.

- Do an activity outdoors, weather permitting. Even if it's a cloudy day you will still receive the serotonin boosting effect of light. And warm up the indoor lights by changing the light bulbs, when possible, to a warm incandescent light. Listen to some inspirational music during your quiet time or your walk, and do ten minutes of inspirational reading.

- Experiment with the meal ideas and recipes in Chapters 12 and 13 and break out of your rut! Add pizzazz by selecting at least three recipes you intend to try this week. Boost your B6 and magnesium intake by including some of the foods from the lists on page 100, and try to have cold-water fish or flaxseed at least twice this week.

- Practice releasing/relaxing breathing for five minutes each day using the exercises on page 189 as your guide. Add in rhythmic two/one breathing.

- Continue to exercise, increasing your time to thirty-five minutes. Continue your conditioning work two days a week, and add in the flexibility exercises on pages 177-178 on two other days.

WEEK SIX:
TAKE CHARGE OF YOUR APPETITE

Work toward proper portions of the foods you eat—and letting food be food: nourishment for your body. Slow down your eating and dine; don't inhale your meals.

ACTION STEPS

- How do you feel after eating? If you still feel hungry, or are craving something sweet, examine your food diary for the timing of the day's meal. Become a student of the setback; longer hours without eating will turn on your appetite and crank up cravings. Also, review "Learning Your Hunger Signals" on page 103, and begin following the ten tips to stay satisfied.

- If you've not yet begun to write, choose a day this week to write or reflect for ten minutes. Examine how you're "feeling" using the questions on page 363. Are your feelings fueling your appetite? What are some ways to express them that treat yourself well?

- Try some variety in your power snacks and breakfasts. Look at the "grab and go" suggestions in Chapter 13 for some fresh ideas.

- Continue to walk, increasing the time to forty minutes, five times a week. Check your heart rate according to the chart on page 164. If you are not reaching your target zone for burning fat, pick up the pace and think about adding in some light (three-pound) hand-held weights, or cross train, adding in some new activities. If you are doing another form of aerobic exercise, monitor your heart rate to stay in the fat-burning zone.

WEEK SEVEN:
STRENGTHEN YOUR IMMUNE SYSTEM

Eat power foods—try to include each food on the Nutritional Top Ten in your daily eating plan. Keep exercising, breathing, and taking care of yourself. Add a time to connect spiritually and to connect with others.

ACTION STEPS

- Review the Nutritional Top Ten on page 140 and assess last week's eating. Are there immune-boosting power foods that you do not normally choose? Plan to include each of these foods in at least one meal or snack this week. You might begin with broccoli or salmon. If you are not a fish eater, plan to visit a natural foods store to pick up some flaxseed. Grind them, and sprinkle them over your cereal or salad. While shopping, look through the refrigerated and frozen sections to familiarize yourself with the many different products made from soybeans. Pick one to try as your protein source at a meal or snack.

- Add in calistenics to your aerobic, conditioning, and flexibility exercises. Use the abdominal exercises on pages 174-175 as a guide.

- Make a list of friends in whose company you feel more alive, happy, and optimistic. Pick one with whom to spend some time with this week. In your quiet time, read about the power of spiritual connection on page 364. Identify some ways that you may begin to receive a new level of peace and power.

ACCEPT PROCRASTINATION, SOMETIMES

When we procrastinate, we are failing to get started on something—or to finish the thing we want to do. By definition, the very word procrastination appears condemning. Yet not all delay comes from poor discipline or lousy work habits. In some circumstances, procrastination may be necessary and may actually serve you well by postponing action to a time when you're more likely to be successful.

> **SMART WEIGH TIP**
>
> *Don't compare yourself to others or adopt their standards—set your own goals for wellness.*

Don't set yourself up for failure by trying to improve your lifestyle if you're distracted by other major problems. It takes a lot of mental and physical energy to change habits. If you're having marital or financial problems or if you're unhappy with other major aspects of your life, you may be less likely to follow through on your good intentions. Timing is critical, and sometimes procrastination can be a good thing.

But if procrastination is not helping you, you can overcome it without beating yourself up. Ask yourself these questions to examine the WHY behind it:

(1) WHAT AM I NOT DOING, AND WHERE HAVE I COME TO A HALT?

- Have you never gotten started?
- Did you stop at the first obstacle?
- Have you run out of steam before the finish?

(2) DO I HAVE A HIDDEN PAYOFF IN PROCRASTINATING?

- Are you being protected from a bigger hurt, like failure or grief?
- Are you fearful of something?

(3) AM I JUST NOT READY TO DO IT?

- Are you still incubating the idea, allowing your mind to work out the solution?
- Is it just not a priority at this time?

(4) CAN I COMBINE IT WITH SOMETHING I LOVE TO DO?

- Make your challenge easier to embrace by inviting your best friend to work it out with you.
- Listen to your favorite CD while planning a meal.

(5) CAN I CHANGE MY ENVIRONMENT?

- Get away, or walk around a lake, for a fresh perspective.
- Rearrange the pantry and fridge to give healthy choices center stage.

(6) CAN I DO IT A DIFFERENT WAY?

- Think about how Jane Fonda would exercise.
- Think about how Julia Child would plan dinner.

(7) DOES MY GOAL NEED TO BE CHANGED?

- Did you try to run too far and too long for your current fitness level?
- Did you plan to lose fifty pounds this winter rather than five pounds over the next month?

THE BIG PICTURE

As you begin to make healthy changes in your lifestyle, be sure to keep your focus on the big picture of looking better and feeling better *for life*. You are not on a diet. You are choosing to take care of yourself and become the best you can be.

Ask yourself more important questions than just what weight you are striving for and how quickly you can get there. Ask yourself where you would like to be in the areas of:

HEALTH _____

ENERGY _____

MOOD _____

APPEARANCE _____

MUSCLE TONE _____

WEIGHT _____

CLOTHING SIZE _____

FITNESS LEVEL _____

EMOTIONAL WELL-BEING _____

SPIRITUALITY _____

This is how one of my female clients answered these questions:

MY HEALTH: I want to stop getting sick every season—and lower my cholesterol and blood pressure.

MY ENERGY: I want to wake up feeling energized and rested, and I want to have energy through my 3:00 PM slump time.

MY MOOD: I want to manage my moods, rather than allowing my moods to manage me. I no longer want to feel like "Ms. Jekel/Ms. Hyde," positive one minute and cranky the next.

MY APPEARANCE: I want to have firmer skin, strong nails, shinier, fuller hair—and less fullness in my midsection.

MY MUSCLE TONE: I want to get a "gravity" lift so that things aren't so saggy!

MY WEIGHT: I think I want and need to weigh about 148. I'm 5'7" and that's been a good weight for me in the past when I'm fit. But I really don't care about numbers on the scale as much as the size of my clothes.

MY CLOTHING SIZE: I want to be back into size 8s and 10s again—I'm in big 12s and 14s now.

MY FITNESS LEVEL: I want to be able to walk/run around the neighborhood and go up my stairs without getting winded.

MY EMOTIONAL WELL-BEING: I want to feel emotions fully, and express them in healthy ways. I no longer want food to be my substitute for connecting with my own emotions or with others—I want to let food be food, not an emotional or relational gap-filler.

MY SPIRITUALITY: I want to operate with a full spiritual tank—with a reservoir of peace and joy. I want to feel connected spiritually.

Remember, *The Smart Weigh* plan is intended to create a healthier lifestyle—not just shed pounds (though you'll do that, too).

You may be thinking, *But this will take too long! I want to be thin now!* Well, the truth is, it *will* take longer, but the results will last this time. You won't be fighting the same battles day after day, month after month, year after year. This is a strategy *gradually* to change the habits and attitudes that may have sabotaged your past efforts. It's not enough to eat healthful foods and exercise for only a few weeks or even several months. Remember, it's not a diet—it's a new way of living.

Breaking free of the diet trap takes thought, planning, and action. But living *The Smart Weigh* builds a powerful momentum that will support healthy goals for a lifetime. But this momentum will only be maintained through establishing practical strategies for living *The Smart Weigh*—while traveling, eating out, grocery shopping, and preparing foods at home.

PART FOUR ■ **PRACTICAL SRATEGIES FOR LIVING *THE SMART WEIGH***

CHAPTER 12 ■ *Smart Weigh* Meal Plans

We live in a society that sends mixed messages. You are supposed to live on fast food and have a figure like Twiggy. That's not possible.

—PAMELA SMITH

My *Smart Weigh* meal-planning guides give you a detailed strategy for fueling your body with the right foods at the right time. The emphasis is not on just what to eat, but how, when, and how much.

The weight-loss meal plan for women of normal activity provides approximately 1,500 calories a day; the weight-loss meal plan for men and very active women provides approxi-

> **SMART WEIGH TIP**
>
> *We all want to lose it yesterday, but it just doesn't work.*

mately 1,800 calories per day; the weight-loss plan for very active men provides 2,200 calories per day. I have also provided tips for boosting your energy quickly, and even a weight-gain plan for those who want to build up—not fluff up!

Portion sizes in each of these plans may need to be adjusted for individual caloric needs. Remember, the number of calories you need depends on your age, size, weight, level of activity, and even stress levels. So don't get caught up in counting every calorie you eat. Instead, focus on eating great foods, prepared in great ways, that will work with your metabolism to release your body's natural ability to burn those calories!

You'll be eating plenty of food at meals, plus two or three snacks, properly balanced in whole-food simple and complex carbohydrates, proteins, and fats. But if you get really hungry at other times of the day, have a piece of fruit with 1 ounce low-fat or soy cheese or 1/2 cup skim or soy milk. Drink as much water and seltzer as you like—but definitely get in 64 ounces every day. Attempt to limit your intake of caffeinated beverages such as coffee, tea, or soda.

> **SMART WEIGH TIP**
>
> *Start fresh, ASAP. If you have a slip, don't wait until Monday or even tomorrow to get back on track—start with the very next power snack.*

It will take two to three days for your body to stabilize—and for you to feel an increase in energy and to regulate your appetite. In about ten to twelve days, you will notice when your body reminds you that it's time for a power snack or meal—every two to three hours. This is a very good thing—a sign that your body chemistries are stabilizing.

As you familiarize yourself with the meal plans below, refer to the lists of healthy carbs and proteins on pages 127-128 to refresh your memory about your best choices. The power snack choices on page 125 will give you direction in converting the following snack guidelines into a variety of minimeals. I've also provided a *Smart Weigh* grocery list (page 263) with many specific suggestions of what to bring home from the market so you'll always have handy the makings for healthy meals.

MEAL-PLANNING TIPS

- **Go for color, go for grains.** Go for blueberries, raspberries, mangoes, papayas, watermelon, honeydew, cantaloupe, apples, oranges, or grapefruit. Go for broccoli, spinach, romaine lettuce, sweet potatoes, and carrots. And vary your breads: try whole-grain English muffins, pita pockets, tortillas, or rolls.

- **Eat beans five or more times a week.** Legumes are one of the highest-fiber foods you can find. Beans are especially high in soluble fiber, which lowers cholesterol levels, and folate, which lowers levels of another risk factor for heart disease, homocysteine. (Quick Tip: To reduce sodium in canned beans by about one-third, rinse off the canning liquid before using. Or look for canned beans with no added sodium.)

- **Have a soy food every day.** This could be soy milk, soy protein isolate powder added to a power shake, soy cheese, tofu, soy nuts, a boca burger, or tempeh.

- **Eat fish four times a week.** To get the most omega-3s, choose salmon, canned white albacore tuna in water, rainbow trout, anchovies, herring, sardines, and mackerel. Or get a plant version of omega-3 fat in flaxseed and canola oil.

- **Eat nuts five times a week.** Learn to incorporate these luscious morsels into your diet almost every day. The key to eating nuts healthfully is not to eat too many; they're so high in calories that you could easily *gain* weight. To help avoid temptation, keep nuts in your fridge—where they are safe from oxidizing and turning rancid and where they are out of sight. Sprinkle 2 tablespoons a day on cereal, yogurt, veggies, salads, or wherever the crunch and rich flavor appeal to you.

The Smart Weigh Weight-Loss Meal Plan for Women

BREAKFAST (WITHIN 1/2 HOUR OF RISING)

SIMPLE CARB: 1 serving fresh fruit

COMPLEX CARB: 2 slices whole-wheat toast OR 1 whole-grain English muffin/bagel (may top with 1 teaspoon all fruit jam, the melted cheese or lite cream cheese from protein, or use the optional 1 teaspoon butter) OR 2 homemade whole-grain low-fat muffins OR 1 1/2 cups whole-grain cereal with added bran/flaxseed★

PROTEIN: 2 ounces low-fat cheese or 1/2 cup low-fat cottage/ricotta cheese OR 4 tablespoons lite cream cheese OR 2 eggs (three times/week) or 2 egg whites or egg substitute OR 1 cup skim milk or nonfat yogurt for cereal

OPTIONAL FAT: 1 teaspoon butter for toast or muffin OR 1 teaspoon olive or canola oil for cooking OR 1 tablespoon chopped nuts as topping for cereal or yogurt

MORNING SNACK (2 TO 3 HOURS AFTER BREAKFAST)

As a whole power snack, may have 1/4 cup trail mix (page 125) OR choose a combination of:

SIMPLE CARB: 1 piece of fresh fruit

PROTEIN: 2 ounces part-skim or soy cheese OR 1 cup nonfat yogurt OR 8 ounces skim or soy milk OR 1/2 cup low-fat cottage/ricotta cheese

LUNCH (2 TO 3 HOURS AFTER MORNING SNACK)

SIMPLE CARB: Begin your meal with 1 piece fruit OR 1 cup cooked vegetables OR 1 cup low-fat vegetable soup

COMPLEX CARB: 1 slice whole-grain bread OR 1 baked potato OR 1/2 whole-wheat pita OR 1 whole-wheat tortilla OR 1/2 cup brown rice/whole-grain pasta

PROTEIN: 3 ounces cooked poultry, fish, seafood, lean beef, or low-fat cheese OR 3/4 cup cooked legumes

HEALTHY MUNCHIES: Raw vegetables as desired (up to 2 cups) with lemon juice, vinegar, mustard, salsa, or no oil salad dressing

OPTIONAL FAT: May use 1 tablespoon salad dressing OR 1 teaspoon olive or canola oil to make your own salad dressing or to cook with OR 1 teaspoon butter for bread or potato OR 2 tablespoons sour cream on potato OR 1 tablespoon light mayo on a sandwich OR 1 tablespoon chopped nuts sprinkled on foods

AFTERNOON SNACK (2 TO 3 HOURS AFTER LUNCH)

COMPLEX CARB: 5 whole-grain crackers OR 1/2 whole-wheat pita OR 1 ounce baked tortilla chips (with salsa, if desired) OR 1 slice whole-wheat bread OR 1 whole-wheat tortilla

PROTEIN: 1 ounce part-skim or fat-free cheese (on bread) OR 1 ounce lean meat OR 1/3 cup low-fat bean dip (with chips above or wrapped in tortilla) OR 1/2 cup nonfat yogurt OR 1/4 cup low-fat cottage/ricotta cheese

DINNER (2 TO 3 HOURS AFTER AFTERNOON SNACK)

SIMPLE CARB: Begin with 1 piece of fruit or 1/2 cup mixed fruit OR 1 cup low-fat vegetable soup AND then enjoy another serving of fruit OR 1 cup nonstarchy vegetables with dinner

COMPLEX CARB: 1/2 cup cooked brown rice or whole-grain pasta OR 1/2 cup starchy vegetables OR 1 small baked sweet potato

PROTEIN: 2 to 3 ounces cooked skinless poultry, seafood, fish, lean beef OR 1/2 cup cooked legumes

HEALTHY MUNCHIES: Raw vegetables (up to 2 cups) as desired with lemon juice, vinegar, salsa, or no-oil salad dressing

OPTIONAL FAT: May use 1 tablespoon salad dressing OR 1 teaspoon olive or canola oil to make your own salad dressing or to cook with OR 1 teaspoon butter for bread or potato OR 2 tablespoons sour cream on potato OR 1 tablespoon light mayo on a sandwich OR 1 tablespoon chopped nuts sprinkled on foods

NIGHT SNACK (AT LEAST 1/2 HOUR BEFORE BEDTIME)

COMPLEX CARB: 3/4 cup whole-grain cereal OR 1 slice whole-grain bread

PROTEIN: 1/2 cup skim or soy milk or nonfat yogurt (with cereal) OR 1 ounce lean meat OR 1 ounce low-fat or soy cheese (melted atop bread)

★Begin adding 1 tablespoon oat bran, 1 tablespoon of wheat bran, and 1 tablespoon flaxseed to cereal; gradually increase to 2 tablespoons of each.

The Smart Weigh Weight-Loss Meal Plan for Men and Very Active Women

BREAKFAST (WITHIN 1/2 HOUR OF RISING)

SIMPLE CARB: 1 serving fresh fruit

COMPLEX CARB: 2 slices whole-wheat toast OR 1 whole-grain English muffin (may top with 1 teaspoon all fruit jam, the melted cheese, or lite cream cheese from protein, or use the optional 1 teaspoon butter) OR 2 homemade whole-grain low-fat muffins OR 1 1/2 cups whole-grain cereal with added bran/flaxseed★

PROTEIN: 2 ounces low-fat cheese or 1/2 cup low-fat cottage/ricotta cheese OR 4 tablespoon lite cream cheese OR 2 eggs (three times a week) or 2 egg whites or egg substitute OR 1 cup skim milk or nonfat yogurt for cereal

OPTIONAL FAT: 1 teaspoon butter for toast or muffin OR 1 teaspoon olive or canola oil for cooking OR 1 tablespoon chopped nuts as topping for cereal or yogurt

MORNING SNACK (2 TO 3 HOURS AFTER BREAKFAST)

As a whole power snack, may have 1/2 cup trail mix (page 125) OR choose a combination of:

SIMPLE CARB: 1 piece of fruit

COMPLEX CARB: 5 whole-grain crackers OR 1/2 whole-wheat pita OR 1 ounce baked tortilla chips (with salsa, if desired) OR 1 slice whole-wheat bread OR 1 whole-wheat tortilla OR 2 pieces whole-grain Crispbread

PROTEIN: 2 ounces part-skim or soy cheese OR 1 cup nonfat yogurt OR 1/2 cup low-fat cottage/ricotta cheese

LUNCH (2 TO 3 HOURS AFTER MIDMORNING SNACK)

SIMPLE CARB: Begin your meal with 1 piece fruit or low-fat vegetable soup AND then enjoy another serving fruit OR 1 cup cooked vegetables with your lunch

COMPLEX CARB: 2 slices whole-grain bread OR 1 baked potato OR 1 whole-wheat pita/tortilla OR 1 cup brown rice/whole-grain pasta

PROTEIN: 3 ounces cooked poultry, fish, seafood, lean beef, or low-fat cheese OR 1 cup cooked legumes

HEALTHY MUNCHIES: Raw vegetables as desired (up to 2 cups) with lemon juice, vinegar, mustard, salsa, or no-oil salad dressing

OPTIONAL FAT: May use 1 tablespoon salad dressing OR 1 teaspoon olive or canola oil to make your own salad dressing or to cook with OR 1 teaspoon butter for bread or potato OR 2 tablespoons sour cream for potato OR 1 tablespoon light mayo on a sandwich OR 1 tablespoon chopped nuts sprinkled on foods

AFTERNOON SNACK (2 TO 3 HOURS AFTER LUNCH)

SIMPLE CARB: 1 piece of fruit

COMPLEX CARB: 5 whole-grain crackers OR 1/2 whole-wheat pita OR 1 ounce baked tortilla chips (with salsa, if desired) OR 1 slice whole-wheat bread OR 1 whole-wheat tortilla OR 2 pieces whole-grain Crispbread

PROTEIN: 2 ounces part-skim or soy cheese (on bread) OR 2 ounces lean meat OR 2/3 cup low-fat bean dip (with chips above or wrapped in tortilla) OR 1 cup non-fat yogurt OR 1/2 cup low-fat cottage/ricotta cheese

DINNER (2 TO 3 HOURS AFTER AFTERNOON SNACK)

SIMPLE CARB: Begin with 1 piece of fruit or 1/2 cup mixed fruit OR 1 cup low-fat vegetable soup AND then enjoy another serving of fruit OR 1 cup nonstarchy vegetables with dinner

COMPLEX CARB: 1 cup brown rice or whole-grain pasta OR 1 cup starchy vegetables OR 1 baked sweet potato

PROTEIN: 3 ounces cooked skinless poultry, seafood, fish, lean beef OR 3/4 cup cooked legumes

HEALTHY MUNCHIES: Raw vegetables as desired (up to 2 cups) with lemon juice, vinegar, mustard, salsa, or no-oil salad dressing

OPTIONAL FAT: May use 1 tablespoon salad dressing OR 1 teaspoon olive or canola oil to make your own salad dressing or to cook with OR 1 teaspoon butter for bread or potato OR 2 tablespoons sour cream for potato OR 1 tablespoon light mayo on a sandwich OR 1 tablespoon chopped nuts sprinkled on foods

NIGHT SNACK (AT LEAST 1/2 HOUR BEFORE BEDTIME)

COMPLEX CARB: 3/4 cup whole-grain cereal or 1 slice whole-grain bread

PROTEIN: 1 cup skim or soy milk or nonfat yogurt (with cereal) OR 2 ounces lean meat OR 2 ounces low-fat or soy cheese (melted atop bread)

★ Begin adding 1 tablespoon oat bran, 1 tablespoon of wheat bran, and 1 tablespoon flaxseed to cereal; gradually increase to 2 tablespoons of each.

The Smart Weigh Weight-Loss Meal Plan for Very Active Men
(Weight Maintenance Plan for Men of Normal Activity and Very Active Women)

BREAKFAST (WITHIN 1/2 HOUR OF RISING)

SIMPLE CARB: 2 servings fresh fruit

COMPLEX CARB: 2 slices whole-wheat toast OR 1 whole-grain English muffin (may top with 1 teaspoon all fruit jam, the melted cheese, or lite cream cheese from protein, or use the optional 2 teaspoons butter) OR 2 homemade whole-grain low-fat muffins OR 1 1/2 cups whole-grain cereal with added bran/flaxseed★

PROTEIN: 3 ounces low-fat cheese or 3/4 cup low-fat cottage/ricotta cheese OR 6 tablespoons lite cream cheese OR 3 whole eggs (times a week) or 3 egg whites or 3/4 cup egg substitute OR 1 1/2 cups skim milk or nonfat yogurt for cereal

OPTIONAL FAT: 2 teaspoons butter for toast or muffin OR 2 teaspoons olive or canola oil for cooking OR 2 tablespoons chopped nuts as topping for cereal or yogurt

MORNING SNACK (2 TO 3 HOURS AFTER BREAKFAST)

As a whole power snack, may have 1/2 cup trail mix (page 125) OR choose a combination of:

SIMPLE CARB: 1 piece of fruit

COMPLEX CARB: 5 whole-grain crackers OR 1/2 whole-wheat pita OR 1 ounce baked tortilla chips (with salsa, if desired) OR 1 slice whole-wheat bread OR 1 whole-wheat tortilla OR 2 pieces whole-grain Crispbread

PROTEIN: 2 ounces part-skim or soy cheese (on bread) OR 2 ounces lean meat OR 2/3 cup low-fat bean dip (with chips above or wrapped in tortilla) OR 1 cup non-fat yogurt OR 1/2 cup low-fat cottage/ricotta cheese

LUNCH (2 TO 3 HOURS AFTER MORNING SNACK)

SIMPLE CARB: Begin your meal with 1 piece fruit or low-fat vegetable soup AND then enjoy another serving fruit OR 1 cup cooked vegetables with your lunch

COMPLEX CARB: 2 slices whole-grain bread OR 1 baked potato OR 1 whole-wheat pita/tortilla OR 1 cup brown rice/whole-grain pasta

PROTEIN: 4 ounces cooked poultry, fish, seafood, lean beef, or low-fat cheese OR 1 cup cooked legumes

HEALTHY MUNCHIES: Raw vegetables as desired (up to 2 cups) with lemon juice, vinegar, mustard, or no-oil salad dressing

OPTIONAL FAT: May use 2 tablespoons salad dressing OR 2 teaspoons olive or canola oil to make your own salad dressing or to cook with OR 2 teaspoons butter for bread or potato OR 4 tablespoons sour cream for potato OR 2 tablespoons light mayo on a sandwich OR 2 tablespoons chopped nuts sprinkled on foods

AFTERNOON SNACK (2 TO 3 HOURS AFTER LUNCH)

Repeat earlier snack choices

DINNER (2 TO 3 HOURS AFTER AFTERNOON SNACK)

SIMPLE CARB: Begin with 1 piece of fruit or 1/2 cup mixed fruit OR 1 cup low-fat vegetable soup AND then enjoy another serving of fruit and 1 cup nonstarchy vegetables with dinner

COMPLEX CARB: 1 1/2 cups brown rice or whole-grain pasta OR 1 1/2 cups starchy vegetables OR 1 baked sweet potato

PROTEIN: 4 ounces cooked skinless poultry, seafood, fish, lean beef OR 1 cup cooked legumes

HEALTHY MUNCHIES: Raw vegetables (up to 2 cups) as desired with lemon juice, vinegar, or no-oil salad dressing

OPTIONAL FAT: May use 2 tablespoons salad dressing OR 2 teaspoons olive or canola oil to make your own salad dressing or to cook with OR 2 teaspoons butter for bread or potato OR 4 tablespoons sour cream for potato OR 2 tablespoons light mayo on a sandwich OR 2 tablespoons chopped nuts sprinkled on foods

NIGHT SNACK (AT LEAST 1/2 HOUR BEFORE BEDTIME)

SIMPLE CARB: 1 piece of fruit

COMPLEX CARB: 3/4 cup whole-grain cereal or 1 slice whole-grain bread

PROTEIN: 1 1/2 cups skim or soy milk or non-fat yogurt (with cereal) OR 2 ounces lean meat OR 2 ounces low-fat or soy cheese (melted atop bread)

★ Begin adding 1 tablespoon oat bran, 1 tablespoon of wheat bran, and 1 tablespoon flaxseed to cereal; gradually increase to 2 tablespoons of each.

BUT I NEED TO GAIN WEIGHT

"People absolutely hate me, but my problem has always been that I can't *gain* weight. I've always been naturally thin, but I'm all of a sudden feeling very scrawny—and I'm tired of people looking at me like I'm anorexic."

Nicole is thirty-two, extremely active, but always a bit fatigued. She had come to me after three months of doing "gainer" shakes, and actually losing two pounds rather than gaining. She had been sick three times in the three months, and she was mad about that—"Here I'm taking great steps to get healthier and I'm just getting thinner, sicker, and more tired. How can I gain weight and get healthy at the same time?"

Nicole's plea is not such an unusual one; many of my clients find it as difficult to gain weight as it is for others to lose it. Why? Their metabolisms are on high burn, and they've developed patterns that rev it up even more. When they seek to gain weight, they want the extra pounds to be muscle, not fat. And that's just more difficult to achieve—especially since many people who have bodies that tend to burn fat rather than store it have never paid much attention to nutrition. Nicole said it this way: "I know there's been a lot of information out there about how to eat right, but I just never bothered with it. Now I'm in terrible shape, thin but exhausted, and what I'm doing isn't working for me. I *want* to meet the needs of my body the best way I can. But I clearly don't have a clue how to do that."

Nicole needed a lot more than a weight-gaining meal plan, she needed a crash course in nutrition. She needed some firm directions for a new way of living her daily life. These are some of the tips I gave her for gaining weight *The Smart Weigh*:

■ **MAKE EVERY BITE COUNT.** Eat power meals and power snacks *every 2 hours*, and choose foods that are nutrient-dense, low-fat, and healthy. Eat by the clock, not by your appetite.

- **DON'T START OFF MEALS WITH FILLERS LIKE SOUP OR SALAD.** Eat the high-calorie part of the meal first.
- **ADD NUTRIENT-RICH FOODS TO YOUR MEALS.** Increase your intake of dried fruit, peas, carrots, baked potatoes, lean beef, bananas, peanut butter on crackers, and low-fat milkshakes.
- **EXERCISE DIFFERENTLY.** Limit your cardiovascular workouts to thirty minutes, and add strength-training at least twice a week to build muscle. You can also do upper body strength-training two days per week and work on the lower body on two different days. Just provide time for recovery.
- **GET YOUR CALORIES FROM PROTEIN AND CARBOHYDRATES.** Hold fat to 30 percent of your daily calories. Have your fat sources be good-for-you choices such as olive oil, nuts, and fish.

This last point about fat can be a confusing one, especially if your weight-gain attempts have centered on shakes, ice cream, gravies, and fried foods the way Nicole's had. Even if you have a metabolism that allows you to maintain your weight easily, excess fat and sugar intake can nonetheless cause big problems with your immune system and energy levels.

When counseling even the thinnest people, I develop a meal plan that, though high in calories and focused on protein, is nonetheless very low in fat. I've worked with professional athletes who have needed to build up additional muscle mass. Sometimes their *Smart Weigh* meal plans include 9,000 calories! But this very high-calorie plan is still low in fat. High-fat eating doesn't add up to healthy, muscle-mass weight gain for an athlete, and it doesn't work to increase performance and stabilize energy for you. By choosing the low-fat versions of protein foods, you will get all of their goodness without the risk.

The Smart Weigh Weight-Gain Meal Plan

ON RISING

8 ounces unsweetened juice

BREAKFAST (WITHIN 1/2 HOUR OF RISING)

SIMPLE CARB: 2 servings fresh fruit

COMPLEX CARB: 3 slices whole-wheat toast OR 1 1/2 whole-grain English muffins (may top with 1 teaspoon all fruit jam, the melted cheese or lite cream cheese from protein, or use the optional 2 teaspoons butter) OR 3 homemade whole-grain low-fat muffins OR 2 cups whole-grain cereal with added bran/flaxseed★

PROTEIN: 3 ounces low-fat cheese or 3/4 cup low-fat cottage/ricotta cheese OR 6 tablespoons lite cream cheese OR 3 whole eggs (twice a week) or 3 egg whites or 3/4 cup egg substitute OR 1 1/2 cups skim milk or nonfat yogurt for cereal

OPTIONAL FAT: 2 teaspoons butter for toast or muffin OR 2 teaspoons olive or canola oil for cooking OR 2 tablespoons chopped nuts as topping for cereal or yogurt

1ST MORNING SNACK (2 HOURS AFTER BREAKFAST)

SIMPLE CARB: 1 piece of fruit

COMPLEX CARB: 10 whole-grain crackers OR 1 whole-wheat pita OR 2 ounces baked tortilla chips (with salsa, if desired) OR 2 slices whole-wheat bread OR 2 whole-wheat tortillas OR 4 pieces whole-grain Crispbread

PROTEIN: 2 ounces part-skim or soy cheese (on bread) OR 2 ounces lean meat OR 2/3 cup low-fat bean dip (with chips above or wrapped in tortilla) OR 1 cup non-fat yogurt OR 1/2 cup low-fat cottage/ricotta cheese

2ND MORNING SNACK (2 HOURS LATER)

Choose from first morning snack options OR 1 cup trail mix (page 125)

LUNCH (2 TO 3 HOURS AFTER 2ND MORNING SNACK)

SIMPLE CARB: Begin your meal with 2 pieces fruit OR 12 ounces unsweetened juice AND then enjoy another serving fruit OR 1 cup cooked vegetables

COMPLEX CARB: 4 slices whole-grain bread OR 1 large baked potato OR 2 whole-wheat pitas OR 4 whole-wheat tortillas OR 2 cups brown rice/whole-grain pasta

PROTEIN: 4 ounces cooked poultry, fish, seafood, lean beef, or low-fat cheese OR 1 cup cooked legumes

HEALTHY MUNCHIES: Raw vegetables as desired (up to 2 cups) with lemon juice, vinegar, mustard, or no-oil salad dressing

OPTIONAL FAT: May use 2 tablespoons salad dressing OR 2 teaspoons olive or canola oil to make your own salad dressing or to cook with OR 2 teaspoons butter for bread or potato OR 4 tablespoons sour cream for potato OR 2 tablespoons light mayo on a sandwich OR 2 tablespoons chopped nuts sprinkled on foods

1ST AFTERNOON SNACK (2 HOURS AFTER LUNCH)

Repeat earlier snack choices

2ND AFTERNOON SNACK (2 HOURS AFTER FIRST SNACK)

Repeat earlier snack choices OR 1 power shake (page 273)

DINNER (2 HOURS AFTER 2ND AFTERNOON SNACK)

SIMPLE CARB: Begin with 2 pieces of fruit or 1 cup mixed fruit OR 12 ounces unsweetened juice AND then enjoy another serving of fruit AND 1 cup nonstarchy vegetables with dinner

COMPLEX CARB: 2 cups brown rice or whole-grain pasta OR 2 cups starchy vegetables OR 1 large baked sweet potato

PROTEIN: 4 ounces cooked skinless poultry, seafood, fish, lean beef OR 1 cup cooked legumes

HEALTHY MUNCHIES: Raw vegetables (up to 2 cups) as desired with lemon juice, vinegar, or no-oil salad dressing

OPTIONAL FAT: May use 2 tablespoons salad dressing OR 2 teaspoons olive or canola oil to make your own salad dressing or to cook with OR 2 teaspoons butter for bread or potato OR 4 tablespoons sour cream for potato OR 2 tablespoons light mayo on a sandwich OR 2 tablespoons chopped nuts sprinkled on foods

NIGHT SNACK (AT LEAST 1/2 HOUR BEFORE BEDTIME)

COMPLEX CARB: 1 1/2 cups whole-grain cereal or 2 slices whole-grain bread

PROTEIN: 1 1/2 cups skim or soy milk or nonfat yogurt (with cereal) OR 2 ounces lean meat OR 2 ounces low-fat or soy cheese (melted atop bread)

★ Begin adding 1 tablespoon oat bran, 1 tablespoon of wheat bran and 1 tablespoon flaxseed to cereal; gradually increase to 2 tablespoons of each.

BOOST YOUR ENERGY *THE SMART WEIGH*

If you are in need of immediate energy, working to stabilize your blood sugars due to hypoglycemia (or just trying to break the sugar habit), trying to overcome gastric distress (even morning sickness), or dealing with high stress levels, follow your appropriate meal plan with these adjustments:

■ Have 4 to 6 ounces unsweetened juice (if citrus is "hard" on your stomach first thing in the morning, try "soft" juices like unsweetened apple or white grape juice) immediately on rising; follow with breakfast within the next half-hour.

■ Add in an extra power snack (see page 125) both morning and afternoon so that you are eating more often—every two hours. Adjust the timing based on your day's schedule (if you are up earlier or later). Follow this plan for two to three days—up to three weeks is advised. By then, you may be energized enough to maintain the basic *Smart Weigh* meal plan that's right for you.

■ Drink more water, but after meals and snacks rather than on an empty stomach.

■ Always have your meal's simple carbohydrate at the beginning of the meal or snack to get the quicker energy release that it provides.

WHAT ABOUT ALCOHOL?

You may have watched it on *60 Minutes*; you may have read about it in the newspaper. It's called "The French Paradox," and it's all about wine, particularly red wine, being good for you. You read that a moderate amount of alcohol, in any form, actually extends life, and may help to offset the negative health effects of a high-fat diet. Your friend's cardiologist recommended that she drink a glass of Merlot

WHAT ABOUT POWER BARS AND ENERGY SHAKES?

The question is, are nutritional bars and canned shakes the nutrition panacea they are touted to be? Well... they are certainly better choices than downing a cola and fries and calling it lunch, but they are a much worse choice than a grilled chicken salad. Better than no lunch at all—but not better than the real McCoy. A can a day won't keep the doctor away!

The problem with manufactured nutrition in a can—or a bar—is that they simply can't duplicate naturally the collection of nutrients in real food. They lack adequate fiber and valuable phytochemicals such as isoflavones, carotenoids, and other plant-derived compounds that get you well and keep you well. Even fruit and dairy-based shakes don't comprise a whole healthy diet—but they can be great as a snack or part of a meal.

And it's not just about nutrient needs—it's also about pleasure. When people turn to liquid lunches or a bar, they deprive themselves of the pleasure of real food, with all its varied textures and smells. In addition, although an energy bar or shake may provide the calories of a chicken sandwich, a bowl of strawberries, and a glass of milk, you're not getting any of the nutrients naturally found in those foods. And that's the long-term problem when these energy bars become chronic substitutes for meals or when eaten in large quantities.

The average person, even the moderately active one, doesn't need energy to come from an engineered bar—he or she simply needs to eat, and to eat often and well. Yet, the "energy" term is very seductive; people feel they're getting more than they are. What you get from one of these bars is really calories, but the term "calorie bar" wouldn't gross the same sales!

Still, if push comes to shove, and the choice is an energy bar over a candy bar, or no meal at all, then choose those that have about 220 to 250 calories, less than 2 grams of fat per 100 calories, over 10 grams of protein, and about 45 to 50 grams of carbohydrate—a snack for a would be weight-gainer, a meal for a would be weight- loser or maintainer. Just be sure to get real food at the next stop.

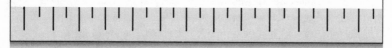

every night to raise her HDL cholesterol; it would be good for her. But is it true? And, if so—how does that advice fit into *The Smart Weigh* meal plan?

It is true that a moderate intake of alcohol has been found to have some positive health benefits, and the research is strong and promising enough that many physicians actually recommend a glass of wine to their patients. But also true is that, over time, excessive alcohol can result in a chronic energy drain; its impact on blood sugars increases appetite, interrupts sleep, and interferes with nutrient absorption. The extra calories it adds to your diet can contribute to weight gain, or prevent weight loss. And more than moderate intake can damage your internal organs (such as your liver, intestines, and heart) and increase risk of cancer, particularly that of the liver and breast.

The fact is, the medical benefits of wine or other spirits are just not compelling enough to encourage people who don't drink to begin. The U.S. dietary guidelines say this: "If you drink, do so in moderation." But what is moderation? It's considered to be a 4 to 6 ounce glass of wine, one light beer, or 1 1/2 ounces of hard liquor a day. Because of the impact of alcohol on your blood sugars, it's best to fit it into *The Smart Weigh* meal plan as a simple carbohydrate, substitut-

WHEN BIGGER ISN'T BETTER!

The next time you add that economy-sized box of cornflakes to your shopping cart, think twice. A recent University of Illinois study asked women to take enough spaghetti from a box to make dinner for two—no measuring allowed. When the women were given a standard one-pound box, they grabbed an average of 234 strands of pasta, enough to make two 350-calorie servings. Not bad. Yet, when they were given a two-pound box, they averaged 302 strands—a 29 percent increase, and a whopping 102-calorie difference per serving.

Researchers got the same result with cooking oil. The women poured 192 more calories' worth into a pan when they used a 32-ounce bottle as opposed to a 16-ounce bottle.

The lesson? If you're buying the family pack, be sure to measure!

ing it for one of your pieces of fruit at a meal. But before you go out and buy more booze, how about a refreshing mineral water with lime instead?

WHAT ABOUT SWEETS?

Reserve for special occasions. *The Smart Weigh* meal plan is designed to load every calorie with life-enhancing nutrition. High-sugar foods bring you lots of empty calories and little else. People who avoid all sugar for a month or two often find that they lose their craving for it. It's worth trying!

Use the guidelines in Chapter 15 if you need help to kick the sugar habit. But remember not to make *any* food absolutely forbidden. That could just set you up for a binge on what you "can't" have.

WHAT ABOUT FASTING?

As a nutritionist I am asked as many questions about wise fasting as about wise eating. These are the answers I give:

- ■ **PURIFY YOUR FAST.** In my opinion, fasting is a physical act of great spiritual significance: It is a commitment and a decision not to look to the world for physical food, but instead to look to God for spiritual food. Don't let the spiritual power that comes through fasting be nibbled away by the wrong motives: to jump-start weight loss, to lose weight quickly, or to rid the body of toxins. Actually, research shows that going without food for prolonged periods of time produces many more toxins than those that come through eating; plus, the metabolism slows drastically, causing fat cell lock-down.

> **SMART WEIGH TIP**
>
> *Go back to basics—are you getting the right portions.*

- ■ **PREPARE FOR YOUR FAST.** Eat smaller meals and snacks every two-and-a-half to three hours the day before a fast. To increase your body's store of energy, eat extra complex carbohydrates (whole-grain bread, pasta, rice) at each of these meals and snacks, along with low-fat proteins. Include a bedtime snack of cereal with milk or yogurt and fruit.

- ■ **CONSIDER YOUR TYPE OF FAST.** I recommend a juice fast for busy people desiring to fast for spiritual reasons. Citrus juices should be avoided when fasting because their citric acid is difficult on an empty stomach, but "soft" juices like unsweetened apple juice, apple-cranberry, or white grape juice are fine. Drink 12 ounces of juice at mealtimes and 6 ounces of juice every 2 hours between meals, along with 2 or 3 quarts of water evenly throughout the day. Avoid caffeine beverages and strenuous exercise. I recommend a water fast only if you are going into a retreat, withdrawing totally from the physical demands of daily life. Drink lukewarm or cool water throughout the day and exercise moderately.

- ■ **CONSIDER YOUR HEALTH STATUS.** Some people should never fast, not even for a day: women who are pregnant or breast-feeding; anyone who is diabetic or hypoglycemic; anyone with liver or kidney problems; anyone who is malnourished. A better choice if you are in one of these groups is, with the same spirit of fasting, to sacrifice a particular favorite food.

- ■ **BREAK THE FAST WISELY.** Don't break your fast with a huge meal or a feeding frenzy but with a small snack, then your first meal two hours later. Your metabolism has slowed down in response to no food, and it will quickly store away large amounts of food taken in after the fast. This is why any weight lost during fasting is quickly regained. Guard against "fasting" breakfast, working through lunch, then going out for a huge meal in the evening. By following sound guidelines, your fast can be a wise—and meaningful—one.

GREAT AND GREAT FOR YOU!

For food to be enjoyable, it needs to taste great; if it doesn't taste good, it has limited power to satisfy. But let's face it: time is short. On weeknights, especially, spending less time in the kitchen becomes a clear necessity if we are to spend more time enjoying our food, friends, and family, in addition to some quiet time for personal recharge. But too often, in our catch-as-catch-can way of doing things, something is compromised: taste, health, or the entire satisfaction of making and enjoying a home-cooked meal. Yet, many interesting and delicious meals can be made in short order.

> **SMART WEIGH TIP**
>
> *Don't toss those measuring cups. It's a good idea to measure out portions once a month to be sure those sizes haven't enlarged.*

Most cooks spend 16 to 45 minutes preparing dinner, according to a recent survey by market research firm The NPD Group. Small wonder that there's a boomlet in convenience foods, recipes that rely on pantry staples, and cookbooks and magazines promising to cut kitchen time. Studies show that people want to make a contribution to the meal they've made their families, but they don't necessarily want to make the whole thing.

That's where convenience products that call for minimal kitchen work, such as chopping fresh herbs for a rice mix or adding chicken strips to a frozen pasta-and-vegetable entrée, come in. Most people don't really hate to cook; what they hate is the stress and spending more time in the kitchen. They hate having to clean up more mess and to feel overwhelmed.

But it needn't be so! The key to great foods that are great for you is being equipped—with a well-stocked kitchen and the knowledge of how to put meals together that are quick and easy. Learning to shop and cook meals *The Smart Weigh*.

WHAT ABOUT SALT?

Although salt is certainly not the number one nutritional evil, it is a concern. The main problem is the amount we use—way, way too much. The average American consumes more than eight times his or her daily requirement—about fifteen pounds per year. This is the equivalent of two to four teaspoons of salt each day. Hypertension, fluid retention, and kidney dysfunction are just a few of the health problems to which those little white granules contribute.

In America today, approximately sixty million people have abnormally high blood pressure, and two million more are adding to the ranks each year. This means that one out of five people are predisposed to high blood pressure—and salt's impact. However, it's not possible to identify who is at risk, so it's wise to practice prevention and cut back on excess salt-even before a doctor tells you that you must.

Salt is made up of 60 percent sodium and 40 percent chloride. In the human body, excess sodium becomes a troublemaker, creating a temporary buildup of fluids, making it harder for the heart to pump blood through the system, and causing a rise in the blood pressure (hypertension). Other factors besides salt intake, such as heredity, a low intake of fruits and vegetables, a high saturated fat intake, and obesity, can also contribute to hypertension.

Unlike heredity, salt consumption is a factor within our control; unfortunately, for the majority of Americans, it is out of control. Shaking the salt habit can be difficult because salt plays a big part in the enjoyment of food. It serves as a catalyst for flavor, enhancing the taste of other ingredients. The key to making this good-for-you cutback is to learn to prepare foods in ways that naturally enhance flavor so less salt is needed for good taste. You'll notice *The Smart Weigh* recipes in the next chapter use herbs and spices which allow you to drastically reduce the amount of salt.

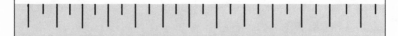

CHAPTER 13 ■ *Smart Weigh* Shopping Guide and Recipes

Our problem is not in knowing what is right, it is doing it.

—ANONYMOUS

Healthy home cooking is still possible—even in the express lane. Keeping a well-stocked pantry, planning a week's worth of healthy menus, and knowing some shortcuts can simplify weekday meal preparation enough to make it, if not a joy, at least less of a hassle. Healthy home cooking is cheaper, and you can control the calories and fat a lot better.

With that said, here are some suggestions to beat the last-minute dinnertime blues and to put together meals that are destined to satisfy the taste buds and the time-budget:

> **SMART WEIGH TIP**
>
> *Plan ahead. An empty fridge after a stressful day begs for pizza. Don't leave meals to chance.*

- ■ **SET ASIDE FIFTEEN MINUTES A WEEK WITH YOUR FAMILY TO PLAN DINNERS.** After a couple of weeks, you'll have menus that you can use over and over.
- ■ **STREAMLINE SHOPPING.** With a week's worth of menus in hand, it's easy to cut back on last-minute trips to the store. Choosing recipes with fewer ingredients will speed you through the checkout lane.

■ **USE THE SUPERMARKET SALAD BAR FOR DICED OR CUBED FRESH VEG-GIES—YOU BUY EXACTLY THE AMOUNT YOU NEED.** Also stock up on bags of precut salad greens from the produce section—they are dated for freshness, so go for the latest date possible.

■ **GET PEELED, FRESHLY COOKED SHRIMP AT THE SHRIMP COUNTER, GRILLED CHICKEN BREASTS FROM THE DELI.** Instead of cooking turkey breast, buy 8 ounces of unsliced cooked turkey breast, then dice at home.

■ **KEEP YOUR CUPBOARDS WELL STOCKED AND ORGANIZED.** Besides canned broth, canned tomatoes, and whole grain pastas, have a few nonperishables on hand to add interest to those basics: chutneys, dried mushrooms, flavored vinegars, etc. It's time-savvy to group similar items together and always restock in the same way. Knowing what's on hand saves rummaging through cabinets when cooking and making shopping lists.

THE WELL-STOCKED KITCHEN

Take a long look at what typically is in your grocery cart. If it's a grease and sugar trap loaded with butter, bacon, and Twinkies, chances are you're not going to be producing slim fixings on the home front. A well-stocked kitchen makes the difference between efficiently putting together healthy flavorful foods versus a meal-time-blues headache or a fast-food nightmare. Now is a good time to strengthen and streamline your grocery shopping, your fridge, and, thereby, your body.

Here are some guidelines for adding the health advantage to your shopping cart—and your *Smart Weigh* grocery list to be sure you bring home "the right stuff:"

■ **CHOOSING CEREALS AND BREADS:** Whole grain is a must for fiber and nutrition. The word "whole" should be the first word of the ingredient list, such as "whole wheat," and "whole oats." Also check labels for hidden fats and sugars; some cereals, like granola, are nutritional nightmares in a bowl. Cereals should have less than 5 grams of added sugar, excluding that from any dried fruit it may contain. Also, remember the now-available variety of whole-grain English muffins, bagels, tortillas, pitas, and crackers— your natural foods store is most apt to have 100 percent whole wheat in these bread varieties.

> **SMART WEIGH TIP**
>
> *Stock frozen veggies. With pasta or stir-fry sauces, they are quick and healthy meals.*

- **BUYING THE BASICS:** Stock up on whole wheat or artichoke pastas and brown rice. Incorporate barley, oats, cracked wheat, and cornmeal into recipes. Include dried or canned beans, split peas, lentils, and chickpeas.

- **FENDING AGAINST FATS AND OILS:** Do not use polyunsaturated oils, but instead use olive or canola oil in small amounts. Select reduced fat or light mayonnaise rather than the fat-free (chemical-filled) varieties. Avoid hydrogenated fats whenever possible—label-reading is a must here.

- **PICKING PRODUCE:** For the best produce, choose what is in season—a good price and an abundant supply will tell you a fruit or vegetable is at it's peak. Ask at your grocery store or farmer's market which are the freshest buying days and where the produce is grown; search for locally grown and in-season fruits and vegetables. Out-of-season produce is more expensive and often imported. If it's imported, it may be only spot-checked for pesticide residues. When fresh is not possible, frozen is the next best choice—but avoid vegetables prepared with butters or sauces, or fruits packed with sugar. Freezing foods doesn't destroy their nutrients and quality as readily as canning does.

SHOPPING *THE SMART WEIGH*

I advocate "real foods" rather than highly processed packaged food. For example, real orange juice or frozen concentrate is far superior to fortified orange-flavored drink. Think "Mother Nature" when you shop. Your grocery store is crammed full of healthful foods, and you don't have to shop at a health food store to get them.

Follow these "trim the fat" tips when you're ready to shop for, plan for, and prepare food that looks great, tastes great, and is great for you:

- Switch from whole milk dairy products to skim or 1 percent milk, buttermilk, and nonfat plain yogurt. Look for fat free or lower fat versions of favorite cheeses such as ricotta, pot, or farmers cheese; skim-milk mozzarella; cottage cheese; and fat free or "light" cream cheese. Check the label to be sure they have less than five grams of fat per ounce. You may also want to try some of the new soy food versions of dairy. You'll get more than you're bargaining for—they are loaded with substances that bless you with disease protection.

- At the deli, go for the leanest cuts. Select sliced turkey or chicken, lean ham, and low-fat cheeses instead of the usual "lunch meats." Limit use of high-fat, high-sodium, processed sausages and meats, hot dogs, bacon, and salami.

- Use this formula for figuring the fat percentage of calories when assessing whether food products are as good as they claim: 9 calories per gram of fat X grams of fat divided by calories per serving. Buy foods that derive less than 25 percent of their calories from fat.

- Buy whole-grain and freshly baked breads and rolls. They have more flavor and do not need butter or margarine to taste good.

- Use the new all fruit jams on breads or toast, rather than fat spreads like butter or margarine.

■ Keep an abundant supply of fresh fruits and cut, munchy vegetables on hand for snacking. Buy light popcorn, breads, and
low-fat crackers rather than chips and cookies. Substitute sorbet or frozen juice bars for ice cream.

THE SMART WEIGH GROCERY LIST

GRAINS AND BREADS
❑ Barley

Brown rice:
❑ Instant
❑ Long-grain
❑ Basmati
❑ Wild rice

❑ Buck wheat
❑ Bulgar
❑ Cornmeal
❑ Couscous

Tortillas, flour:
❑ Mission
❑ Buena Vida fat-free

❑ whole-wheat bagels
❑ 100% whole-wheat
bread *("whole" is the
first word of the ingredients)*
❑ whole-wheat
English muffins
❑ whole-wheat
hamburger buns

Whole-wheat or
artichoke pasta:
❑ Angel hair
❑ Elbows
❑ Flat
❑ Lasagna
❑ Orzo
❑ Penne

❑ Spaghetti
❑ Rotini (spirals)

❑ whole-wheat
pastry flour
❑ whole-wheat pita
bread

CEREALS *(whole grain
and less than 5 grams of
added sugar excluding dried
fruit):*
❑ All Bran With
Extra Fiber
❑ Cheerios
❑ Familia Müesli
❑ Bran Buds
with psyllium
❑ Grape-Nuts
❑ Grits
❑ Kashi
❑ Kellogg's Just
Right
❑ Kellogg's Low-
Fat Granola
❑ Kellogg's Nutri-
Grain Almond
Raisin
❑ Kellogg's Raisin
Squares
❑ Kellogg's Special K
❑ Nabisco Shredded
Wheat
❑ Ralston Müesli

❑ Post Bran Flakes
❑ Shredded Wheat
'N Bran
❑ Wheatena

Oats:
❑ Old-fashioned
❑ Quick-cooking

Unprocessed bran:
❑ Oat
❑ Wheat
❑ Rice

CRACKERS
Crispbread:
❑ Kavli
❑ Wasa
❑ Crispy cakes
❑ Health Valley
graham crackers
❑ Harvest Crisps
5-Grain *(not all whole
grain, but good for variety)*
❑ Ryvita Wholegrain
crispbread
❑ Ry Krisp

DAIRY
❑ Butter
❑ Light butter

Cheese: *(low-fat — fewer than 5 grams of fat per ounce)*

Cheddar:
❑ Kraft Fat-Free
❑ Kraft Natural
  Reduced Fat
❑ Cottage cheese
  (1% or nonfat)

Cream cheese:
❑ Philadelphia
  Light (tub)
❑ Philadelphia Free

❑ Farmer's
❑ Jarlsberg Lite

Mozzarella:
❑ Nonfat
❑ Part-skim
❑ String cheese

Soy Cheese:
❑ Veggie Slices

Nonrefrigerated:
❑ Laughing Cow
  Light
❑ Parmesan

Ricotta:
❑ Nonfat
❑ Skim milk

❑ Sun-Ni Armenian
  String
❑ Egg substitute
❑ Eggs
❑ Egg whites
❑ Milk (skim or 1%)
❑ Reduced fat sour
  cream
❑ Nonfat plain yogurt
❑ Stonyfield Farm
  yogurt

CANNED GOODS

Chicken broth:
❑ Swanson's
❑ Natural Goodness

❑ Evaporated skim
  milk
❑ Hearts of Palm

Soups:
❑ Healthy Choice
❑ Pritikin

❑ Progresso:
❑ Hearty Black Bean
❑ Lentil
❑ 99% Fat-Free
  Chicken Noodle

Tomatoes:
❑ Paste
❑ Sauce
❑ Stewed
❑ Whole
❑ Fresh Cut

CONDIMENTS

❑ Honey

Hot pepper sauce:
❑ Pickapeppa sauce
❑ Shriracha Chili
  Sauce
❑ Jamaican Hell Fire
❑ Tabasco

Mayonnaise:
❑ Light
❑ Miracle Whip Light

Mustard:
❑ Dijon
❑ Spicy hot

❑ Pepperoncini
  peppers

Salad dressing:
❑ Bernstein's
  Reduced Calorie
❑ Good Seasons
❑ Kraft Free
❑ Jardine's fat-free
  Garlic
❑ Vinaigrette
❑ Pritikin

❑ Soy sauce
  (low sodium)

❑ Salsa or
  picante sauce

Spices and herbs:
❑ Allspice
❑ Basil
❑ Black pepper
❑ Cayenne
❑ Celery seed
❑ Chili powder
❑ Cinnamon
❑ Creole seasoning
❑ Curry
❑ Dill weed
❑ Five spice
❑ Garlic powder
❑ Ginger
❑ Mrs. Dash Original
  Blend
❑ Mrs. Dash
  Garlic and Herb
  Seasoning
❑ Mustard
❑ Nutmeg
❑ Oregano
❑ Onion powder
❑ Paprika
❑ Parsley
❑ Pepper, cracked
❑ Rosemary

❏ Saffron
❏ Salt
❏ Thyme

Fresh herbs:
❏ Basil
❏ Chives
❏ Cilantro
❏ Ginger
❏ Parsley
❏ Rosemary
❏ Thyme

❏ Vanilla extract
❏ White wine
   Worcestershire
   sauce

Vinegars:
❏ Balsamic
❏ Cider
❏ Red wine
❏ Rice wine
❏ Tarragon
❏ White wine

FRUITS

Fresh fruits:
❏ Apples
❏ Apricots
❏ Bananas
❏ Berries
❏ Cherries
❏ Dates (unsweetened, pitted)
❏ Grapefruit
❏ Grapes
❏ Kiwi
❏ Lemons
❏ Limes
❏ Mango
❏ Melon
❏ Nectarines
❏ Oranges

❏ Papaya
❏ Peaches
❏ Pears
❏ Pineapple
❏ Plantains
❏ Plums

Dried fruits:
❏ Apricots
❏ Peaches
❏ Pineapple
❏ Raisins (dark and golden)
❏ Mixed

VEGETABLES
❏ Asparagus
❏ Beets
❏ Bell peppers
❏ Broccoli
❏ Brussels sprouts
❏ Cabbage
❏ Carrots
❏ Cauliflower
❏ Celery
❏ Corn
❏ Cucumbers
❏ Eggplant
❏ Garlic
❏ Green beans
❏ Greens
❏ Hot peppers
❏ Kale
❏ Mushrooms
❏ Okra
❏ Onions
❏ Peas
❏ Red Potatoes
❏ Radicchio
❏ Romaine lettuce
❏ Salad greens
❏ Shallots

❏ Simply Potatoes
   hash browns
❏ Spinach
❏ Squash (yellow, crookneck)
❏ Sugar snap peas (frozen)
❏ Sun-dried tomatoes
❏ Sweet potatoes
❏ Tomatoes
❏ Whole potatoes
❏ Zucchini

BEANS AND MEATS

Beans and peas:
❏ Black
❏ Chickpeas/ garbanzo beans
❏ Cannelini
❏ Kidney
❏ Lentils
❏ Navy
❏ Pinto
❏ Split peas

❏ Garden Burger

Beef (lean):
❏ Deli-sliced
❏ Ground round
❏ London broil
❏ Round steak

Fish and seafood:
❏ Clams
❏ Cod
❏ Grouper
❏ Mussels
❏ Salmon
❏ Scallops
❏ Shrimp
❏ Snapper
❏ Swordfish
❏ Tuna

Lamb:
❑ Leg
❑ Loin chops

Pork:
❑ Canadian bacon
❑ Center cut chops
❑ Tenderloin

POULTRY

Chicken:
❑ Boneless breasts
❑ Legs/thighs
❑ Whole fryer

Turkey:
❑ Bacon
❑ Breast
❑ Ground, extra lean
❑ Deli-sliced
❑ Whole

Veal:
❑ Chops
❑ Cutlets
❑ Ground

Water-packed cans:
❑ Chicken
❑ Salmon
❑ Tuna
❑ Charlie's Lunch Kit

Soy:
❑ Tofu

❑ Silk (milk)
❑ Boca Burgers
❑ Tempeh

MISCELLANEOUS

All-fruit spreads and
pourable fruit:
❑ Knudsen
❑ Polaner
❑ Smucker's Simply
 Fruit
❑ Welch's Totally
 Fruit

❑ Baking powder
❑ Baking soda

Bean dips:
❑ Jardine's
❑ Guiltless Gourmet

❑ Bread crumbs

Cooking oils:
❑ Canola
❑ Olive
❑ Cornstarch

Fruit Juices
(unsweetened):
❑ Apple
❑ Cranberry-apple
❑ White grape
❑ Orange

❑ Nonstick cooking
 spray

Nuts/seeds
(dry-roasted, unsalted):
❑ Flaxseed
❑ Peanuts
❑ Sunflower kernels
❑ Pecans
❑ Pumpkin seeds
❑ Walnuts

Pasta sauce:
❑ Pritikin
❑ Classico Tomato
 and Basil
❑ Ragú Chunky
 Gardenstyle

❑ Peanut butter
 (natural)

Popcorn:
❑ Orville
 Redenbacher's
 Natural
❑ Light or Smart Pop
 microwave popcorn
❑ Plain kernels

Tortilla chips:
❑ Baked Tostitos
❑ Guiltless Gourmet

❑ Water *(spring or
 sparkling)*

Wine:
❑ Dealcoholized
❑ Red
❑ White

NOTES: _____

_____

_____

_____

_____

_____

_____

_____

_____

_____

_____

_____

_____

_____

_____

_____

_____

_____

_____

_____

_____

_____

_____

_____

_____

_____

_____

_____

_____

Once your pantry and fridge are stocked with the "right stuff," you're equipped to put together meals in short order. These tips will help to stream-line your time in the kitchen.

- **USE YOUR FREEZER AS A PANTRY AS WELL.** If you're grilling two chicken breasts, why not grill twelve and store ten? Besides storing defrost and serve meals and leftovers, use the freezer for quick-to-thaw meal makers such as frozen veggies, extra cooked brown rice, and freezer-to-oven proteins, such as your advanced grilled chicken or meats.

- **WORK ON MORE THAN ONE RECIPE AT A TIME.** People tend to do one recipe, finish it, and go on to the next. And that just takes too much time. Whatever takes longest, do first. That way, the rest of the meal prep falls into place at the right time.

- **USE SPEEDIER COOKING METHODS.** Forget roasting or braising and go with broiling, sautéeing, or steaming. And try pressure cooking—particularly for preparing whole grains. It can cut cooking time by a third.

- **INVEST IN GOOD SHARP KNIVES.** You may not even need to haul out the food processor or chopper.

- **QUICK-THAW WITH YOUR MICROWAVE.** Stick frozen chicken breasts in the microwave on defrost, cook them at full power for 2 to 3 minutes, then slice the still partially frozen chicken into strips. Throw them into a skillet—they will be thin enough to heat through quickly.

- **CUT DOWN ON CLEANUP.** Try to keep the number of utensils to a minimum and use nonstick pans whenever possible. And my best tip: get someone else to wash the dishes!

- **DESIGNATE A FALL-BACK RECIPE.** Find one recipe you love and tape it into your cupboard door nearest your stove. Keep the

ingredients for the recipe on hand at all times. You'll make it
when time is crunched to the max. My favorite quick meal is
Baked Spaghetti. (See recipe on page 276.)

When you're planning meals and cooking *The Smart Weigh,*
remember to pay attention to added fat in preparation. Follow these
tips for trimming the fat from your diet:

■ **EAT MORE FISH AND SKINLESS POULTRY, AND
FEWER RED MEATS.** If you eat red meats,
buy lean and trim well (before and after
cooking)—and cook them in a way that
diminishes fat, such as grilling, broiling,
or roasting on a rack.

> **SMART WEIGH TIP**
>
> *Don't give in to peer
> pressure. If the cookies,
> chips, or ice cream you
> buy for the rest of the
> family is sabotaging
> your efforts, stop buy-
> ing it.*

■ **USE MARINADES, FLAVORED VINEGARS, PLAIN
YOGURT, OR JUICES WHEN GRILLING OR BROILING TO TENDERIZE
LEANER CUTS OF MEAT AND SEAL IN THEIR MOISTURE AND FLAVOR.**
Mix these marinades with fresh or dried herbs such as basil,
oregano, and parsley to add flavor.

■ **LIMIT PROTEIN PORTIONS TO 5 OUNCES PRECOOKED.** After cooking,
the size will resemble that of a deck of cards. This is the typical lunch portion of fish or chicken served in a restaurant. (The
typical dinner portion is 9 ounces.) Let brown rice, whole-
grain pastas, potatoes, and vegetables become the centerpiece
of your meals.

■ **USE NONSTICK COOKING SPRAYS AND SKILLETS.** These will enable
you to brown meats without grease; and sauté ingredients in
stocks and broths rather than in fats and oils. If a recipe calls
for basting in butter or "its juices," instead, baste with tomato,
lemon juice, or stocks.

■ SKIM THE FAT FROM SOUPS, STOCKS, AND MEAT DRIPPINGS. Refrigerate and remove the hardened surface layer of fat before reheating. As you do, think about that fat hardening in your body, and the great favor you are doing for yourself by getting rid of it!

■ USE LEGUMES (DRIED BEANS AND PEAS) AS A MAIN DISH. These meat substitutes can be a high nutrition, low-fat meal. Attempt a switch at least twice each week. If beans have been gaseous in the past, try Beano (available from your pharmacy or health food store); it's a natural enzyme that works wonders for digestion of beans and other gas-forming foods while your body is becoming more tolerant on its own.

■ SUBSTITUTE PLAIN, NONFAT YOGURT OR FAT-FREE RICOTTA CHEESE IN DIPS OR SAUCES CALLING FOR SOUR CREAM OR MAYO. Also, use these as toppings for baked potatoes and chili. (And don't forget low-fat, flavorful salsa, a great low-cal topping for almost anything.)

■ USE TWO EGG WHITES IN PLACE OF ONE WHOLE EGG. Egg whites are pure protein; egg yolks are pure fat and cholesterol.

In the pages ahead are suggested menus that incorporate all of my principles for preparing specific dishes and meals *The Smart Weigh*. Each menu is made up of recipes that have been designed to form a pleasing whole of contrasting flavors, textures, and colors. Each meal is designed with the proper balance of protein, complex carbohydrates, simple carbohydrates, and fat as outlined in *The Smart Weigh* meal plans in Chapter 12.

The nutrient balance and calorie count is roughly the same for each breakfast, lunch, and dinner. If you really like one of the meals, or don't care for another, just mix and match meals from one day to the next. A tuna sandwich is fine for breakfast, and an egg-white omelet works just fine for dinner. Substitute green beans if you're not craving asparagus; leave out a spice or herb if you don't have it available. You can also use healthy foods you have on hand to create something new and personally yours.

I have analyzed each recipe for its nutritional value. Besides the calories, carbohydrate, protein, and fat grams, I have included information about sodium and cholesterol for those of you watching these numbers as well. The fat grams are also expressed in terms of the percentage of calories derived from fat in each particular dish. My meals are designed to give less than 25 percent of the calories from fat, with the average dish yielding 17 percent.

Individual recipes that are higher in percentage of fat calories are paired with those having low or no fat to balance the whole meal properly. I have used these profiles to plan balanced meals that give appropriate levels of nutrients. Portion sizes may need to be adjusted to fit caloric needs according to your own individualized meal plan. Don't get caught up in counting every calorie or fat gram—just focus on eating great foods, prepared in great ways, that are great for you.

Most of the recipes in the pages ahead have been my favorites, many are those I've developed for restaurants interested in healthier menu offerings. Many have been passed on to me by friends (often chefs) and family. Some have been developed, others "made over" for *The Smart Weigh*. There is an endless array of cooking tricks—part art, part science—to turn unhealthy, full-of-fat dishes into tasty, nutritious ones. I have used them all in these recipes, and you may want to use them on some of your favorites as well.

Basically, I use four methods to reduce the amount of fat, calories and other detrimental substances in a recipe.

- I reduce the amount of high-fat, high-salt ingredients and look for ways to enhance flavor, texture and nutritive value.
- I replace a high-fat, high-salt ingredient with a different one that is lower in fat and sodium and higher in flavor.
- I use smaller amounts of fattier foods that pack a powerful flavor punch: feta cheese, Parmesan, coconut, toasted nuts, sesame oil, and turkey bacon or sausage made from turkey. I cut the quantity to less than fifty percent of what is called for in the typical recipe.
- I use a cooking method that reduces fat yet enhances moisture and flavor. This reduces or eliminates the need for fats, oils, and rich sauces. Some of the techniques I use most in cooking *The Smart Weigh* are grilling and broiling, parchment cooking, poaching, sautéing and stir-frying, steaming or boiling, and microwaving.

GETTING STARTED

You'll find that these meals are fresh, fun, and flavorful—they will fill you with good food and good health. The key is getting started—and remember it's progress, not perfection that counts. You may start with some of the following "grab 'n go" breakfasts. Or you may start packing a more interesting lunch that's healthier and more energizing. It may be one fabulous dinner a week or elements of *The Smart Weigh* cooking sprinkled throughout all your meals. Wherever you choose to begin—get cooking and have fun!

MY QUICKEST BREAKFASTS

Don't resort to the food industry's versions of "instant" breakfasts, like toaster fruit pies, granola bars (just candy with oats), and artificially flavored and colored powdered drink mixes. Instead of going for breakfast in the fast lane—and getting much more fat, calories, and sodium than you've bargained for—grab and go with your own quick and easy breakfast:

POWER BREAKFAST SHAKE
SERVES 1

You can put all these together in the blender container and place the whole thing in your fridge before bed. In the morning pull it out and place it on the blender apparatus and zap: you've got a drinkable "instant" breakfast that's loaded with whole food nutrients.

1/2 cup frozen fruit

1 cup skim milk

1 coddled egg white, or 1/4 cup egg substitute

2 teaspoons honey

1 teaspoon vanilla

1 tablespoon wheat germ

Blend together until smooth and frothy.

Gives 1 complex carbohydrate (wheat germ), 2 ounces protein (milk and egg whites), and 1 simple carbohydrate (fruit).

NUTRITIONAL PROFILE PER SERVING: 37 GRAMS CARBOHYDRATE; 17 GRAMS PROTEIN; 0 GRAMS FAT; 0 CALORIES FROM FAT, 2 MILLIGRAMS CHOLESTEROL, 88 MILLIGRAMS SODIUM, 216 CALORIES.

SCRAMBLED EGGS BURRITO
SERVES 1

Heat a nonstick pan or griddle over medium-high heat. Add the tortilla to heat and soften, turning it over after 15 seconds. After another 15 seconds, remove the tortilla from the pan and wrap it in foil to keep warm. Spray the pan with nonstick spray, continuing to heat. Beat together the eggs, grated cheese, and creole seasoning.

1 10-inch whole wheat flour tortilla

1 egg, lightly beaten, or 1/4 cup egg substitute

2 tablespoons (1 ounces) 2-percent milk cheddar or soy cheese, grated

1/4 teaspoon creole seasoning (or salt and pepper to taste)

2 tablespoons salsa

1/4 cantaloupe, sliced

Add to the pan and scramble. Place the egg mixture on the tortilla and spoon on the salsa. Wrap it up burrito-style. Serve with the sliced cantaloupe. Gives 1 complex carbohydrate (tortilla), 2 ounces protein (eggs and cheese), and 1 simple carbohydrate (cantaloupe).

NUTRITIONAL PROFILE PER SERVING: 32 GRAMS CARBOHYDRATE; 13 GRAMS PROTEIN; 5 GRAMS FAT; 20 PERCENT CALORIES FROM FAT (WITH EGG SUBSTITUTE), 8 MILLIGRAMS CHOLESTEROL, 613 MILLIGRAMS SODIUM, 223 CALORIES.

4 egg whites
1 cup nonfat ricotta cheese
2 tablespoons canola oil
1 teaspoon vanilla
2/3 cup old-fashioned oats, uncooked
1/4 teaspoons salt
nonstick cooking spray
4 tablespoons all-fruit jam or pourable all-fruit syrup
2 cups mixed berries

HOT OATCAKES WITH BERRIES
MAKES 12 3-INCH PANCAKES

Measure the egg whites, ricotta cheese, oil, vanilla, oats, and salt into a blender or food processor and blend for 5 to 6 minutes. Spoon 2 tablespoons batter into a hot skillet sprayed with nonstick spray. Turn the pancakes when bubbles appear on the surface; cook for 1 more minute.

For one serving, spread 3 pancakes with all fruit jam or fruit syrup. Top with mixed berries. Freeze any leftovers in individual freezer bags. When ready to use, toast the pancakes to thaw and heat. Each serving gives 1 1/2 complex carbohydrate (oats), 2 ounces protein (ricotta and eggwhites), and 1 simple carbohydrate (fruit and fruit jam)

NUTRITIONAL PROFILE PER SERVING: 35 GRAMS CARBOHYDRATE; 12 GRAMS PROTEIN; 7 GRAMS FAT; 26 PERCENT CALORIES FROM FAT, 3 MILLIGRAMS CHOLESTEROL, 97.5 MILLIGRAMS SODIUM, 251 CALORIES.

2 egg whites, lightly beaten
2 tablespoons skim milk
1 teaspoons vanilla
1 10-inch whole wheat flour tortilla
nonstick cooking spray
2 tablespoons Grape-nuts or low-fat granola
1/2 cup mixed berries
1 tablespoon all-fruit pourable syrup

SOUTHWESTERN FRUIT TOAST
SERVES 1

Beat together the egg whites, milk, and vanilla. Dip the tortilla into the mixture, letting it absorb the liquid for a minute or so. Coat a nonstick skillet with nonstick spray and heat. Gently lift the tortilla with a spatula, place it in the skillet and cook until it is golden brown on each side. Sprinkle one half of the tortilla with cereal and berries. Fold the tortilla over omelette style and slide it onto a plate. Drizzle it with all-fruit syrup. Gives 2 complex carbohydrates (tortilla and cereal), 2 ounces protein (milk and egg whites), and 1 simple carbohydrate (fruit and fruit syrup)

NUTRITIONAL PROFILE PER SERVING: 44 GRAMS CARBOHYDRATE; 13.5 GRAMS PROTEIN; 2 GRAMS FAT; 7 PERCENT CALORIES FROM FAT, 8 MILLIGRAMS CHOLESTEROL, 266 MILLIGRAMS SODIUM, 249 CALORIES.

ORANGE VANILLA FRENCH TOAST

SERVES 4

4 egg whites, lightly beaten

1/2 teaspoon ground cinnamon

1/2 cup skim milk

4 slices whole wheat bread

2 tablespoons frozen, unsweetened orange juice concentrate, undiluted

4 tablespoons all-fruit jam or pourable syrup

1 teaspoons vanilla

nonstick cooking spray

Beat together the egg whites, milk, orange juice concentrate, vanilla, and cinnamon. Add the bread slices one at a time, letting the bread absorb the liquid; this may take a few minutes. Coat a skillet with nonstick cooking spray and heat. Gently lift each bread slice with a spatula and place it in the skillet; cook on each side until golden brown. Serve each slice of toast topped with 1 tablespoon all-fruit jam or all-fruit pourable syrup. Freeze the leftovers in individual freezer bags. When ready to use a slice, toast it to thaw and heat. Each serving gives 1 complex carbohydrate (bread), 1 ounce protein (egg whites and milk), and 1 simple carbohydrate (juice and all-fruit jam).

NUTRITIONAL PROFILE PER SERVING: 28 GRAMS CARBOHYDRATE; 8 GRAMS PROTEIN; 1.5 GRAMS FAT; 11 PERCENT CALORIES FROM FAT; 2 MILLIGRAMS CHOLESTEROL; 250 MILLIGRAMS SODIUM; 152 CALORIES

BAKED BREAKFAST APPLE

SERVES 1

1 small Golden Delicious apple, cored

1 tablespoon raisins

2 tablespoons old-fashioned oats

2 tablespoons apple juice

1/4 teaspoon cinnamon

1/2 cup nonfat ricotta cheese

Place the apple in a microwavable bowl. Mix together oats, cinnamon, and raisins. Fill the cavity of the cored apple with the mixture. Pour the apple juice over the apple, and cover it with plastic wrap. Microwave on high for 1 minute. Turn the dish around halfway and microwave for 1 minute more. Spoon the ricotta cheese onto a plate, and top it with the apple and the heated juice mixture. Gives 1 complex carbohydrate (oats), 2 ounces protein (ricotta), and 1 simple carbohydrate (apple, juice, and raisins).

NUTRITIONAL PROFILE PER SERVING: 30 GRAMS CARBOHYDRATE; 14 GRAMS PROTEIN; 1 GRAMS FAT; 6 PERCENT CALORIES FROM FAT; 23 MILLIGRAMS CHOLESTEROL; 100 MILLIGRAMS SODIUM; 183 CALORIES

1/2 banana, quartered lengthwise

1/4 cup crushed unsweetened pineapple

1/2 cup nonfat ricotta cheese

2 tablespoons Grape-Nuts or low-fat granola

1/4 cup strawberries, sliced

1 teaspoon honey or all-fruit pourable syrup

BREAKFAST SUNDAE SUPREME

SERVES 1

Place the banana quarters star-fashion on a small plate. Scoop ricotta cheese onto the center points. Surround with the other fruit; then sprinkle with cereal. Drizzle with honey or all-fruit syrup. Gives 1 complex carbohydrate (cereal), 2 ounces protein (ricotta), and 2 simple carbohydrates (fruit).

NUTRITIONAL PROFILE PER SERVING: 42 GRAMS CARBOHYDRATE; 15 GRAMS PROTEIN; 1 GRAM FAT; 4 PERCENT CALORIES FROM FAT; 5 MILLIGRAMS CHOLESTEROL; 111 MILLIGRAMS SODIUM; 224 CALORIES

2/3 cup old-fashioned oats

1 teaspoon vanilla

1 1/2 cups skim milk

1/2 teaspoon cinnamon

1/2 cup apple or white grape juice, unsweetened

1/2 teaspoon pumpkin pie spice

2 tablespoons raisins, dark or golden

HOT APPLE CINNAMON OATMEAL

SERVES 2

In a small pot, bring the oats, milk, and juice to a boil. Cook for 5 minutes, stirring occasionally. Add raisins, vanilla, cinnamon, and pumpkin pie spice. Remove from heat, cover the pot and let the oats sit for 2 to 3 minutes to thicken. Combine all ingredients and cook for 5 to 6 minutes on high. Gives 1 complex carbohydrate (oats), 1 ounce protein (milk), and 1 simple carbohydrate (juice and raisins).

NUTRITIONAL PROFILE PER SERVING 29 GRAMS CARBOHYDRATE; 11 GRAMS PROTEIN; 1 GRAM FAT; 5 PERCENT CALORIES FROM FAT; 3 MILLIGRAMS CHOLESTEROL; 97 MILLIGRAMS SODIUM; 169 CALORIES

MY QUICKEST LUNCHES

(1) CHEESE QUESADILLAS: Fat-free whole wheat tortilla sprinkled with 2 ounces shredded part-skim cheddar cheese and drizzled with salsa—folded and browned in a nonstick skillet until cheese melts. Serve with apple slices.

(2) BAKED SPAGHETTI: Cooked whole wheat angel hair pasta in a sheet pan—topped with one jar of Classico Tomato Basil Sauce, sprinkled with 1 pound shredded mozzarella cheese, and baked for 8 to 10 minutes on 375 degrees. One 3x5 (index card size) is approximately one serving. Serve with "salad in a bag" with low-fat vinaigrette.

(3) VEGETABLE TORTILLA PIZZA: Large whole wheat flour tortilla brushed with Classico Tomato Basil Sauce, topped with chopped veggies of choice, and sprinkled with grated mozzarella. Bake until lightly browned and crisp (about 5 minutes) at 450 degrees. Serve with baby carrots to munch on.

(4) GRILLED CHICKEN SANDWICH: Grilled marinated chicken breast (from your freezer) on whole-grain bun with lettuce, tomato, salsa, or Dijon mustard. Serve with fresh fruit.

(5) TURKEY AND WHITE BEAN SOUP: Smoked turkey breast (precooked) made into soup with chicken stock and cannelini beans. Serve with raw veggies and fruit.

(6) QUICK TACO SALAD: Canned black beans, rinsed, then spiced with creole seasoning and sprinkled with shredded part-skim cheddar cheese. Heat and serve over mixed greens and crumbled baked Tostitos with salsa. Serve with sliced oranges.

> **SMART WEIGH TIP**
>
> *Enlist professional help. Registered dietitians, certified personal trainers, and psychologists can help you deal with problems that may be hindering your efforts. If you feel like you can't do it on your own, seek help.*

(7) EVEN QUICKER GREEK SALAD: Mixed greens (from a bag), topped with crumbled feta cheese and shredded Boar's Head turkey or ham, and drizzled with low-fat vinaigrette. Serve with toasted petite whole wheat pita and a piece of fruit.

(8) CHEESE BAKED POTATOES: Microwave potatoes for 4 minutes each, then cut open and top with cooked broccoli florets and Laughing Cow Lite Wedges (2 per potato) or 2 ounces of another part-skim cheese. Microwave again until cheese melts. Top with nonfat sour cream or salsa. Serve with salad and low-fat vinaigrette.

DELICIOUSLY SIMPLE DINNERS

PASTA SHRIMP POMODORO WITH FRESH BROCCOLI SALAD
SHRIMP (PROTEIN) • PASTA (COMPLEX CARBOHYDRATE)
BROCCOLI (SIMPLE CARBOHYDRATE)

1 1/2 pounds shrimp, peeled and deveined

1/4 cup white wine Worcestershire sauce

8 ounces dry angel hair pasta

2 teaspoons olive oil

2 cloves garlic, minced

1 small red onion, chopped

1 each yellow, orange, and red bell peppers, cut into strips

1 teaspoon Mrs. Dash seasoning

1 teaspoon creole seasoning

1 teaspoon dried oregano

1/2 teaspoon dried basil

1 can (32 ounces) whole tomatoes

2 tablespoons grated Parmesan cheese

PASTA SHRIMP POMODORO
SERVES 4

Marinate shrimp in Worcestershire sauce for at least 15 minutes.

In a large saucepan, cook pasta in salted water until done. Drain.

Spray a nonstick skillet with cooking spray. Lightly sauté half of the garlic and half of the onions. Add shrimp and sear on one side for 1 minute; then turn and sear on other side.

Spray another skillet with cooking spray and add olive oil; heat. Add remaining garlic and onions, sauté. Then add peppers, seasonings and herbs. Allow peppers to soften, then add tomatoes, breaking up tomatoes with spatula while heating. Allow to simmer and reduce for about 4 to 5 minutes. Add shrimp, stirring all together. Sprinkle with Parmesan cheese. Serve over cooked pasta.

2 bunches fresh broccoli, trimmed and cut into small pieces

1 cup chopped fresh parsley

2 to 3 green onions, sliced

1/2 cup nonfat cottage cheese (or ricotta)

1/4 cup light mayonnaise

1/2 cup skim milk

2 cloves garlic, minced

1 teaspoon Mrs. Dash seasoning

1/2 teaspoon creole seasoning

3/4 teaspoon dill weed

FRESH BROCCOLI SALAD
SERVES 8

Blanch broccoli for 5 minutes in boiling water. Immerse quickly in ice water to chill; drain. Toss with parsley and green onions.

Make dressing by blending cottage cheese, mayonnaise, milk, garlic, and seasonings in blender until smooth. Stir in dill. Toss with vegetables and chill well.

HERB CRUSTED ORANGE ROUGHY WITH HERB ROASTED POTATOES

FISH (PROTEIN) • POTATOES, BREAD CRUMBS (COMPLEX CARBOHYDRATE)
BROCCOLI (SIMPLE CARBOHYDRATE)

HERB-CRUSTED ORANGE ROUGHY

SERVES 4

Marinate orange roughy in Worcestershire sauce for at least 15 minutes, or up to 1 hour.

Preheat oven to 375 degrees.

Season fish with seasoning and roll in bread crumbs. Spread mustard on top of fish and roll in bread crumbs once more.

Spray a nonstick skillet with cooking spray; heat. Sear fish in hot skillet on both sides, then transfer to oven and roast until done and browned.

Serve on bed of tomato basil sauce with steamed broccoli. Sprinkle with chopped parsley.

4 orange roughy fillets (5 ounces each)

1/4 cup white wine Worcestershire sauce

1 teaspoon creole seasoning

1/2 cup dried bread crumbs (purchased)

2 tablespoons chopped fresh herbs (cilantro, basil, rosemary, thyme)

1/4 cup Dijon mustard

2 cups broccoli florets, steamed until crisp tender

1/2 cup Tomato Basil Sauce (recipe follows)

1 tablespoon parsley, chopped

TOMATO BASIL SAUCE

MAKES 14 1/2-CUP SERVINGS

Sauté onions, garlic, shallots, and herbs in olive oil until onions are transparent, about 3 to 4 minutes.

Add fresh and canned tomatoes. Cook for 5 minutes at full heat. Lower heat and continue cooking until sauce has reduced by one-third.

Add seasonings. Cook for about 1 1/2 hours, stirring occasionally. Leave chunky; do not grind or blend.

This sauce may be made in large quantities and frozen (after cooling) in zip-top bags for later use. Microwave or place in refrigerator to thaw.

1 tablespoon olive oil

2 white onions, diced medium

2 teaspoons minced garlic

1/2 cup minced shallots

1 tablespoon chopped fresh thyme

1 teaspoon chopped fresh rosemary

1 tablespoon chopped fresh oregano

2 tablespoons chopped fresh basil

5 tomatoes, skinned, seeded, and diced★

1 can (32 ounces) whole tomatoes

1 tablespoon creole seasoning

1 tablespoon Mrs. Dash Garlic and Herb seasoning

★*Tomatoes are easily skinned by immersing them in boiling water for 10 seconds. Remove with slotted spoon. Skins will "slip off."*

2 pounds (about 5 large) red-skinned potatoes, scrubbed and quartered

2 cloves garlic, minced

2 teaspoons olive oil

1/2 teaspoon creole seasoning

1 teaspoon Mrs. Dash seasoning

1 tablespoon chopped fresh rosemary (or 1 teaspoon dried)

HERB-ROASTED POTATOES
SERVES 4

Preheat oven to 450 degrees.

Spray a shallow roasting pan with cooking spray. Add potatoes, garlic, olive oil, seasonings, and rosemary, and spread in an even layer. Bake until the potatoes begin to brown, 20 to 30 minutes, turning them once midway through roasting.

SEARED PORK TENDERLOIN WITH CINNAMON SWEET POTATOES AND FRESH ASPARAGUS
PORK (PROTEIN) • SWEET POTATOES (COMPLEX CARBOHYDRATE) ASPARAGUS (SIMPLE CARBOHYDRATE)

1 1/2 pounds pork tenderloin, trimmed of all visible fat

1/2 cup white wine Worcestershire sauce

1/2 teaspoon creole seasoning

2 tablespoon chopped fresh herbs (cilantro, basil, rosemary, thyme)

1 teaspoon Mrs. Dash seasoning

2 garlic cloves, minced

1 large red onion, sliced thin

SEARED PORK TENDERLOIN
SERVES 4

Preheat oven to 400 degrees.

Marinate pork tenderloin in Worcestershire sauce, seasonings, herbs, and garlic for at least 1 hour.

Sear pork on both sides in hot ovenproof skillet, then top with sliced onions. Place whole skillet in oven for 15 minutes or until internal temperature reaches 150 to 170 degrees. May pour on additional marinade while roasting.

4 sweet potatoes

cinnamon

CINNAMON SWEET POTATOES
SERVES 4

Preheat oven to 400 degrees.

Wash and scrub sweet potatoes. Place in oven for 35 minutes. (You may add the skillet of pork tenderloins to the oven after 20 minutes.)

Cut open sweet potatoes and push ends together to "mash" toward center and fluff. Sprinkle with cinnamon.

FRESH ASPARAGUS
SERVES 4

Microwave asparagus in chicken stock and seasonings for about 7 to 8 minutes or until crisp tender.

1 pound fresh asparagus, trimmed
1/4 cup chicken stock (fat-free/low salt)
1 teaspoon Mrs. Dash seasoning
1/2 teaspoon creole seasoning

CHICKEN LAURENT WITH BROWN RICE PILAF
CHICKEN (PROTEIN) • RICE (COMPLEX CARBOHYDRATE)
ASPARAGUS, RED ONION (SIMPLE CARBOHYDRATE)

CHICKEN LAURENT
SERVES 4

Preheat oven to 375 degrees.

Marinate chicken breasts in Worcestershire sauce for at least 15 minutes.

Place asparagus spears with 1/4 cup water in a glass baking dish; cover with vented plastic wrap. Microwave on high to blanch for 3 to 4 minutes.

Spray nonstick ovenproof skillet with cooking spray. Add olive oil and heat. Add garlic and shallots to pan; lightly sauté. Add marinated chicken breasts and brown on both sides, sprinkling with seasonings. Lay asparagus and red onion slices on top of chicken.

Stir together wine and chicken stock in a small stock pot; add cornstarch mixed with 1 tablespoon cold water. Stir over moderate heat until thickened. Pour over chicken and vegetables.

Bake in oven for 30 minutes.

4 boneless, skinless chicken breast halves (1 pound)
1/4 cup white wine Worcestershire sauce
2 teaspoons olive oil
2 cloves garlic, minced
2 teaspoons shallots, minced
1 teaspoon Mrs. Dash seasoning
1/2 teaspoon creole seasoning
1 pound asparagus, trimmed
1 red onion, sliced thin
1/3 cup white wine★
2/3 cup chicken stock (fat-free/low salt)
2 teaspoons cornstarch
★ or substitute dealcoholized wine or more chicken stock

1 teaspoon olive oil

1/2 red onion, diced

2 cloves garlic, minced

1 3/4 cups chicken stock (fat-free/low salt)

1/2 teaspoon creole seasoning

1 tablespoon chopped fresh herbs (cilantro, basil, rosemary, thyme)

2 cups instant brown rice

BROWN RICE PILAF
SERVES 6

Spray a medium saucepan with cooking spray; add olive oil and heat. Add diced onion and garlic, and lightly sauté about 1 to 2 minutes; then add chicken stock, seasoning and herbs.

Let mixture come to a boil, then stir in brown rice. Let boil for 1 minute, turn down heat to low and cover. Let simmer for 5 minutes, uncover skillet, and fluff rice with fork. Cover again. Let sit for another 5 minutes.

CHICKEN PAELLA WITH SPICY TOMATO AND CUCUMBER SALAD
CHICKEN (PROTEIN) • RICE, PEAS (COMPLEX CARBOHYDRATE)
TOMATO, CUCUMBERS (SIMPLE CARBOHYDRATE)

1 pound boneless, skinless chicken breast, trimmed of fat and cut into chunks

1/4 cup white wine Worcestershire sauce

2 teaspoons olive oil

2 cloves garlic, minced

1 small onion, diced

1 cup arborio (or medium grain) rice

2 cups chicken stock (fat-free/low salt)

1/4 teaspoon crushed saffron threads (or 1/8 teaspoon powdered)

1/2 teaspoon creole seasoning

1 teaspoon Mrs. Dash seasoning

1 cup frozen peas, thawed

1/3 cup jarred, roasted red peppers, drained and cut into strips

CHICKEN PAELLA
SERVES 4

Marinate chicken breasts in Worcestershire sauce for up to 1 hour.

Spray a large nonstick skillet with cooking spray. Add olive oil and heat over medium-high heat. Add garlic and onions and sauté 30 seconds, then add marinated chicken chunks. Sauté until slightly browned on the outside and opaque inside, 3 to 4 minutes. Remove chicken from skillet and set aside.

To skillet, add rice and stir to coat well. Stir in chicken stock, saffron, and seasonings. Cover and cook over low heat for 20 minutes. Gently stir in cooked chicken, green peas, and roasted red peppers. Cover again and cook, stirring occasionally, until rice is tender, about 5 minutes more. Serve immediately.

SPICY TOMATO AND CUCUMBER SALAD

SERVES 6

In a medium-sized bowl, mix together all ingredients. Cover and refrigerate about 2 hours or until chilled.

2 large tomatoes, cut into wedges

1 cup diced cucumber

1/2 cup finely chopped red onion

1 clove garlic, minced

2 tablespoons chopped fresh cilantro

2 tablespoons red wine vinegar

2 teaspoons chopped fresh hot green chili pepper (or 1/4 teaspoon crushed red pepper)

1 teaspoon honey

1/2 teaspoon creole seasoning

POACHED SALMON OVER BLACK BEANS AND CORN WITH APPLE WALNUT SALAD

SALMON, BLACK BEANS (PROTEIN) • CORN, BLACK BEANS (COMPLEX CARBOHYDRATE) • VEGETABLES, FRUIT (SIMPLE CARBOHYDRATE)

4 SALMON FILLETS (5 OUNCES EACH)

POACHED SALMON

SERVES 4

In a large nonstick skillet, bring poaching stock to boil. Add salmon and asparagus spears; simmer 5 to 7 minutes until done.

Spoon Black Bean and Corn Salsa onto plate. Add fresh spinach leaves and place poached salmon and asparagus spears on top of the leaves.

Sprinkle with chopped chives and garnish with twisted lemon slice.

POACHING STOCK:

1 cup white wine★

2 cups chicken stock (fat free /low salt)

1 whole shallot, quartered

2 cloves garlic, minced

2 sprigs fresh thyme

2 bay leaves

1/4 teaspoon cracked black pepper

1/2 teaspoon creole seasoning

1 pound asparagus, trimmed of tough stalks

2 cups Black Bean and Corn Salsa (recipe follows)

2 cups fresh spinach leaves, washed and stemmed

1 tablespoon chopped chives

1 lemon, sliced

★or substitute dealcoholized wine or more chicken stock

2 cups black beans, drained and rinsed

1 cup frozen corn kernels, thawed

2 plum tomatoes, diced

1/2 red onion, minced

1 serrano pepper, minced

1 tablespoon chopped fresh cilantro

1 tablespoon olive oil

4 cloves garlic, minced

juice of 2 limes

1 tablespoon balsamic vinegar

1 teaspoon cumin

2 teaspoons hot pepper sauce

1 teaspoon creole seasoning

BLACK BEAN AND CORN SALSA
MAKES 10 1/3-CUP SERVINGS

In a large bowl, combine all ingredients and mix well. Allow to marinate at least one hour before serving.

2 Granny Smith apples, cored and sliced thin

2 tablespoons chopped walnuts

2 tablespoons chicken stock (fat free/low salt)

1 tablespoon white wine vinegar

2 teaspoons walnut oil (or olive oil)

1 tablespoon finely chopped shallots

1 teaspoon Dijon mustard

1/4 teaspoon salt

1/4 teaspoon cracked black pepper

8 cups washed, dried, and torn mixed greens (red leaf, romaine, frisee, radicchio, arugula, or bibb)

APPLE WALNUT SALAD

In a small, dry skillet over low heat, stir walnuts until lightly toasted, about 3 minutes. Transfer to a plate to cool.

In a large salad bowl, whisk together chicken stock, vinegar, oil, shallots, mustard, salt, and pepper. Add greens and apples and toss thoroughly. Sprinkle with the toasted walnuts.

RED LENTIL CHILI WITH SOUTHWEST CORNBREAD AND CRUNCHY JICAMA AND MELON SALAD
LENTILS, CHEESE (PROTEIN) • LENTILS, CORNBREAD (COMPLEX CARBOHYDRATE)
VEGETABLES, SALAD (SIMPLE CARBOHYDRATE)

RED LENTIL CHILI
SERVES 10 (1 1/2 CUPS EACH)

In food processor, finely chop carrots, zucchini, squash, eggplant, and onion. Spray nonstick skillet with cooking spray. Add olive oil. Heat over medium high heat. Add chopped vegetables. Sauté for 5 minutes. Add lentils, chicken stock, seasonings, herbs, spices, garlic, jalapeño peppers and tomatoes. Simmer for 2 hours.

1/2 pound carrots

1 small zucchini

1 small yellow squash

1/2 large eggplant

1/2 large red onion

3/4 tablespoon olive oil

12-ounce bag red or brown lentils, rinsed

2 cups chicken stock (fat free /low salt)

1 teaspoon Mrs. Dash seasoning

1 teaspoon creole seasoning

2 bay leaves

1/2 tablespoon oregano

1/2 teaspoon cumin

1 teaspoon chili powder

3/4 teaspoon cayenne

3/4 teaspoon nutmeg

2 cloves garlic, minced

1 jalapeño pepper, chopped

2 cans (32 ounces each) plum tomatoes

2 tablespoons canola oil
1/2 cup finely chopped onion
1 egg, lightly beaten
1 tablespoon honey
1 cup skim milk
1 cup whole wheat pastry flour
1 cup yellow cornmeal
1 tablespoon baking powder
1/2 teaspoon salt
1 cup fresh or frozen corn
1/2 cup shredded part-skim cheddar cheese

SOUTHWEST CORNBREAD
SERVES 16

Preheat oven to 375 degrees.

Heat oil in a small skillet. Add onion and sauté for 5 to 8 minutes or until onion is soft.

Beat together egg, honey, and milk; set aside.

In a separate bowl, combine flour, cornmeal, baking powder, and salt. Add to liquid mixture. Add corn, shredded cheese and onions along with all excess oil. Mix well. Spread into an 8-inch square pan coated with cooking spray.

Bake for 25 to 35 minutes or until brown and firm on top. Cut into 16 pieces.

1 medium jicama, julienned
1 medium cantaloupe, cut into 1/2-inch cubes
3 tablespoons lime juice
3 tablespoons chopped fresh mint (or 1 tablespoon dried)
1 teaspoon grated lime peel
2 teaspoons honey
1/4 teaspoon salt

CRUNCHY JICAMA AND MELON SALAD
SERVES 4

In a medium-sized bowl, mix together all ingredients. Cover and refrigerate 2 hours or until chilled.

RISOTTO WITH SPRING VEGETABLES AND MIXED GREENS WITH CITRUS VINAIGRETTE

CHEESES (PROTEIN) • RICE (COMPLEX CARBOHYDRATE) • SALAD (SIMPLE CARBOHYDRATE)

RISOTTO WITH SPRING VEGETABLES

SERVES 4

In a medium-sized stockpot, bring chicken stock to boil over medium heat. Add carrots and cook 3 to 5 minutes until almost tender. Add asparagus and snap peas, and cook 1 minute longer. Remove vegetables with slotted spoon and place in bowl to cool. Reduce heat and keep stock simmering.

Spray a nonstick skillet with cooking spray. Add olive oil; heat. Add garlic and onions, and sauté until translucent, about 3 minutes. Add rice and stir to coat grains. Add wine and cook until most of liquid has been absorbed, about 2 to 3 minutes. Add 1/2 cup simmering chicken stock and cook another 2 to 3 minutes.

Continue adding stock, 1/2 cup at a time, until rice begins to soften, about 15 minutes.

Stir in the seasoning and basil, adding more stock to keep mixture creamy. Stir in reserved vegetables and cheese. Sprinkle with herbs.

5 1/2 to 6 1/2 cups chicken stock (fat free/low salt)

16 baby carrots, shaved and cut in half

8 medium stalks asparagus, trimmed and cut into 2-inch pieces

1 cup sugar snap peas (thawed if frozen)

1 red bell pepper, cut into strips

2 teaspoons olive oil

2 cloves garlic, minced

1 red onion, diced

1 cup arborio or medium grain rice, uncooked

1/2 cup white wine★

1/2 teaspoon creole seasoning

1 1/2 tablespoons chopped fresh basil

1/2 cup grated Parmesan cheese

2 tablespoons chopped fresh herbs (cilantro, basil, rosemary, thyme)

★or substitute dealcoholized wine or more chicken stock

MIXED GREENS WITH CITRUS VINAIGRETTE

SERVES 4

Just before serving, toss lettuce leaves with Citrus Vinaigrette. Top with curly-leaved onion and sprinkle lightly with herbs and diced tomatoes.

12 cups washed, dried, and torn mixed greens (red leaf, romaine, frisee, radicchio, arugula, or bibb)

1/2 cup Citrus Vinaigrette (recipe follows)

4 green onions, leaves curled

2 tablespoons chopped fresh herbs (cilantro, basil, rosemary, thyme)

2 plum tomatoes, diced

2 tablespoons olive oil

2/3 cup rice wine vinegar

1/3 cup orange juice

1 tablespoon Dijon mustard

1 teaspoon honey

2 teaspoons minced garlic

1 tablespoon minced shallots

1/2 teaspoon creole seasoning

2 tablespoons chopped fresh cilantro

CITRUS VINAIGRETTE
SERVES 12

Mix all ingredients together. Refrigerate.

CHAPTER 14 ■ *Smart Weigh* Dining Out and Travel Guide

Do what you can, with what you have, where you are.

—THEODORE ROOSEVELT

f it seems as if you hardly eat at home anymore—you're right. The home-cooked meal is not yet an endangered species, but meals prepared and eaten at home are at an all-time low, according to the fourteenth annual NPD Group report on Eating Patterns in America. The newest statistics show that 47 percent of U.S. food dollars are spent eating away from home.

In the last decade of the twentieth century alone, dining in restaurants increased by 14 percent—and fast food restaurants captured more than 80 percent of that growth in the past five years. Every day 160 million people eat out at restaurants and 2 million children eat at one of the three major burger joints. Each day, 100 million M&Ms are downed, along with 30 million hot dogs. No wonder we're in the shape we're in!

But I can't always eat at home, you might be thinking. No, most of us in the twenty-first century are on the run, and having every meal at our own dining room table is unrealistic. But the typical scenario when dining out is to eat too much of the wrong foods prepared in unhealthy ways. In a small study of 129 women, researchers at the University of Memphis and Vanderbilt University found that those who ate out more than five times a week consumed an average of 2,056 calories per day, compared with an average of 1,768 calories for those who ate out five or fewer times a week. That may not sound like much, but that higher calorie consumption could add up to two to three pounds on your body every month.

The challenge before the person choosing to dine out *The Smart Weigh* is to enjoy fine food without compromising health and weight. The main threats to healthy dining out lie mostly in the "hidden fats" of restaurant preparation. A typical restaurant meal packs in the equivalent of twelve to fourteen pats of butter. To sidestep some of the land mines of eating out, follow these guidelines.

DINING OUT *THE SMART WEIGH*
Plan Ahead

When you're in charge, choose a restaurant that you know and trust for quality food and a willingness to prepare foods in a healthful way upon request. Many progressive and responsible restaurants have begun to offer healthy menu selections—recognizing that healthy eating is not a passing fad.

Order Smart

Never be timid about ordering foods prepared according to your needs. After all, you are paying (and paying well) for the meal and service. You also have a right to know the content of what you are going to eat. Remember, it's your health, your money, and your waistline—so speak up! Don't be intimidated by the waiters or chef; they generally want to please you.

Most foods can be prepared without fat and butter; just order meats, poultry, or fish grilled without butter or oils, and request sauces on the side. Good choices: marinated, grilled breast of chicken, grilled or broiled fish or seafood, and steamed shellfish. Entrées that are poached in wine or lemon juice are good options as well as those simmered in tomato sauces.

When fresh vegetables are available, order them steamed without added butter or sauces. When ordering salad dressing for salads, mayonnaise for sandwiches, butter or sour cream for a potato, ask for it on the side, and apply them in limited quantities. For example, lightly drizzle 1 tablespoons of dressing on your salad for flavor, and use extra vinegar or lemon juice for moisture.

Restaurant menus give you plenty of clues about what the selections contain. Avoid items with these words attached:

FAT LADEN WORDS		
à la mode (with ice cream)	bisque (cream soup)	escalloped (with cream sauce)
au fromage (with cheese)	buttered (with extra fat)	pan-fried (fried with extra fat)
au gratin (in cheese sauce)	casserole (with extra fat)	hash (with extra fat)
au lait (with milk)	creamed (with extra fat)	hollandaise (with cream sauce)
basted (with extra fat)	crispy (means fried)	sautéed (fried with extra fat)

If you see these words, be bold enough to ask for the entrée prepared in a healthful way; that is, if the description says "buttered," ask for it without added butter; if the description says "pan-fried," ask for it grilled or poached instead.

Watch Your Portions

The typical restaurant serves twice as much as you need. And believe me, as an adult there are no rewards for cleaning your plate. You can make better choices: ordering appetizers instead of entrées, lunch portions at dinner, sharing a meal with a willing partner, or taking home leftovers for a great meal tomorrow.

Remember not to give meat the starring role in your meal choices. A healthy serving of meat is the size of a computer mouse or a deck of cards. You'll get the right foods in the right proportions for a healthy meal every time if half of your plate holds veggies, one quarter holds the protein serving, and the other quarter holds the starchy foods (rice, pasta, or potatoes).

Have a carbohydrate and a protein at each meal, never just a salad. You may order a chef's salad with extra turkey rather than ham, or a shrimp cocktail with your salad; but be sure to include a protein. Many salad bars offer protein sources in cottage cheese, grated cheese, or chopped eggs. Your carbohydrate may be a roll, crackers, or baked potato.

Finally, guard against the desire to eat all you can at all-you-can-eat brunches, buffets, or even salad bars. Your overeating ("I want to get my money's worth") is not going to cheat the restaurant out of anything, but it can cheat you out of many healthy years.

EAT-SMART IDEAS

Let's look at the good and bad qualities of various cuisines and restaurants. Use this guide to help you make better choices when eating away from home.

Mexican

> **EAT-SMART MEXICAN**
> black bean soup; chili or gazpacho; chicken burrito, tostada, or enchilada; soft chicken tacos; chicken fajitas (without added fat).

Ask that a salad be served immediately (with dressing on the side) in place of the chips. It will help prevent the "munch a bunch" syndrome. And don't eat the fried tortilla shell your salad may be served in; those shells are grease sponges with upwards of twenty-two grams of fat per shell.

Always order à la carte rather than a combo plate, which is often laden with high-fat side dishes such as refried beans (refried beans are made with pure lard). You can also request that the sour cream and cheese toppings be omitted from your dish. These carry ten grams of fat per ounce.

And beware of the margaritas—they are loaded with both salt and sugar, to say nothing of alcohol!

Asian

Chinese, Korean, Thai, or Vietnamese food is an excellent choice for dining out, as stir-frying is the main method of cooking. This terrific technique cooks the vegetables quickly, retaining the nutrients, and, if requested, uses very little oil.

> **EAT-SMART ASIAN:** bamboo-steamed vegetables with chicken, seafood, or fish; Moo Goo Gai Pan; shrimp or tofu with vegetables (with no MSG and little oil); wonton, hot and sour, or miso soup; udon noodles with meat and vegetables; Yakitori (meats broiled on skewers).

Order dishes that have been lightly stir-fried (not deep-fried like egg rolls) and are without heavy gravies or sweet and sour sauces. Half a dinner portion is appropriate, with steamed brown or white rice; fried rice is just that—fried!

Many restaurants will prepare food without MSG if you ask, and be careful to watch the soy sauce you add. Both are loaded with sodium.

Sushi is awesome for the enthusiast, but be sure you are eating it at a high-quality restaurant that is serving the freshest fish from the best sources. If in doubt, have grilled teriyaki instead.

Italian

Controlling the size of the portion is especially important here; the typical plate of spaghetti is five times too much. Although pasta with red sauce is a relatively low-fat choice, order it in a side dish or appetizer

EAT-SMART ITALIAN:
grilled chicken with a pasta side dish or bread; fresh fish with pasta side dish or bread; clam linguine with red sauce (be careful about the amount of pasta); grilled shrimp on fettucine with red sauce; Cioppino (seafood soup); minestrone soup and salad (dressing on side), with à la carte mozzarella cheese or meatballs for protein; side dish of spaghetti with two à la carte meatballs.

EAT-SMART SEAFOOD:
fresh fish of the day—grilled when possible, without butter, sauce on the side; steamed oysters, shrimp, or clams; lobster/crabmeat/crab claws; seafood kabobs; mesquite grilled shrimp; blackened fish or seafood from the grill, prepared without butter.

portion topped with steamed or grilled seafood, chicken, or fish. Ask for your salad with dressing on the side, and never hesitate to request a red sauce rather than a butter or white sauce.

Seafood

When possible, order fresh fish/seafood—steamed, boiled, grilled, or broiled without butter. A small amount of cocktail sauce is a better choice for dipping than butter (two dips in butter = fifty calories). Remember that small seafood items such as shrimp, oysters, etc., are deadly in terms of fat and calories when fried; the surface area is so high that more breading adheres and absorbs more fat.

Steak Houses

Portion control is also crucial here. A 16-ounce steak or prime rib will give you far more protein and fat than you need. Order the smallest cut available, and plan on taking some home.

Health/Natural Food Restaurants

Do not feel "safe" here by any means! Although you will have an opportunity to get whole grains and nicer fresh vegetable salads, you still need to avoid the fats and sodium. Many foods are prepared in the same way at "health food" restaurants as at the drive-through; they just have healthier sounding names. Beware of sauces and high-fat cheeses smothering the foods, as well as high-fat dressings on salads and sandwiches. If you have a cheese dish, be sure to use no other added fats in the meal; the cheese will contain enough for the day.

Fast Food Restaurants

If you have to eat in a hurry and can't request special preparation for a sit-down meal, at least become more aware of the hidden fats in the foods you consider while you're on the run.

- Special sauces: it's the mayonnaise, special sauces, sour cream, etc., that triple the fat, sodium, and calories in fast foods. Always order your take-out without them.
- Stuffed potatoes may seem a healthy addition to the fast food menu, but not if they're smothered in cheese sauce (equivalent to nine pats of butter per potato). Ask for grated cheese, and no butter, instead.
- Chicken is a lower-fat alternative than beef, but not when it's batter-fried. One serving of chicken nuggets has the equivalent of five pats of butter—more than twice what you would get in a regular hamburger. And the fat it's soaked in is purely saturated—usually just melted beef fat. A chicken sandwich is no health package either—it usually has enough fat to equal eleven pats of butter, unless the chicken is grilled.
- Croissant sandwiches aren't a whole lot more than a meal on a grease bun. Most take-out croissants have the equivalent of

EAT-SMART STEAK HOUSE: petite cut filet; shish-ka-bob or brochette; slices of London broil (no sauces); Hawaiian chicken or marinated grilled chicken breast; char-broiled shrimp (grilled without butter).

EAT-SMART HEALTH/NATURAL: vegetable soup and 1/2 sandwich (avoid tuna/chicken salad due to mayo); "chef"-type salad (no ham) and whole grain roll; stir-fry dishes, asking for "light" on oil; marinated breast of chicken; fresh fish of the day, grilled when possible; vegetable omelet with whole-grain roll; pita stuffed with vegetables and cheese; fruit plate with plain yogurt/cottage cheese and whole-grain roll.

more than four pats of butter, and the toppings add insult to injury.

■ Salad bars can add fiber and nutrients to a meal, but it's only salad vegetables that do so. The mayonnaise-based salads, the croutons, and the bacon bits should be left on the bar, and dressing used sparingly. Use extra lemon juice or vinegar instead.

■ Frozen yogurt, although lower in fat and cholesterol than ice cream, contains more sugar—so it is not a perfectly healthy substitute. This also applies to frozen tofu desserts. Substitute one of the new sorbet-like frozen desserts that are primarily fruit. They will contain some sugar, but usually not in such high amounts.

While many unhealthy foods await you in the fast food lane, some are also available that can make eating "fast" a part of your *Smart Weigh* plan. Use this guide to help you eat smarter at the take-out counter.

BURGER KING: Although no burger is truly lean, the smaller the portion, the less fat you get. A Whopper Jr. without mayo is filling and tasty and delivers twenty-eight fewer grams of fat than the Big King. Also try the B.K. Broiler Chicken Sandwich (without dressing or mayo; try BBQ sauce for a bit of extra flavor) or Chunky Chicken Salad with reduced-calorie Italian Dressing and your own whole-grain crackers or whole-grain bread.

WENDY'S: Order a plain baked potato (without cheese sauce—get a side of chili instead as a topping). Or try the salad bar, filling up on raw vegetables rather than potato or macaroni salad, etc; use garbanzo beans or chili for protein. Other smart choices include the Jr. Hamburger (without mayonnaise), Grilled Chicken or Spicy

Chicken Filet Sandwich, Chicken Caesar Pita (without the dressing), Garden Veggie Pita (without the dressing), or Caesar Side Salad (without the dressing) topped with Grilled Chicken using reduced-fat and low-calorie Italian dressing instead of the Caesar.

MCDONALD'S: Choose the Grilled Chicken Deluxe Sandwich (try it with barbeque sauce); Grilled Chicken Salad Deluxe (with lite vinaigrette dressing and your own whole-grain crackers or bread for carbohydrate); or a small hamburger.

CHICK-FIL-A: CharGrilled Chicken Garden Salad (with no-oil salad dressing) is a smart choice, as is the CharGrilled Chicken Deluxe Sandwich without mayonnaise and the Hearty Breast of Chicken Soup with a side salad with no-oil dressing.

> **SMART WEIGH TIP**
>
> *Tackle buffets. You don't have to eat "all you can eat" because it says you can.*

TACO BELL: Order a Grilled Chicken or Grilled Steak Taco. You may also order a Bean Burrito, but it has an extra five grams of fat.

BOSTON MARKET: Don't think "safe" here, even though this spot gives a sense of healthier fast food. The best choices are the Quarter Chicken (without skin), the BBQ Chicken (without skin), or the Skinless Rotisserie Turkey Breast served with low-fat new potatoes and green beans, steamed vegetables, or zucchini marinara. The best sandwiches are the Turkey Breast Sandwich or Chicken Sandwich, both with no cheese or sauce, with fruit salad or low-fat steamed vegetables. A great main-dish soup is their Chicken Chili; have it with fruit salad.

KFC: Tender Roast Breast of Chicken without skin, with green beans or Mean Greens. Another choice is the value BBQ chicken sandwich.

ARBY'S OR RAX: Try the Rax Turkey Sandwich (without mayonnaise) or the Rax Roast Beef Sandwich (no sauce). Or try these items from Arby's lite menu: Light Grilled Chicken, Light Grilled Chicken

Salad, Light Roast Chicken Deluxe, Light Roast Chicken Salad, or Light Roast Turkey Deluxe.

SUB SHOPS OR DELIS: Get a small six-inch sub (turkey or roast beef, no oil or mayo). Subway's Roasted Chicken on whole wheat, Tuna with light mayo, Seafood and Crab with light mayo, or the Subway Club on wheat are also good choices.

PIZZA PLACES: Order the personal-size pizza, with vegetable toppings if desired. Eat only half the pizza and save the remaining half for another meal. Or, if you're sharing the pizza with others, try a thin crust cheese pizza (topped with veggies, banana peppers, or chicken, if desired—no sausage or pepperoni). One slice for women, two slices for men.

BALLPARKS AND ARENAS: You may not know about all the positive culinary changes that have taken place at the Big League ball parks and arenas. Don't worry, you can still warble "Take me out to the ball game" and "Buy me some peanuts and Cracker Jacks," but now you can add, "Buy me some veggie wraps and carrot juice." Lower-fat foods are tentatively establishing a toehold in the Majors. Some hardcore fans—guys with protruding bellies and painted faces—may stick with beer and foot-longs, but others can choose to eat from the smart parts of the food pyramid while cheering the home team.

For example, at Edison International Field, home to the Anaheim Angels, health-conscious fans can pick three-bean salad over French fries and sausage sandwiches. At the Cleveland Indians' Jacobs Field, garden burgers and turkey breast on whole-wheat compete against fried fish, chips, and pepperoni pizza.

Of course, not all ballparks are into soy burgers and granola. At the Toronto Blue Jays' SkyDome, McDonald's serves as the main food vendor. And a typical SkyDome dessert is funnel cake—deep-fried dough covered with confectioner's sugar. But for the most part, the new foods are catching on—Subway is there providing their low-fat-on-multigrain-roll subs, and salads with grilled chicken are standard. Water—even sparkling spring varieties—is sold right next to flowing beer.

Your eat-smart strategy is not to go into the stands starving and parched, but to top off the tank before you go—and go for the best choices you can while you're there.

Appetizers

Many restaurants specialize in appetizers: fried cheese; nachos; fried potato skins loaded with bacon, sour cream, and cheese; fried zuc-chini and mushrooms; those gigantic onion "blossoms." These are cardiovascular nightmares when you consider that two potato skins or two pieces of fried cheese are basically the fat calories of a whole meal (and should be used as such). Many restaurants are offering raw vegetable plat-

> **EAT-SMART APPETIZERS:** chicken burritos or fajitas; grilled seafood; marinated chicken breast; non-creamed soup.

ters, but the dip will negate the value of the veggies. If you indulge, do so very carefully.

Breakfast

Breakfast can be a special meal out because most restaurants offer safe and easy choices. If breakfast is later than normal, energize with a snack when you arise, then the later meal. You also may choose to have your larger lunch portions for breakfast and a smaller lunch three to four hours later. Follow these guidelines in ordering:

- Order whole wheat toast or grits unbut-tered; then add one teaspoon of butter, if desired.

> **EAT-SMART BREAKFAST:** Eggs scrambled (without fat), or egg substitute, and whole wheat toast or English muffin; French toast (with whole wheat bread) and berries; fresh vegetable and egg-white omelet and toast; whole-grain cereal with skim milk and fruit; Fresh fruit bowl with cot-tage cheese and whole wheat toast.

- Ordering à la carte is usually safer so that you are not tempted by the abundance of food in the "breakfast specials" or buffets.
- Be bold and creative in ordering. Rather than accepting French toast with syrup and bacon, ask for it prepared with whole wheat bread, no syrup, and a side of fresh berries or fruit instead. Some restaurants will substitute cottage cheese or one egg for the meat. Many also serve oatmeal and cereal even though it's not always on the menu. It's a nice carbohydrate with milk and fresh fruit, especially strawberries or blueberries.
- Always look for a protein and a carbohydrate source. A Danish doesn't do it!

SMART WEIGH SNACKS

Your best eat-smart snack strategy is to keep wisely prepared power snacks wherever you are. Human nature is such that if the right food isn't available, we're apt to reach for the wrong thing—or push through on fumes with no fuel at all. Instead, keep power snacks in your desk drawer, briefcase, or suitcase (refer to the power snack suggestions on page 125).

If the best-laid plans fail and you find yourself face-to-face with the vending machine, wondering which buttons to push, think of this chart below—and go for the tasty, easy-to-find, low-fat yet high-voltage alternatives to all your favorite "sure-to-burn-out-quick" treats.

TRAVELING THE SMART WEIGH

Traveling is stressful and depleting in the best of times—even if you're on your way to a week in the sunny Caribbean. And for the road warrior—the one who does business "by air"—there seems to be no end to travel. While your friends and neighbors might think your job is glamorous, we both know traveling is exhausting. It's not unusual to arrive at your destination dehydrated, drained, and disoriented—surely unfit to be productive or even to have fun. This is especially the case when traveling by air.

Flying causes anxiety. So does rushing to the airport at the last minute, unloading those bags, and lugging that briefcase. Try to arrive at the airport with enough time to relax for a few minutes. Give yourself (and the ticket counter staff) adequate time to get you checked in and your luggage safely on board.

EAT-SMART IDEAS: INSTEAD OF...	CHOOSE...
Snickers bar (280 calories/14 grams fat/6 grams protein)	Crisp apple, mozzarella string cheese (115 calories/ 4 grams fat/ 7 grams protein)
1.74 ounces bag peanut M & M's (250 calories/13 grams fat/5 grams protein)	2 whole-wheat Wasa crisp breads with 8 ounces Stonyfield Farm nonfat yogurt (270 calories/1 gram fat/12 grams protein)
60 Ruffles potato chips (560 calories/35 grams fat/7 grams protein)	24 Baked Lays potato crisps, 1 ounces part-skim cheddar cheese (300 calories/6 grams fat/11 grams protein)
16 ounces Coca-Cola Classic, 6 Ritz crackers (299 calories/5 grams fat/2 grams protein)	Bottle of water; turkey sandwich with 1 slice bread, 1/4-pound turkey, lettuce, tomato, mustard (214 calories, 5 grams fat/24 grams protein)
4 cups microwave popcorn, 1 bottle Snapple Iced Tea (240 calories/7 grams fat/3 grams protein)	4 cups light microwave popcorn, tall Starbucks Frappuccino (248 calories/4 grams fat/6 grams protein)
1 jelly doughnut (220 calories/9 grams fat/4 grams protein)	1/2 whole-grain bagel with 2 tbsp light cream cheese, 1 teaspoons all fruit jam (141 calories, 4 grams fat, 8 grams protein)
Wendy's medium Frosty (440 calories/11 grams fat/11 grams protein)	1/2 cup vanilla yogurt and fresh berries sprinkled with 1/4 cup low-fat granola (205 calories/1 gram fat/6 grams protein)

Use these tips to help keep you in tip-top shape for the rest of the trip: energized, strong, and healthy.

Drink Up

Water, that is. Flying is dehydrating; the pressurized cabin air is ten times more arid than the desert, causing you to lose fluid through your skin. This leads to puffy hands and ankles, fatigue, and a bloated feeling. So drink lots of water—the suggested 8 glasses a day plus an additional 8 to 12 ounces for each hour in the air. And limit your consumption of alcohol on planes; it is a major dehydrator and has more impact in the air than on the ground. Hint: When the flight attendant asks what you want to drink, ask for water.

Jet Fuel for Jet Travel

Whether a business traveler or a vacationer, you want to be bright-eyed when you arrive at your destination. So don't forget to maintain good nutrition while you're traveling. To short-circuit the stress sequence that accompanies you on your trip, eat adequate pre-flight complex carbs (some whole-wheat bread, cereal, or a banana) with low-fat proteins. Moderate your intake of refined carbohydrates and sugars before and during the trip. Eat more protein and low-fat fare (low-fat dairy products, grilled meats, eggs) to boost your alertness.

On travel days, try not to go more than three hours without a healthy meal or snack. Carry a few convenient power snacks (like trail mix or dried fruit with Laughing Cow Lite Wedges) in your briefcase or purse. While everybody else is eating salted peanuts, you'll be stoking your own furnace with protein and good calories.

Pack some power snacks to keep you on track once you arrive at your destination, too. Eating on some kind of an even schedule will necessitate having your own power snacks available—enabling you to eat the right foods at the right time regardless of where you find yourself during the day. Power snacks will help you accomplish "smart eating on the move" and will keep your stressed and lagging metabolism burning high. Pack foods that don't need refrigeration, such as the trail mix or dried fruits and cheese mentioned above. I take along boxed milk as well.

Airport and airline food can do real damage to your energy and your plan to eat *The Smart Weigh*. Stay away from caffeine in colas and coffee, and don't get trapped by the high-fat, spicy, and sweet foods throughout the airport. Generally it's wise to order a special meal for air travel (give your airline twenty-four hours' notice). Diabetic meals are highest in protein, fiber, and freshness, and you can enjoy them at no extra cost.

Car Travel

When you drive to your destination, don't be seduced into stopping at the first fast food restaurant or stockpiling a bunch of high-fat, high-sugar snacks when you stop for gas. Surprise everyone—maybe even yourself—by bringing along a bag of healthy snacks. Also make brief stops to stretch, exercise, and breath deeply so you arrive relaxed rather than stiff and bloated.

Rub in Relaxation

During the trip, put your fingers to your shoulder muscles or temple, and massage. If it hurts, it probably means your muscles are tight. If you're flying, use some of the flight time to relax your muscles and to breathe deeply. You'll arrive at your destination that much more rested. If you are at an exit row or by the aisle, use the space to stretch your legs and do some ankle rotations.

Stay in Shape

How many times have you packed your workout clothes but never made it to the hotel's spa or gym? What about those times you attended a conference at a beachfront hotel or golf course, but you never set foot outside the doors once the meetings started? At the very least, plan on a brisk walk each day during your stay, and make time to use the pool or exercise room. You'll be surprised how changing into workout clothes, taking a walk, and breathing deeply will recharge you for the next event or meeting.

Even if you're sightseeing, and are beat from all the walking, you'll still receive an energy and metabolic boost from a focused ten-minute walk that doesn't have you stopping for traffic or great buys.

Give Yourself a Break

Resist the temptation to schedule every moment with activities and people. Leave some quiet time in which to be recharged and revitalized without interruptions. Just a ten-minute time-out—even a power nap—in the middle of your day can restore your alertness and enhance performance.

Finally, Sleep

Road warriors probably know the inside of hotels better than their travel agents. Though there is nothing like your own bed, try to get the same number of hours of sleep at the hotel as you usually get at home. If there's room in your luggage, packing your own pillow will give you a better chance of good shut-eye. And don't use that room minibar for a nightcap as you unwind at day's end. Watch out for those chocolate mints and sweet amenities hotels like to give as your good-night kiss, too.

TIME ZONE BLUES

Jet lag is more than just a sense of being tired; it is an actual discrepancy in the body's intrinsic biological sleep cycle, or "circadian rhythm." Your body's sleep cycle is controlled by the daily alternating sunlight and darkness patterns you experience. When you travel to a new time zone, your circadian rhythm remains on its original biological schedule for several days—so your body's internal clock and the external clock are saying two different things. Your body is telling you to sleep in the middle of the afternoon or turn on in the middle of the night.

Symptoms of time zone blues are fatigue, insomnia, headaches, indigestion, disorientation, and metabolic slowdown—adding up to a serious drain on your enjoyment—not to mention your body's natural ability to process the food you eat efficiently.

Here are some anti-jet lag tips to help reduce the strain:

- Get plenty of sleep during the days and weeks before traveling across time zones, or when daylight-saving time begins (the first Sunday in April) and ends (the last Sunday in October). Starting your trip fully rested will ease the transition.

  Change your bedtime three nights before you depart. If you're traveling west, go to bed one hour later for each time zone difference you experience (up to three hours). If you're traveling east, do the opposite: start going to bed one hour earlier for each time zone (again, up to three hours). Limit your intake of stimulants such as caffeine and alcohol, particularly three hours before you plan to go to bed.

- Get into the day/night cycle of the time zone you're going to as quickly as possible after you arrive. Don't hide in dark museums or hotel rooms upon arrival at your destination—

stay out in the daylight. Light acts as a powerful cue to your body, telling your internal clock where you are and what schedule to keep. So does exercise. When you fly east, attempt to exercise at least thirty minutes in the morning sun. When you fly west, attempt to exercise at least thirty minutes in the late afternoon sun.

This is one time to resist napping; instead try to keep moving during the day and go to bed in the evening.

■ Be careful with sleep medications; they don't resolve the biological imbalance caused by jet lag. Melatonin supplements *can* be used to correct circadian disorders, but don't take this hormone without first consulting a doctor, and definitely not for long periods of time. Other than occasional use as an anti-jet lag measure, melatonin taken at the wrong time or in high doses can *cause* sleepiness, sleep disturbance, and impaired work or driving performance—and it may actually shift circadian rhythms in the wrong direction. Moreover, since the Food and Drug Administration doesn't regulate melatonin and other "dietary supplements" for safety and efficacy, there are no standards for purity or dosages.

Don't be discouraged and think you can't ever eat out or travel healthfully. You can have healthy meals away from home; it's just a matter of learning to make good choices. The trick is to learn what you *can* eat, and then follow through. Rather than feeling dismayed or overwhelmed about everything on a menu that doesn't fit into eating *The Smart Weigh*, use your creativity and knowledge to find good things that do.

PART FIVE ■ **LIVING FREE FROM THE TRAP**

CHAPTER 15 ■ Kicking the Habit: Sugar and Caffeine

The man who believes he can do something is probably right, and so is the man who believes he can't.

—ANONYMOUS

Mary had been counseling with me for seven months when her birthday rolled around. Although rejoicing in her new healthy life (and a weight loss of over forty pounds), she was now gripped with fear that birthday treats would sabotage all the progress she'd made.

"Honestly, Pam," Mary confided, "I feel like an addict—and my drug of choice has always been sweets. It may start as just a little piece of birthday cake, but it's a bowl of Haagen-Dazs before I go to bed. And, history has shown that

> **SMART WEIGH TIP**
>
> *Don't deprive yourself. There is no forbidden food, just some you may choose not to have.*

once I've started, it doesn't stop. I just *have* to do it differently this year."

Mary's experience is a familiar one. Sweets do taste great, but for many the pull is much stronger than a taste bud tickle. The craving for sugar takes on an unnatural drive.

One of the biggest blunders we make in eating isn't about eating at all. It's about depending on food for a chemical brain boost to get us through the rough times when energy is low and we're being dealt some bad cards. The two prime examples of substances we give too much power to are sugar and caffeine. Let's take a look at breaking their grip.

OUT OF THE SUGAR TRAP

A heavy sugar intake brings a pleasurable rise in feel-good brain chemicals that will be followed by a quick fall a few hours later. That dip often triggers "eating for a lift" to relieve the fatigue, brain fog, and mood drop. Usually the chosen food is again high in sugar, and the seesaw effect continues. Then the guilt tapes begin to play: *You've already blown it, so go ahead and finish the cookies before you get "back" to healthy eating.* And the more you eat, the more you crave, trying to get that same boost.

Equalizing your brain chemistries is a key to living *The Smart Weigh* because too-low levels of serotonin and endorphins trigger the craving for a drug that will provide fuel for these neurotransmitters. Not everyone is as sugar sensitive as Mary—not everyone turns a bite of chocolate into an addictive drug. But there is evidence that some people use sweet foods and refined carbohydrates as powerful mood-altering drugs—and experience the similar roller-coaster of behavior and thoughts of an addict.

People without such an inflammatory chemical response will experience a pleasurable feeling from the rise in brain chemicals that follows eating refined carbohydrates and sweets. But people with a heightened sensitivity will experience a powerful euphoria—not just feeling good, but feeling *great.* These people can be trapped in a vicious cycle of highs and lows controlled by soaring and plummeting body chemistries. Even those who violently oppose drinking or the use of street drugs can get on a different addiction—sugar, ice cream, chocolate, and soda. And the dependency can be just as strong. In fact, if you have used alcohol or drugs in an addictive way some time in your life, it's very likely that your body's chemistry responds more intensely to these chemicals than other people's. This body chemistry doesn't change in sobriety from, say, alcohol; it often just finds another "drug of choice"—and that is often sweets.

The amount of sugar added to foods eaten by an average American in one day? Nineteen teaspoons, or 304 calories. That includes sugars added by manufacturers to foods like soda, flavored yogurts, and cookies—as well as those added directly by the consumer, such as to iced tea or cereals. The amount of weight you'll lose in one year if you cut that added sugar in half? Sixteen pounds for an average adult.

If sugar is affecting your well-being, make it your goal to cut back on your daily use of sweets and other refined carbs and eat whole carbohydrates and fruits to stabilize your body chemistries and satisfy your natural craving for sugar. Sweets are not worth robbing yourself of your precious energy and stamina.

For help in kicking the sugar habit, use these tips:

KNOW YOUR ENEMY. Sugar is called by many names—honey, brown sugar, corn syrup, fructose, and so on—but it's all sugar. Much of our problem with sugar lies in the fact that it is hidden in nearly every packaged product on the grocer's shelf. American consumption has risen to 146 pounds per person per year, mainly from prepared foods.

Beware if sugar, or another name for sugar (like any word ending in –ose), is in the top three ingredients in a packaged product. If it is, you're getting more than you're bargaining for. Also realize that sugar is hidden in refined carbohydrates that have been stripped of their fibers and nutrients, giving a quick "rush" into your bloodstream, followed by a rush of feel-good chemicals from your brain. No wonder it can seem to have such power.

KNOW YOURSELF. How much is enough for you—and how much triggers the desire for more? Does nibbling a little bit of sweets lead to a lot? Mary found that even occasionally eating high-sugar foods was difficult for her—she *was* hurt by "just a little bit." It wasn't about the calories or sugar's health risk, it was the effect it had on her body. The seesaw effect resulted in a "more she has, more she wants" syndrome.

If this sounds familiar, it may be necessary for you to "just say no" to sugar-laden foods for long enough (twelve to fourteen days) to allow your blood sugar and brain chemical levels to stabilize, and to allow your energy and appetite for healthy foods to return. Only then can you assess the impact sweets can have on your body—and on your resolve.

KNOW THAT WITHDRAWAL IS REAL. If you are sugar sensitive, you are apt to experience physical symptoms of drug-deprivation. You may feel shaky, nauseous, edgy, or experience headaches or diarrhea.

As you embark on any healthy lifestyle change—especially as chemically impacting as pulling back from a high intake of sugar— your body needs time to adjust physiologically and emotionally. It will take at least five to six days before the change begins to feel comfortable physically. You can expect the following:

> **DAY 1 AND 2:** You may feel slightly sluggish, irritable, and dissatisfied with your eating.
>
> **DAY 3:** This will be one of your most difficult days as your body begins to feel the chemical change. It may seem that every cell in your body is crying out for food, particularly something sweet. But the urge for sweets is not impossible to overcome.

DAY 4: If you make it through the third day without overeating or homicide, this one won't be so difficult.

DAY 5: This may be a day of a ravenous appetite; you can expect to be hungry for food—not sweets necessarily, just food. You can eat a full meal and still think: *That was a good appetizer—what else is there to eat?*

DAY 6 AND 7: By now it should be getting easier and easier; you have more energy, and you have more control over your appetite. You are now on the road to a lifetime of good eating. The surprise of feeling good makes it all worth the effort.

I know these symptoms may sound more like withdrawal from hard drugs than simply allowing your body to adjust to a wonderfully healthy way of eating. But let's face reality: putting in healthy foods means leaving out the unhealthy, and that means a chemical change—a withdrawal of sorts. If you recognize that the chemical changes are necessary, but temporary, it will be easier for you to break through to a lifetime of good eating.

KNOW WHEN YOU'RE VULNERABLE. Identify—and avoid—resolve-breakers like fatigue, hunger, anger, or loneliness. If you need something when you're tired, to "get through," break for a nap even if it is more difficult rather than reaching for the cookies. If you have spent a lifetime pushing down anger with food you should switch to the more difficult but healthier choice—write away your anger in a journal or discuss its cause with someone.

KNOW THE DRILL. Resist the "I've Already Blown It" Syndrome. Even when you succumb to temptation and consume foods you know interfere with your health, be assured that a lapse in healthy eating doesn't ruin all the health you have attained over weeks of wellness.

A lapse is just that—a lapse. Don't let it become a relapse, another relapse, and finally a collapse. Look at each meal and snack as an event—don't wrap it all into one bad day or one unhealthy weekend. Instead, get right back on track with the next meal or snack. Your body will stabilize quickly, you'll feel great, and you'll be thanking yourself the next day.

KNOW THAT IT WILL GET EASIER. Although we are born with a natural preference toward foods with a sweet taste, these preferences have been overdeveloped and fueled by a lifetime of high sugar intake and erratic eating patterns. As you cut back, over time, your cravings diminish and your taste buds regain their ability to pick up the sweetness in a carrot or piece of fruit.

"POWER SNACK" THROUGHOUT THE DAY. Just in case it hasn't sunk in yet: eating every two to three hours throughout the day keeps your energy okay and a ravenous appetite away. Go for energy-boosting combos like fresh fruit or a box of raisins with low-fat cheese or yogurt, a half sandwich, or a trail mix of dry roasted peanuts and sunflower seeds mixed with dried fruit. Keep power snacks available wherever you are—they will serve as a lift to your body and prevent the drowsiness and sweet cravings that often follow meals.

RELY ON THE NATURAL SWEET TREAT. Fruit naturally fulfills our sweet desires. And remember to go for the fruit, not the fruit juice; the fiber slows the release of the fruit's simple carbohydrate, which prevents blood sugar spikes and insulin surges.

CONSUME ENOUGH FIBER. Remember that water-soluble fibers—found in oats, barley, brown rice, apples, dried beans, and nuts—serve as a "time-release capsule," releasing sugars from digested carbohydrates slowly and evenly into the bloodstream. This helps keep your energy levels up and even and your cravings down.

SAVE THE BEST FOR LAST. If you do have sweets, add a dessert to the end of the meal rather than having the treat *as* your meal, or your snack. This allows the balanced meal to temper the insulin surge, keeping blood sugars more stable.

WHAT ABOUT ARTIFICIAL SWEETENERS?

As you become aware (and possibly alarmed) about your intake of sugar, you may be tempted to use sugar substitutes. Don't. There are no absolutes in the safety of chemicals—saccharin, aspartame, or any new one to come along. The long-term effects of their use will not be known for years.

For example, in the short time since aspartame has appeared on the market (as Nutrasweet), cautions concerning its use have accelerated. Questions have been posed about its allergic reaction in some; its impact on brain chemistry due to its crossing the blood barrier of the brain; its danger with possible breakdown in hot foods; its effect on children and the unborn; and it's connection to the rise in brain tumor incidence. The verdict is not in.

And the battle will continue, for even though aspartame is made from natural sources, it is still made in a laboratory and is not found in nature. The possibility that problems might occur from frequent use is real, as, for example, hindering the brain's formation of serotonin, causing the let-down that follows an aspartame intake to bring anxiety and depression—and an increased appetite.

Also consider that aspartame is made from phenylalanine, which is an amino acid. High doses of a single amino acid can throw off the balance of amino acids in your brain and body. Because phenylalanine is a precursor to dopamine and norepinephrine, which are stimulating neurotransmitters, high usage of aspartame can create a "speed-like" effect. There is also concern about aspartame's potential to keep insulin levels elevated, thereby heightening the risk of disease and adding to the obesity problem. Remember, foods alone don't make insulin rise; just the sight, smell, and taste of food can do it. But, in the case of artificially sweetened beverages, there are no calories for the insulin to work with—so the blood sugar level drops, stimulating hunger.

Finally, understand that as long as you continue to use sugar-laden foods or sugar substitutes, you will keep your taste buds trained for sugar. The goal is to cut back on its use so you no longer need everything to taste sweet. Allow your taste buds to change so that the desire for sweetness can be met in a safe way—from fruits and other naturally sweet foods.

TAKING BACK YOUR POWER

As important as it was for Mary to come to understand the chemical power of sweets, it was also crucial that she identify the emotional war going on within her related to food—particularly sweets. Because, for Mary, the trap was two-pronged: physical and emotional.

Her personal war was rooted in her chemical sensitivity and physical reaction to the foods she ate, as well as in the powerful emotional charge she had placed on food. Breaking free of its grip was going to take more than just a diet, more than just an attitude change. It meant shining light on the real issues: the need to stabilize body chemistries for physical stability, along with demystifying the emotional charge food can have. You'll read more about making peace with food in Chapter 18.

Mary made both of these moves toward freedom, and she was ultimately able to take back the power she had given to sweets, looking at a dessert as just what it was—food. And, yes, she did have a piece of birthday cake at her party. She enjoyed it for the moment but was surprised at how sickeningly sweet it was. She was also surprised at how great it made her feel—almost elated. But it didn't set her up to eat the whole cake—nor to finish it off with a pint of ice cream—because she was now alerted to the drop that would inevitably follow. Sugar no longer had power over her.

How about you? Do you have a sweet that seems to call your name? If chocolate is your sugar seductress, you may be hooked on more than the sugar alone. In addition to the chemical impact of chocolate on the brain's neurotransmitters (research shows it to release similar substances as those released in romantic love), chocolate packs a one-two punch with a double hit of sugar *and* caffeine. Not so different from that double mocha-cappucino that may woo you at midafternoon. Or maybe it's that caffeine/aspartame-pumped diet soda—the equivalent of rocket fuel to many.

ARE YOU A JAVA JUNKIE?

Caffeine is among the world's most widely used and addictive drugs. Ironically, caffeine remains a relatively acceptable way of artificially stimulating the brain at a time when society is being exhorted to "Just Say No" to drugs.

> **SMART WEIGH TIP**
>
> *It's not the Last Supper. This is not your last chance in life to have a particular food.*

Caffeine works to keep you alert by blocking one of the brain's natural sedatives, a neurotransmitter called adenosine. It stimulates the central nervous system, increases your pulse rate and heartbeat, and can even give quite a boost to your mood. A single cup of coffee can seem to work energy miracles when needed—even helping athletes to push a little farther. All in all, it's powerful stuff.

But, like other drugs, there is a downside to caffeine: too much causes a surge of adrenaline. But when the spurt is over, power levels plummet and stress hormones are produced. Even small amounts of caffeine may cause side effects, including restlessness and disturbed sleep, heart palpitations, stomach irritation, fibrocystic breast disease, and diarrhea. It can promote irritability, anxiety, and mood disturbances. Caffeine can also aggravate premenstrual syndrome and mood swings in women. And studies have shown that the stress hormones still circulate, elevating blood pressure, up to eight hours after the last caffeine hit. And those stress hormones play a key role in fat cell lock-down.

The stimulant effect is thought to kick in with consumption of 150 to 250 mg of caffeine—the amount in one mug of brewed coffee or three glasses of iced tea. And because caffeine is also found in soda (regular and diet), chocolate, and even decongestant cold pills, it adds up quickly. The levels soar when you get java from a gourmet coffee shop. New analysis shows that these specialty brews can contain two to three times the caffeine found in a cup made from your typical supermarket brands. These specialty coffees are stronger because more grounds are used to give the brew its rich flavor and the beans are often roasted, making the coffee even more potent. In fact, one large cup of specialty coffee packs a walloping 280 mg of caffeine, and some have been found to contain 550 mg. It's at these higher levels of intake, about 600 mg, that you can get too energized and start to feel the java jitters: frazzled nerves, the shakes, insomnia, and ultimately, fatigue.

Do you need to cut out caffeine altogether? Not necessarily. Despite its drawbacks, it's definitely an energy boost. My concern is when caffeine becomes your very best friend. I do encourage you to cut back slowly to a ceiling of 250 mg. And if, after cutting back to this amount, you still experience any of the above-mentioned effects, I would suggest withdrawing altogether. You'll also get more of an energy boost from the caffeine you do consume if you have cut back on your intake.

Pain is the word that best characterizes cutting back on caffeine consumption, and that is why you must do so gradually. Again, caffeine is a powerfully addictive drug that will bring withdrawal symptoms as you give it up. Many people experience zombie-like fatigue, irritability, lethargy, and headaches from going "cold turkey," and the symptoms may last for up to five days. They expect to feel better by nobly giving up espresso, but end up feeling horrible instead. Then they drag back to caffeine saying this "healthy thing" just didn't work for them.

Let me tell you about Greg. He is an on-site supervisor for a large development company. He is on the job at 5:30 every morning, and his breakfast used to be a Big Gulp of coffee (that's right, 64 ounce of java). He'd get the crews started and check in at the office by 8:00 AM, then stop for a refill of coffee on the way (another 64 ounce)—and then again on the way back to the job site. In the afternoon, he switched to diet Mountain Dew for his jet-fuel.

Then Greg came to the first session of my *Smart Weigh* series, recommended by his physician to get control of his increasing blood pressure and high cholesterol levels. He listened, targeted the caffeine as his problem, and quit. Cold turkey. He went to the ER three days later thinking he had spinal meningitis because he had an immobilizing headache and felt paralyzed with flu-like fatigue.

Even if you don't drink as much caffeine as Greg, don't put your body through what Greg did. Cut back *slowly* over the course of a week to ten days. Start by cutting back to a safer level of two cups of coffee or three cups of tea. Gradually cut back, a quarter of a cup at a time, until you are down to none. Or substitute a decaffeinated product for the real thing in the same reducing amounts. Withdrawal will be less painful if you follow *The Smart Weigh* meal plan. Eating small, balanced meals throughout the day will stabilize your body chemistries and reduce your reliance on caffeine for energy. And, if you focus on drinking more water than you have in the past, you won't have room for the other beverages. In addition, try to get outdoor exercise every day to get a boost of feel-good endorphins.

Finally, whether it's a mindset you want to break, or the grip of sugar or caffeine, don't set up any food as a forbidden fruit. As Mary learned, there are no good or bad foods; there is no such thing as a legal or a cheat food. Food is simply food. The power it lords over us is the problem. While it's important to assess the physiological power eating may have over our body chemistries and develop a better plan, setting our focus on what we shouldn't do and what we shouldn't eat only sets us up for failure.

A mind filled with worry can fall into the negative—attracting the very thing we are most worried about. Chronic worry can become toxic to us due to the resulting brain chemical surges that ravage the body—hindering the immune system, slowing the metabolism, and affecting our mood. These chemical surges can also take on a life of their own—wreaking havoc with our whole body chemistry and hormonal status. Negative thoughts can spin into a tornado, swallowing us up in an immobilizing state of imbalance called depression. All affect our ability to take charge of our weight.

CHAPTER 16 ■ Energy Drains: Worry, Depression, and Hormones

My problem is not the problem, my problem is my attitude about the problem.

—ANONYMOUS

If you've ever spent hours mentally replaying a conversation or ruined a weekend because you couldn't quite stop fretting about work, you have a glimpse of how much energy chronic worry can drain. Worry is not a passive pursuit; it requires energy and will result in the body slowing down metabolically to conserve—locking into the fat storage mode.

Some worry may actually be good for us, such as concern about our safety and the safety of our family. Some degree of stress and worry can keep us on our toes and boost performance. But when worry takes on a life of its own it can become toxic, obsessive, and chronic.

> **SMART WEIGH TIP**
>
> *Stop worrying. Remind yourself that you only have control over you. If you can't do anything about it, just let it go.*

It's crucial to discern between good worry and draining worry, and to take action—always the positive response to stress. When there is no action to be taken, then continuing to worry is nothing more than spinning wheels. It becomes as self-destructive as nail-biting or smoking, and wears you down, without bringing you any closer to solving the issues that cause it.

To stop your internal wheels from spinning out of control and into obsession, try these quick fixes for your fixations:

CALM YOURSELF. Sit quietly in a comfortable position, eyes closed. Choose an empowering thought, phrase, or word that is rooted in your faith. These are some of my favorites: *I can do all things through God who gives me strength. I am more than a conqueror through Him. Be still, and know that I am God.* Then breathe naturally, and as you do, repeat the affirmation silently as you exhale. When other thoughts come into your mind, push them out by returning to your affirmation. Continue for ten to twenty minutes, as your schedule allows. You may feel better after just one session. Most people get the most benefit from such a calming time if they make room for it at least once a day.

LISTEN TO YOURSELF. Whenever you feel depressed, overtaken by food cravings, or exhausted, you need to stop, take a few slow, deep breaths, and consider what you're thinking or telling yourself. You may find that your internal voice is yakking away about how bad things are going, and how you'll never get this done, and you'll never do it right. You may be feeding yourself irrational drivel that is making you feel worse—or even making you sick. By simply acknowledging that your mind is filled with too much busybody thought, you can start slowing it down and cleaning it out.

SET ASIDE DESIGNATED WORRY TIME. To ward off that free-floating sense of doom, schedule an hour after work—on the ride home, in the tub—to sort out your anxieties. (Bedtime is NOT the time.) For particularly nagging problems, it can be helpful to write in a journal or talk with an understanding friend. If you start worrying during the day, resolve to hold off until your "obsession session." Whatever you do, don't let worries play over and over again in your mind, like a broken record. Instead vent them—get them out.

Inside your head, you constantly work over the content. Outside your head, you can look at it more realistically—and that's vital to both your emotional *and* physical well-being.

GIVE YOURSELF A REALITY CHECK. If you're dreading an upcoming event, consider the absolute worst-case scenario. (*If I do this exactly right, I still won't do it up to the standard of perfection and I'm going to be fired and I'll never be able to get a job again!*) Sometimes when you ask the question, "What's the absolutely worst thing that can happen," you realize that it probably won't. Remind yourself that, even if disaster were to strike, you would and could survive. Then, try to assemble *real* assessments of what is likely to happen. (*My boss may tell me I need to make a few minor changes before sending this report out.*) Tell yourself, "I can handle it." Reining in your runaway thoughts and replacing them with reality will diminish the negative chatter—and you will relax and release it.

IDENTIFY "STINKING THINKING." When you feel overcome by stressful thoughts, recognize that you need to calm down by saying something gentle to yourself like "Oh, there I go again." Just the admission tells you that the stress is from within, from your own thinking, not just the outside world. When you can, write down the thoughts that are bothering you. Then identify the mistakes in your thought patterns. These are the most common:

> **PERFECTIONISM.** Everything must be perfect; everything you do must be right and correct every time.
>
> **AWFULIZING OR CATASTROPHIZING.:** Assuming the worst, that a certain event or happening will be horrible.
>
> **GENERALIZING.** The holidays were bad last year, and they'll be bad every year.

Replace your draining, "stinking thinking" with a positive outlook. If you're worrying about a party you have to go to, then replace, say, the fear of overeating with excitement about the people you will be seeing. Write down, "I'll be happy to see so and so, and I'll spend a lot of time talking to them."

TRY CLASSIC THOUGHT-STOPPING TECHNIQUES. To banish an unwanted thought the moment it occurs, speak to it: say, STOP! Or, wear a rubberband on your wrist and snap it to snap you out of the obsessing moment. Practice the breathing you learned in Chapter 8: inhale slowly through your nose, expanding your diaphragm; hold a moment, then focus on exhaling through your mouth as fully as you can. Taking deep breaths from the abdomen will calm you, and help you to ease out of the panic mode.

DON'T TRY TO CONTROL EVERYTHING. If you have a tendency to obsess, chances are good that you're also a perfectionist. Realize that going over something again and again will not magically produce the "right" answer or perfect solution. More important, accept that you don't always have the power—or the responsibility—to make everything flawless or everyone happy. Some things that weigh you down are way beyond your control or power to change; others just aren't worth the worry. Be more selective about the things you allow to rent space in your mind. Remember, *you* pay the rent with your well-being.

Do look for opportunities to seize what control you can. You may not be able to avoid eating on an airplane, but you can call ahead and order a special meal that tastes better and is better for you.

ZAP YOUR NEGATIVE THINKING WITH POSITIVE ACTION. Instead of staring at your credit-card bill in despair, make an appointment with a financial counselor. Instead of dwelling on how much you hate your job, work on your resume. Instead of agonizing that you may have offended a friend, call her, talk to her about it. Call it "obsession rehab": you replace a virtual addiction to certain fears with productive, restorative activity.

GET MOVING. Because it burns off anxiety-causing adrenaline and allows the blessed release of endorphins, exercise is a sure bet to change your emotional and mental state, right along with the physical. Even a quick walk around the office will help you walk away from your worries.

GET INVOLVED. When you're self-absorbed, you're much more prone to worry. When you strike a good balance of investing in yourself and being involved with others, it brings richness to your life. Trouble in one part doesn't overtake or overcome you because there's much more to life than that one area.

GET HELP. This is critical when you're miserable. If exhaustive and self-abusive worrying persists, seek out a trusted friend, pastor, or a counselor to talk to. Your energy levels and your quality of life are much too precious to be neutralized by worry. Obsessive worry can sometimes spin out of control, and spin you right into a depression of a mountainous sort. You'll need help to find your way down.

OUR EVER-CHANGING MOODS

Mood colors everything we do: what we eat, what we wear, whether we'll make love with our spouse tonight or end up in a disagreement. We all know what it is to be in a great mood: we feel strong and energetic and have a good self-image. We love, we're lovely, our potential is unlimited, and life is bathed in light.

Bad moods are also easy to identify. We're "off," drained of energy, overwhelmed, and irritable. Bad moods hit us all—only 2 percent of us report feeling cheerful every day. Most of us swing in and out of bad moods fairly regularly and predictably. Polls show that the average person spends about three days out of ten trying to lift up and over a bad mood.

As we discussed while looking at the factors involved in equalizing your brain chemistry, your moods probably have more rhyme and rhythm than you realize. They are most often based on natural biological patterns and chemical changes from lifestyle and food choices you make throughout the day. You may blame your funk on the day's frustrations, but chances are it's more related to your daily rises and falls of stress chemicals. Becoming a keen observer of your moods will help you to track them and influence them for the better.

But there are times when a bad mood is more than the blues—it's depression, and it's tough to shake. When you're depressed, you feel out of control, hate yourself, hate life, hate the people in your life, feel hopeless and overwhelmed. Everything is dark and grim.

Because a positive mental attitude is so crucial to living *The Smart Weigh*, and a bright, hopeful perspective is necessary to make the lifestyle upgrades that can lead to vitality, I address the possibility of depression with every one of my clients—particularly those battling overeating and a dependence upon food, sugar, or caffeine.

BEWARE THE DOWNWARD SPIRAL

Depression is both a physical and mental condition marked by sadness, hopelessness, and fatigue. It's a monster of a disorder that causes the entire body to slow down, pulling you down and back from life.

Depression can have many triggers—both internal and external. Internal triggers include brain chemical imbalances, hormonal changes, nutritional deficiencies, or illness. Depression may be caused by certain high blood pressure medications, birth control pills, and the hormonal changes that come with menstruation, menopause, childbirth, or breastfeeding cessation. Depression can also be externally triggered by any loss and its resulting grief. The death of a loved one, financial problems, or life changes such as a move, job loss, children leaving home, or divorce can send you into a downward spiral.

Even the healthiest grieving includes a period of depression, but sometimes losses are compounded or intensified in such a way that you can't resolve them—and you get stuck in the depression. You can also get stuck if you don't give yourself permission to grieve—believing that you are somehow showing weakness or ungratefulness if you give in too much to your sadness. The more you stuff your natural, authentic feelings, the more depressed you get. The converse is also true: the more you allow yourself to grieve, the more rapidly you recover from the loss.

It's not just unprocessed grief that can result in depression. For example, anger that is not released in healthy ways can dam up within you and become depression. This is why depression is often described as "frozen emotion" or "anger turned inward."

When a person gets sucked into a downward spiral, the blues can rapidly progress into clinical depression. The body stuck in depression loses the capability to produce the brain chemicals (neurotransmitters) that fight dark perspectives. Clinical depression is accompanied by several telltale symptoms, including profound sadness; a loss of interest in things once enjoyed; feelings of worthlessness and hopelessness; anxiety; changes in appetite (usually resulting in significant weight loss or gain); sleep disturbances; digestive problems; problems concentrating, thinking, remembering, or making decisions; and recurring thoughts of death or suicide.

Depression is known to exacerbate a range of medical conditions because it is associated with poor compliance to recommended treatment. But it does more than get people off balance emotionally and off track with self-care; it actually affects them *physiologically.* For example, in people with diabetes, depression has also been shown to trigger an adverse physiological response, driving up their blood-glucose levels. How it does this is not yet properly understood; but the theory is that depression alters levels of the hormone cortisol, which can worsen insulin resistance and compromise the immune system, leading to heart disease and other killer diseases. Whether or not this occurs in the normal population without diabetes has not been confirmed through research.

If overeating and poor self-care is rooted in depression, a professional evaluation is critical. Antidepressant medication, often necessary to correct and replenish brain chemistry gone awry, can often avert serious depression—saving lives, families, marriages, and careers. But antidepressant therapy alone is rarely enough to stabilize the body's chemistries for life—it's just a jump start. The long-term answer for depression-related overeating and fatigue comes through getting help to deal effectively with life and hurts, along with embracing a lifestyle of self-care and expressing emotion. A professional evaluation can identify where the real problems are, and help to determine when depression is as much a physical problem as a chemical one. Again, depression can be caused by a variety of physiological imbalances. One of them is fluctuating hormones.

HORMONE HAVOC

As we've discussed, hormone fluctuations can wreak havoc with a woman's metabolism—not just during menopause, but on a monthly basis. And not just a day or two before her menstrual cycle; many women experience lethargy, mood changes, and a raging appetite from ovulation through the end of their period. They barely get a breath of energy before the symptoms begin again.

If a woman is to unlock the fat cell storage mechanism and turn up her fat-burning potential, she must understand and deal with the hormones that play major roles in her energy and well-being. Two of the hormones most familiar to women are estrogen and progesterone. Estrogen not only serves in the regulation of the menstrual cycle, but acts as a mild antidepressant and greatly enhances a woman's sense of well-being. When estrogen is not produced at proper levels, memory, mood, and energy all suffer—which explains the many changes associated with menopause when estrogen production dramatically falls off. Before menopause, estrogen levels peak in the first two weeks of the menstrual cycle and decrease during the two weeks after ovulation.

> **SMART WEIGH TIP**
>
> *Get inspired. Read a lot about other people who have overcome great obstacles.*

Progesterone is also involved in regulating a woman's menstrual cycle, and works to prepare the lining of the uterus for pregnancy. Progesterone begins to increase at ovulation, at the time the estrogen levels decrease, and stays high over the last two weeks of the menstrual cycle. Progesterone is the hormone culprit for PMS-related symptoms: irritability, fatigue, depression, decreased sexual desire, increased appetite, and achiness. Energy and sexual drives are thought to be diminished due to progesterone's suppression of dopamine, the brain neurotransmitter that keeps us alert, motivated, and poised for action.

The hypothalamus, the body's control center, monitors the levels of hormones produced by the ovaries. And this control center is affected by external as well as internal factors. It is the hypothalamus that is battered by the stress chemicals, causing the metabolism, blood sugars, and fluid balance to go awry in times of intense stress. Little wonder that the symptoms of hormone havoc are metabolic slow-down; blood sugar fluctuations resulting in irritability, fatigue, and food cravings; and fluid retention and bloating. And approaching menopause is another hormone struggle altogether. The hormonal fluctuations that tended to intensify once or twice a month can now take on a life of their own.

Proper nutrition, exercise, and sleep can be tremendous stabilizers, but can fuel havoc if they are deficient. Women who skip meals or go long hours without balanced eating are setting themselves up for fatigue, moodiness, and fat storage.

Here are some stabilizers you can count on to help calm the hormone havoc within:

ADD CALCIUM. Recent research shows that menstruating women who supplemented with 1,200 mg of calcium had significantly less intense symptoms of PMS, and some had no symptoms at all.

GO FOR SOY. These foods have been shown to alleviate many of the symptoms of hormone fluctuations—even the hot flashes of menopause. Substitute soy-based foods (tofu, soy cheese, soy beans or soy protein powders) for meat proteins at least once a day. To be effective, soy products must contain 35 to 45 mg of soy protein isolates. Read the product label.

EAT SMART. Go easy on sweets and alcohol. Although most often the object of hormone-related cravings, these substances trigger a response like throwing gas on a fire. Refined sugars have been shown to aggravate just about every symptom of PMS. So focus on eating whole carbohydrates throughout your day to even out your blood sugar response.

If you eat whole grains, you will also get the blessing of vitamin B6 and magnesium—two nutrients particularly helpful in stabilizing brain chemical production. Beyond whole grains, good food sources of vitamin B6 include fish, chicken, turkey, potatoes, and bananas (see page 100). And a daily supplement of 150 mg can help alleviate PMS symptoms for many women. If you supplement with B6, limit yourself to less than 300 mg per day; higher levels have been linked to neuromuscular damage and paralysis.

A magnesium supplement may be helpful as well, although a well-balanced diet including green, leafy vegetables, soy products, and lots of whole grains is apt to fill your magnesium need. The recommendation by most PMS researchers is 350 mg of magnesium per day to lessen the intensity of symptoms. Magnesium gluconate and magnesium aspartate are the most absorbable forms.

LIMIT CAFFEINE. Caffeine aggravates fibrocystic breast pain, and complicates the energy and mood seesaw of PMS.

EXERCISE EVERY DAY. Although this may be the last thing you feel like doing when your hormones are fluctuating, regular exercise can change your entire hormone and brain chemistry makeup. The stress-busting endorphins that exercise releases can calm your personal storm.

CONSIDER HORMONE REPLACEMENT THERAPY. To calm the hormonal hurricane induced by menopause, you have the option of replacing dwindling hormones with synthetic forms of progesterone and estrogen. But certain risks and side effects need to be discussed with your health care provider. Still, don't ignore the hormone replacement issue; more is at risk than moods or hot flashes alone. Hormone deficiency increases the risk of osteoporosis, heart disease, and Alzheimer's—risks that are not worth taking. Find the right choice and balance for you.

THYROID DISORDERS

You may not have identified it as such, but your thyroid gland is also a part of your hormonal system. It's a mysterious gland, most often getting the blame for weight gain, a slowed metabolism, and fatigue. Although less than 2 percent of all cases of obesity can be traced to a metabolic disorder such as low thyroid function, it needs to be considered because a malfunction has such a detrimental impact on energy and weight.

The thyroid gland controls the metabolism of body energy, regulating your metabolic rate and the number of calories you need to keep your body operating. It does so by releasing hormones to regulate your body systems. One of the more important thyroid hormones secreted into your bloodstream is thyroxine, which serves to regulate your heartbeat, metabolic rate, body temperature, and even the rate at which waste moves through your GI tract.

The reason for thyroid dysfunction is unclear. One possibility appears to be a viral infection that triggers the body into an immune response directed against itself. A common target for this autoimmune response is the thyroid gland. If the thyroid gland becomes overactive, it releases too much hormone; if it is underactive, it releases too little. If the hyperactive thyroid gland works too hard, it accelerates the heartbeat and produces an anxious, uncomfortable excess of energy. A sluggish thyroid function, on the other hand, causes low energy, dry skin, hair loss, lowered immunes, poor appetite, intolerance to cold, weight gain, and constipation. Some women may experience an irregularity in their heart rate, and headaches as well.

One out of five women over sixty have hypothyroidism, often unbeknownst to them. What they do know is that they are experiencing overwhelming fatigue, chilliness, and a host of other maladies that may be mislabeled "aging." Because overeating, exhaustion, and depression are often the most pronounced signs of thyroid problems, it's important to get a thorough physical if your body doesn't respond to positive lifestyle changes. Treating an underactive thyroid is not difficult, once diagnosed; it just requires a daily dose of a synthetic thyroid hormone.

Along with the medication, your metabolism can be boosted by treating the symptoms naturally. Keep your slow metabolism revved up to a higher gear by following *The Smart Weigh* eat-right prescription. Eating balanced mini-meals every 2 1/2 to 3 hours and getting quality proteins throughout the day can also help to arrest hair loss and cure skin maladies. And keep your sluggish GI tract on the move with adequate fiber and lots of water.

Hormone levels gone awry affect every part of the body—and soul. Because of the intricate interplay between hormones and the neurotransmitters of the brain, being caught in hormone havoc can bring destructive forces into our lives and distort the very way we look at life and at our bodies. And because a positive body image is such a vital part of living free from the diet trap, it's important to see all of our entrapments clearly—and take charge of what we can.

A negative body image can be a powerful force that neutralizes our energy, vitality, and self-control. It needn't be. Once you see a lamp of hope shining on the physical you, it may be time to look to the soul and evaluate your emotional relationship with your body, eating, and food.

CHAPTER 17 ■ Body Image Battles

Your thoughts and companions are like elevator buttons—they will either take you up, or take you down.

—ANONYMOUS

We live in a culture that has an ideal body type that only a tiny percentage of the population can ever hope to achieve. Trying to live up to that kind of standard is enough to make even the most sensible person a little nuts.

But it may surprise you to know that having a poor body image not only messes with your mind, it can also be one of the major hindrances to losing weight. In a study of 177 men and women, researchers from the Stanford University School of Medicine found those with a healthy body image were more than twice as successful at meeting weight-loss goals—55 percent compared to 26 percent. Those with no history of weight fluctuations also fared well (63 percent versus 35 percent).

> **SMART WEIGH TIP**
>
> *Look in the mirror and say, "I am wonderfully made"—and don't give up.*

Some people who want to be thinner have a reasonable body image in mind—they simply don't want to carry around excess weight. But many people, especially women, do *not* have a healthy body image in mind. Rather, they are seeking to rearrange their figure into perfection.

The crazy thing about body image is that it is often the very thing that lures people into the diet trap—and then becomes the very thing that makes them most miserable about being there. It's also the thing that keeps them stuck. Because with a poor body image, it's never good enough—and neither are you.

People who may be genetically destined to carry more weight than the average person have a particular challenge to their self-image. It's a social challenge because of the abuse and prejudice heaped upon them. It's a personal and vital challenge to overcome, however, because studies show that a poor self-image actually fuels poor health habits. Those who feel uncomfortable with their heavier bodies are less apt to exercise— they don't want people thinking, "You sure need to do more of that!" Or, as one of my clients heard from a car speeding by her while she was walking: "Run, Fattie—it might do that fat some good!" Horribly painful words, and definitely not motivating.

> **SMART WEIGH TIP**
>
> *Quit the numbers game. Forget how much you weigh— go for feeling great and how you fit into the clothes you want to wear.*

Because of this kind of social conditioning, many people put so much emphasis on their looks that they ignore their many other good qualities. They also let their negative body image keep them from vital health-care and social activities. One of my clients, Mary, had not had a gynecological appointment for five years, even though she has a history of irregular pap smears. Why? She didn't want her doctor to see her body or have to stand on the examining room scale. Jim, thirty-two, had not gone to a family gathering for two years for fear of what his family would think when they saw him. Cynthia, forty-one, had stopped undressing in front of her husband and would not let him touch her stomach or thighs— which created distance and hurt in their intimate relationship.

MIRROR, MIRROR ON THE WALL

How about you? Do you ever stand in front of the mirror and dream about where you'd get a few nips and tucks if you could? Do you feel as if life would be better *if only* you had smaller thighs, a flatter tummy, or there was simply less of you?

A critical question for your health and happiness is this: Do you have a healthy image of your body? Answer these questions with "never," "sometimes," "often," or "always," and find out how you measure up. It may be time to give your body image a boost.

1. Do you dislike seeing yourself in mirrors?
2. Do you find shopping for clothes somewhat unpleasant because it makes you more aware of your "weight problem?"
3. Do you ever feel ashamed to be seen in public?
4. Do you avoid engaging in certain activities, sports, or public exercises because of being self-conscious about your appearance?
5. Do you ever feel embarrassed about your body in the presence of someone of the opposite sex?
6. Do you ever think your body is ugly?
7. Do you ever feel that other people must think your body is unattractive, even repulsive?
8. Do you view your shape differently from the way others do?
9. Do you ever feel that family or friends may be embarrassed to be seen with you because of your weight?
10. Do you try to lose weight to look good for someone else?
11. Do you ever compare yourself with other people to see if they are heavier or thinner than you are?
12. Does feeling guilty or uncomfortable about your weight preoccupy most of your thinking?
13. Are your thoughts about your body and physical appearance negative and self-critical?

14. Are you driven by a desire to be thin, equating thinness with success and being in control? Do you think about life in terms of "if only" ("if only I were thinner, then I would be married... have more friends... get a better job...").

15. Do you try to lose weight, thinking that when you shed unwanted pounds, you'll become a wonderful person—forgetting that you are already a wonderful person?

Maintaining negative beliefs—as evidenced by any questions to

---

MEDIA HYPE

This "Did You Know" was sent via e-mail to my seventeen-year-old daughter. I'm hoping it was circulated around the Internet to millions of young girls like her (and those not so young) to put into perspective the truth about our beauty— and the lies that are pervasive in society. Many thanks to the person who put these facts together.

Did you know ...

■ If shop mannequins were real women, they'd be too thin to menstruate.

■ There are 3 billion women who don't look like supermodels—and only eight who do.

■ Marilyn Monroe wore a size 14.

■ If Barbie were a real woman, she'd have to walk on all fours due to her unrealistic proportions.

■ The average American woman weighs 144 lbs. and wears between a size 12 and 14.

■ One out of every four college-aged women has an eating disorder.

■ The models in the magazines are airbrushed, i.e., they're not perfect.

■ A psychological study in 1995 found that three minutes spent looking at models in a fashion magazine caused 70 percent of women to feel depressed, guilty, and shameful.

■ Models twenty years ago weighed 8 percent less than the average woman. Today they weigh 23 percent less.

which you answered "sometimes," "often," or "always"—is a sign of a not-so-hot body image. Answering "often" or "always" to many of these questions can reveal a body image war that can get in the way of your happiness, thwart your success in losing weight and keeping fit, and even lead to depression and eating disorders. But guess what? No matter what "they" tell you—the magazines, Hollywood, your friends and family—looking like Kate Moss or Ally McBeal isn't the cure-all for the woes of life.

In living *The Smart Weigh*, what's most important is that you feel good about who you are. Until you like yourself as is, and understand who you *really* are apart from how you look, trying to change your body shape will be a losing proposition. High self-esteem is crucial for a healthy, balanced lifestyle—and it's a must for successful weight loss. After all, how can you take care of yourself if you don't like yourself? It just doesn't work. Rather than treating yourself well—and improving your health and weight as a result—you end up using "diet" regimes to beat yourself up and literally whip yourself into shape. And when you fail—which you inevitably will—then you've amassed more evidence that you just can't succeed and you'll never be "good enough."

If this vicious cycle sounds familiar, then it's time to smile back at that image in the mirror and value all the wonderful characteristics about the person reflected there.

When each of my daughters turned ten, we went away for a mother-daughter weekend to celebrate the beginning of each girl's "pre-teen" years. We talked about who they were, who they had been created to be—and how difficult it was to "measure up" to the expectations of their peers. We talked about the pain so many teens experience due to never feeling they have enough "brains, bucks, or beauty."

Following the advice of wise family therapists, we spent time listing all of the things we liked about ourselves physically—hair? eyes? height? sense of humor? sensitivity? Then we looked at all the things we didn't like, and wished we could change—nose? hips? teeth? moodiness? too tall? too short? And we looked at all the things that we could reasonably change with better self-care or practical help: braces, better eating, adequate sleep. The rest we wrote on pieces of paper and burned—because all of the wishing and misery in the world would not make one daughter less tall, and the other taller. It was crucial that they appreciate the wonder of who they were and what they looked like—not who they wished they could be or who they thought they should look like.

I took this exercise right back into my counseling. I realized that, as adults, many of us are still struggling with those same issues of bucks, brains, and beauty—and trying desperately to "measure up" in the eyes of others. I realized that no matter what our age—ten, twenty, forty, or sixty—falling in love with our bodies, being thankful for what we do have, recognizing what we cannot change as well as what we can, is a challenge.

You may want to go back and review the ten tips to boost positive perspective on page 84 in Chapter 5, such as practicing positive self-talk, seeing the world realistically, recognizing your special qualities, and putting your body back together. These tips are not a one-time event, but can become daily affirmations in your life as you learn to embrace yourself for exactly who you are.

THE HORROR OF A SWIMSUIT

It's not just healthy habit patterns that get sacrificed to a poor body image; relationships pay the price as well—with yourself and others. That's why one of the strongest aspects of my counseling with overweight clients is my focus on freeing them from self-reproach, end-less rumination about their appearance, and their reluctance to appear in public. The horror of "exposing" yourself to the public eye—especially when that exposure involves bare skin—can keep even the thin among us from good-for-you activities like swimming or walking on the beach. In a recent survey conducted by *Prevention* magazine and NBC, nearly half of American women are so self-con-scious about revealing their bodies that they refuse to be pho-tographed in a swimsuit.

Kay was certainly among them—swimsuits were the reason she started dieting, in her early teens, to begin with. She was a Florida girl and, for the most part, *loves* summer: the hot, hot weather, the long sunny days, trips to the beach, splashing in the pool. "So what is my problem?" Kay asked me at our first session together. "It's that all too often, in the back of my mind, there is this constant nagging thought: *I hate my thighs!*" Actually, it was her "thigh"—the left one.

> **SMART WEIGH TIP**
>
> *Find new measures of success. Use a pair of jeans one size too small —try them on once a month to see how they are fitting.*

Kay explained that she underwent some bone-grafting surgery, due to a congenital leg problem, done at age seven. Surgical tech-nique was not so good then and the resulting huge scar and the scar tissue seemed to become its own special saddlebag. "Ever since I was a teenager, the first hint of cellulite seemed to accumulate around that area," Kay explained. "I've had this creeping self-consciousness about revealing my lower half. I've always wanted to carry a sign to the beach saying, 'I had surgery,'" she said half-laughing, and half-teary. "While my teeny friends were wearing shorts or bathing suits without a care, I was devising ways to cover myself. And shopping for a bathing suit was sheer agony. There was one golden year, when

I was fourteen, when the very in-style suit had a little skirt around the bottom, covering just the right spot on my thigh. I loved that suit; it was pink and white checked.

"Well, that was then. I'm a big girl now, right? And a smart one." Kay is a very smart woman—a professional therapist who, strangely enough, counsels other women on body image. Yet, through the years, she's had to work *very* hard on her perception of her own thigh. Kay has had to learn that who she *really* is has nothing to do with her image in the mirror. It has become very important to her to do the right things for the right reasons. She doesn't want the reason for caring for herself by eating well and exercising to be rooted in her "thigh anxiety." She had worked hard on her perception (*it is not that big*) and her interpretation (*my self-worth is not determined by my thigh*).

As Kay continues to learn to love herself and give herself the gift of health she deserves, she has let her intermittent self-consciousness teach her some valuable lessons. "It still crops up occasionally," she says, "and it makes me mad that I'm bothered by it at all. I mean, who cares, really? Why do I want beautiful thighs? Who am I trying to impress? When those old feelings of self-loathing threaten to undermine my commitment to self-care, I understand that I'm still in need of unconditional love... and I'm thankful for the reminder. Only a spiritual connection will give me that."

Another thing Kay is learning is how to deal effectively with what's really eating her so she won't automatically turn to food to soothe her moods or solve her problems. Like many of us, she has a history of getting caught in a vicious cycle—turning to food as a comfort when she is sad or anxious. So, the more frustrated and panicked she would feel about her thighs, the more she would eat. A clothes-shopping excursion inevitably ended at Baskin-Robbins.

A healthy relationship with food is one of friendship, where food is regarded as the nourishment it was created to be. But food is not simply food in the world today. We live in a nation of people preoccupied with food—obsessed by it.

I grew up believing that there was no problem in life that couldn't be solved with a banana split. Eating, and overeating, was my response to every emotion. As a family we ate to celebrate when we were happy; to feel better when we were sad; to give us something to do when we were bored; to gain control when we felt anxious or frustrated. I ate to stuff my anger and to soothe my nerves. I ate when I felt out of control. Although my eating itself would have looked out of control to others, it actually gave me a sense of being in charge of something.

In order to live free of the diet trap, food needs to be given its proper place in our lives. Food can be healthy nourishment. It can be a source of pleasure. It certainly does more than satisfy hunger. It's time to make peace with food.

CHAPTER 18 ■ Making Peace with Food

Life can only be understood by looking backward, but it must be lived by looking forward.

—ANONYMOUS

W e just talked about accepting our bodies, but in a nation where fashion models average a size two and thin is perpetually in, you don't have to have an eating disorder to spend most of your waking hours—and sometimes, sleeping ones, too—agonizing over food. If you started your day thinking about what you couldn't have for breakfast or kicking yourself for what you ate for dinner last night, then it's time to call it *war*—a food war.

If your mental conversations follow this script—"Have I been good or bad today?" "How many fat grams did I eat today?" "How many calories did I burn off at the gym?" "Is that brownie going to show up on the scale? Or worse, on my thighs?" "I won't eat tonight to make up for it"— then, in addition to the diet trap, you may be struggling with food obsession or dependency, which can destroy you.

See how you answer these questions:

> **SMART WEIGH TIP**
>
> *Challenge the power of food. Determine if you're really eating because you're hungry or eating for other reasons.*

- Do you make promises to control your eating, but break those promises again and again?
- Do you skip meals, especially breakfast, and hope your stomach won't notice?
- Do you feel a sense of power when you skip meals?
- Do you regularly go the whole day with little or no food, yet wonder why you are sick and tired?
- Have you tried to get through the day on coffee, tea, or soda?
- Do you deny the physical damage or complications caused by your eating choices?
- Are you constantly dieting or discussing food and weight loss?
- Do you eat more, or at a more frenzied pace, when under stress?
- Have you found yourself unable to stop eating?
- Have you ever thought, "I was bad today; I won't eat tomorrow"?
- Do you go on a binge the week before going on a diet?
- Do you consume huge quantities of food rapidly and often secretly?
- Do you dispose of or hide the evidence because you are ashamed of what you've done?
- Have you eaten to the point of nausea or vomiting, or until your stomach hurts?
- Do you feel "good" when you are eating, but when you stop eating, are overcome with guilt, remorse, or self-hatred? Do you eat more to relieve those feelings?
- Do you avoid social engagements that involve eating if you are on a diet?
- Does eating, or planning to eat, seem to be a hassle?
- Do you fast or drastically cut and count calories to lose weight?
- Do you have an on-a-diet, off-a-diet mentality, rather than eating moderately and wisely as the norm?

- Do you think of any food as bad or forbidden rather than simply as food?
- Have you relied on diet pills or shakes or any product that promises to do the weight-loss work for you?

If you answered yes to a number of these questions, than the food fight has taken on a life of its own. Pick the top three issues you struggle with on the list and personalize them, such as, "I regularly think, 'I was bad today, so I'll starve tomorrow.'" Now, open your mind to some new revelations about food and your body that might help you make peace with both.

IS THE REFRIGERATOR LIGHT THE LIGHT OF YOUR LIFE?

Most of us have been taught that food "makes us feel better," and we have certainly discovered that it does. When we feel sad or anxious, a candy bar or bag of chips can be very soothing. When we are stressed or angry, chocolate chip cookies reduce the inner tension. Many people go back to their normal, more balanced way of eating once the uncomfortable feeling has passed. But others do not return to "normal" eating patterns. Their logic goes something like this: "If food made me feel good yesterday, then it should do the same today; and if today, then tomorrow."

Food doesn't let us down, even if everything—and everyone—else does. We can become as dependent on food as on any chemical substance, and it can be as destructive as any other addiction.

Millions of Americans are emotionally dependent on food. Food dependency and obsession has nothing to do with your weight; you may be very overweight or quite thin. Rather, it has to do with an improper relationship with food in which food and eating–and often dieting—have assumed an unnatural importance in your life.

In this improper love-hate relationship, food has an unnatural control over you. You may love the way it tastes and makes you feel, but hate it for what it does to your body and how it controls your life. Like any unhealthy relationship, food dependency results in a roller coaster of emotions: gratification and satisfaction, guilt and remorse, being "good" only to be "bad," going "on" a diet only to go "off" a diet. The obsession fills your thoughts and drives your actions, robs you of physical well-being and emotional serenity, and affects your self-esteem. Such captivity has life-damaging consequences.

Food or dieting becomes a trap when it is used as a substitute for love, friendship, or success, or when it's used to cover up more serious emotional issues.

FOOD IS NOT AN EVIL

Human beings must have food to survive and thrive; we are created to depend on it and enjoy it. Food itself is not evil, but many of us use food badly. Sometimes we love eating more than we love ourselves, more than we love other people, and more than we love God.

Take an inventory of your own thoughts about food as you read these commonly held beliefs about food and dieting. Observe how these play out in the lives of Steve, Tori, Karen, Deborah, and Jim.

■ *Food (or dieting) helps me cope with stress, frustration, and the insecurities of life. Overeating seems to smooth away the rough edges and relieve the tension, thus allowing me to cope. It provides a quick fix.*

It sure did for Steve—a man who was the envy of all his friends for his rigid dieting and exercise. And it was not only Steve's willpower that amazed his friends; he had an uncanny expertise in the stock market. The most successful stockbroker in his firm, he had many influential clients with large portfolios. His success had its drawbacks, though: the stress was intense and constant, though he "handled it well"—or appeared to, anyway.

Steve couldn't meet the pressures of his job head-on because the main source of his stress was coming from within—his driving need for perfection. He needed everything to go according to plan, but invariably it didn't. So he resorted to a familiar pattern that would relieve the tensions and fuel his workaholic habits: he would go on a binge of massive quantities of sweets. But those sweet binges tarnished the standard of perfection he'd set for himself—so he would maniacally exercise and diet his guilt away.

■ *Food (or dieting) fills the gaps in my life. Food can be the friend and companion that is with me no matter what. When I'm lonely, eating seems to fill the emptiness. It substitutes for love, attention, and pampering. When I'm happy, it's a way to celebrate—even if I'm not with other people. When I'm working hard with seemingly little recognition or appreciation, food becomes a justly earned reward and comfort.*

Tori saw me during the time she was transitioning into being an empty-nester—and it wasn't coming easy. She had loved motherhood, and had accepted it with joy and a sense of challenge. She had dedicated twenty years to raising her daughter, Meghan. And then Meghan took a job in another state and moved—leaving Tori feeling lost and empty.

Tori felt so abandoned that she demanded appreciation from the very person who could not give it to her—Meghan. Meghan was struggling with her own emotions of breaking away and could not be the support that her mother craved. Since Tori was going to an "empty well" and coming up dry, she turned to food to fill her bucket. And it did, temporarily. But the more Tori ate, the more weight she gained and the more depressed she got—which only ended up isolating and alienating her from the healthy relationships that *were* available.

■ *Food (or dieting) gives me a sense of identity and control. Loving and controlling food is a lot safer than loving people. When life seems most out of control, rigid denial of food or counting every calorie or fat gram—even planning a binge—gives me a sense of being very much in control of at least one area of life.*

At forty-nine, Karen was heavier than she had ever been—yet she had been on a diet for twenty-two years. She was tired of battling food and the scale and wanted to break out of the diet trap.

But Karen was not willing to give up compulsive dieting because she didn't want to give up control. As long as she could control food—her natural enemy—she felt she had control of her world. But the truth was, she wasn't controlling it—it was controlling her. Every time she broke her rigid diet, she saw herself as a failure. When she would reach her "goal weight" and relax a bit, she immediately gained five pounds as the fluid balance restored itself. That led to horror, which led to more restrictions and more failures.

I watched Karen yo-yo like this for three years before she told me that her husband was a practicing alcoholic. Then it all made sense to me. She had been using her compulsive dieting, alternating with compulsive eating, to cover up her pain and shame related to her husband's disease. She believed she didn't have any hope for change, and felt out of control. Food and dieting temporarily restored her balance.

■ *Food (or dieting) helps me sabotage the "perfect image" people expect me to live up to. I was an obedient, people-pleasing child, and now I'm that kind of adult. In my "good-girl" world, food is something to be "bad" with. Even though becoming overweight is the result, overeating is a socially acceptable vice and a passive form of rebellion.*

Deborah is a minister's wife and a minister's daughter. She grew up with a rigid set of rules for "acceptable behavior" and never dreamed of breaking them. She was "Papa's precious," always wearing a smile.

But Deborah didn't always *feel* like smiling. In fact, she sometimes felt quite resentful of being the preacher's daughter and having to be perfect to meet the expectations of the congregation. She would be immediately overwhelmed with shame for these "bad" feelings, and found that she could act out how bad she felt she was by bingeing on food. She did it in secret, so no one would ever know just how rebellious she was.

> **SMART WEIGH TIP**
>
> *Take an emotional inventory. Ask yourself: "What do you feel guilty about? Resent? Fear? Regret? What are you angry about?" Then deal with it— without food.*

When she started gaining weight, she began to make herself sick after overeating—to get rid of the evidence. She developed a secret life-style of overeating and purging that followed her into her marriage. Then one day, she exploded with the truth—when she couldn't contain the secret shame any longer. She couldn't stand the reality that no one—not even her husband—knew who she really was.

> ■ *Food (or dieting) helps me deal with deep-seated emotions and feelings. Keeping my mind on food can keep it off issues of the heart and soul. Overeating seems like a safe way to express my hidden emotions. Stuffing food, or rigidly denying myself food, is a way to stuff feelings, to numb them, to shut them off.*

Eating to stay Mr. Nice Guy is exactly what Jim had done since childhood.

Because he had a high metabolism and weight was never a problem for him, overeating seemed to be the perfect way to deal with the unexplainable rage that would rise up within him. This was such an established pattern that Jim ceased to recognize that he ever even felt angry. He just knew he was tired all the time.

Jim's business was in the midst of great transition when he first came to me for counseling. His commission rate and his sales territory had been changed three times in two months. He had also recently been passed over for a promotion. Jim was vaguely aware he was eating excessive quantities of sweets and vaguely realized that this had increased with the stress at work. But his wife was very aware of Jim's behavior, and was concerned because of his family's proclivity toward diabetes.

Jim had difficulty reporting any set eating patterns; he said his eating was based on availability and the situation he faced at the moment. He was astonished to begin identifying those situations as the ones that made him angry. As long as he could eat a cookie when he began to feel "something" inside, he could avoid dealing with the emotion.

DEALING WITH WHAT'S EATING YOU

The satisfied feeling we get from food *does* fill the gaps—temporarily. But typically, the more we eat, the more depressed we get, and the more we need to eat to feel better. But because food is a quick fix, we never get the chance to fill in the gaps permanently and in healthy ways.

As long as we're eating (or even actively avoiding eating), we don't have to deal with what's eating us. We might appear calm, even happy, on the outside, yet we're crying or raging on the inside.

Remember Sherri, the woman in Chapter 4 who compared herself to a juice box that had its contents sucked dry all day, every day? Sherri's real problem was that she ate to help her deal with what was eating her.

When she was dieting, she would fill her mind with the dieting "rules" and let those become her focus. But, ultimately, she would have a lapse. For all of her hard work, she would reward herself with a doughnut, which would throw her into the "I've-blown-it-now" syndrome. So she would eat six. Her eat-today, diet-tomorrow strategy meant that today she would eat everything she couldn't have when she dieted tomorrow. As is often the case, her momentary lapse became a relapse, which led ultimately to her collapse.

But today Sherri is off that merry-go-round and doing terrifically with *The Smart Weigh*. Two months after her first visit to me, she made many changes. She was eating in a more even and balanced way than ever in her life. She had lost seven pounds, purely as a side benefit of her change in eating—not by starving or "dieting." And because these were seven pounds of fat—not water and muscle—her "thin" clothes were actually too big. And speaking of muscle, Sherri had started walking at lunch time as a powerful stress release, and doing strength and conditioning exercises three mornings a week.

Yet Sherri would occasionally let her eating habits slip out of control. The "binge" was now generally on good foods (although donuts still sneaked in occasionally), but it ended then and there. It lacked the frenzy and desperation of previous years. But it still happened—and it scared her.

So I asked Sherri to keep a week's diary of what she ate and when. I asked her to note what she was feeling when she overate or wanted to. We were trying to discover the triggers that would send her into a binge. Her food diary became a mirror in which she observed her emotional responses and how eating had been the reaction.

Sherri saw that if she was eating the right things at the right time she could usually not overeat, though the desire was still there—particularly when she was pressured for time and incapable of "producing." It wasn't her actual job of producing that was the problem—she was talented and loved the work. It was the daily need to meet others' expectations, depending on others to come through, which they didn't, and playing the political games that seemed to be required at work. And she did it all with an edge of anger and resentment because it pulled her away from her daughters. By the time she got home *to* them, she had nothing left *for* them. Food seemed to fuel her for her tense meetings during the day and get her through her nights.

Up until this moment of insight, Sherri had always claimed that she simply loved food—particularly chocolate and especially doughnuts. She now saw that, in reality, she had an emotional relationship with food, one that had started years before when, as a child, Sherri discovered that eating certain foods made her feel better, and eating a lot of certain foods made her feel a lot better. She had grown up in a perfectionistic family and had used food to dull her sense of failure and relieve the stress. Since she had developed a life pattern of depriving herself of food for her soul, doughnuts became a sweet substitute. It was time to make peace. She had to learn how to truly feed her soul.

CHAPTER 19 ■ Feeding Your Soul

The great thing in this life is not so much where we are, but in which direction we are moving.

—ANONYMOUS

There is more to living well than just caring for and feeding your physical being. I believe we humans are three-parted beings: body, soul, and spirit. I also believe that all three parts need to be nourished. You need to care for and feed your soul and spirit with the right kind of soul food.

Many people get caught in unhealthy habits because they don't get their needs met on all three levels—spiritually, emotionally, and physically. And because legitimate needs are not being met in legitimate ways, it's just a matter of time before they are met in illegitimate ways. Like falling headfirst into food.

> **SMART WEIGH TIP**
>
> *If you feel like you can't do it on your own, seek help to deal with what's eating you.*

Before I embraced nutrition as a profession, I was handicapped in all three areas of my life. I was searching for real answers to my questions about the purpose of life—especially my life. I knew I was spiritually empty, but I didn't have a clue about how to get filled. I was carrying a lot of emotional baggage, and food became the easy way to fill up my vacuums and get the fuel I needed to carry the emotional burden. While overfeeding my physical body, I was starving my soul and spirit.

I could cover my eating dependencies with pendulum swings in my weight. I gained weight—but I always lost it again. And, I could overcome overeating as long as I was trapped in the iron-will discipline of a diet. To cope with my unresolved emotions, I could replace the obsessive use and intense preoccupation with food with an obsessive and intense preoccupation with dieting. But, unfortunately, it always came back up.

As I changed career paths and began to learn more about nutrition and taking care of my physical body, I became strong enough to overcome many of my unhealthy eating patterns. Dieting was no longer an answer for me. It would be some time before I learned about—and responded to—my emotional and spiritual needs, but just meeting my physical needs allowed me to break free enough from food and dieting to see the gaping holes in my life.

Many of my clients experience this also. As they become stronger physically, getting their bodies on an even nutritional keel, they are free to see the deeper emotional and spiritual needs that hinder their health. The goal of *The Smart Weigh* is to live well, free, and whole in all these areas—spirit, soul, and body. The people I see getting free of the diet trap and getting well—and staying that way— acknowledge and care for all three. This is not easy to do, but it is possible.

DEALING WITH ROOT ISSUES

We have been created with an intricate design for our physical growth—no one is born an adult. To grow and thrive, our human body requires certain nutrients; without them, it becomes malnourished and growth is stunted.

A similar design exists for our emotional growth: at birth we are emotionally immature and must be fed love and be nurtured to thrive. Without this food for our souls, our emotional growth is arrested, and we fail to thrive. Even though our bodies may have been clothed and fed, our emotions may have been starved and neglected in our homes. As adults, we may appear to cope well with day-to-day life, until stresses, hurts, and challenges overtake us. Then our childlike emotions reveal themselves, and we respond in an emotionally disabled way.

One woman, who struggled for years with both anorexia nervosa and overeating, described it this way: "I grew up in a single-parent home with a young mother who was understandably overwhelmed by the challenge of caring for me. For many reasons, she was unable to 'be there' for me emotionally, and I learned early that staying 'out of the way' and taking up as little room as possible was the best strategy for survival. Because I was convinced so early that I deserved—and could get—only 'crumbs' emotionally, it seemed natural and desirable literally to starve my body and soul as I grew older.

"Now I'm nearly forty years old, and I'm still 'starving' to some degree. While I no longer starve literally, I still have that mentality: I know I can survive 'just fine' on very little, and so it continues to feel natural to withhold good food, good fun, and good love from myself. And when I can't stand the 'crumbs' anymore, I dive head-first into a whole loaf of bread (with lots of butter) to fill me up.

"I want so much to discover that what happened to me as a child need no longer dictate how I treat myself. I want to know—and live as though—my Creator longs to give me the bread of life."

Not all families, well intentioned as they may have been, planted healthy seeds of love into the souls of their children. Hurts happened, abandonment occurred, shame resulted. As children from these families grow into adulthood, these unhealthy emotional seeds grow into invisible weeds of guilt and fear, poor self-image, and lack of healthy boundaries, limits, and trust. To thrive—not just survive—and walk in freedom from the diet trap or any life trap, we must identify and root out these toxic weeds in our soul.

FACING FEELINGS

A good place to start with nourishing your soul is to begin to identify—and face—your feelings. You were created with feelings that you can't ignore. They don't just "go away" because you deny them. Processing your feelings requires that you understand and celebrate how you were made—as an emotional being who *feels*.

If, as a child, you were discouraged from expressing your feelings—particularly negative ones such as anger, guilt, or frustration—you quickly learned which feelings got positive or negative reactions. Perhaps now, as an adult, your life has become a list of emotional shoulds and should nots, leaving you believing that what you feel is bad, wrong, or unacceptable. But if your emotions can't be expressed, they have to be bottled up some way, somehow. Maybe with business, maybe with a smile—or maybe by stuffing them or soothing them with food.

Emotions produce energy (e-motion = energy in motion), and if we don't release that energy, we must spend energy to keep it in. But like a dam springing leaks, feelings stuffed inside can come out "sideways" through physical ailments—joint and muscle pain, insomnia, ulcers, even cancer. Instead of crying, we get headaches. Instead of saying we don't want to go someplace with someone, we get stomach cramps. Instead of saying no to another work project, we push ourselves to exhaustion and develop fatigue or high blood pressure. Or we overeat.

Our bodies react to repressed emotion whether we like it or not. The unreleased energy robs us of our well-being by causing increased tension, anxiety, or depression. New research is revealing that

---

FAMILY SYSTEMS THAT SET THE TRAP

Eating dependencies most often come out of three types of unhealthy family systems:

THE PERFECT FAMILY. This family places high priority on appearances—the family's reputation, identity, and achievements. Its ruling question is: What will people think? Mistakes are not allowed. This family can appear close, loving, and caring from the outside—a perfect front for a rigid set of rules, many of which govern emotions: don't cry, don't get angry, don't mope, smile when you feel like crying. It takes a lot of eating to hold those emotions in.

THE ENMESHED FAMILY. This family emphasizes the need to be close—very close. There are no boundaries; everyone is community property, with a fence protecting them from the "outside." Secrets stay in. The ruling slogan is: "You can't trust anyone outside of the family." Because of the enmeshment within this family, members have a difficult time developing an independent life or unique personality. As a result, food sometimes becomes the only thing the person feels he or she can control. Overeating becomes the one thing in life that is daring, risky, and rebellious.

THE CHAOTIC FAMILY. There are no rules in this family—or they stay hidden and inconsistent because the parents are emotionally unavailable to their children. It may be alcoholism, workaholism, abuse, or any number of issues that distance the children from their caregivers—but it teaches the children not to talk, trust, or feel. They become well-trained experts at deadening their feelings with food—or any substance of choice.

All of these family systems are the result of unhealthy rules and belief systems that have been passed down from generation to generation; the accompanying pain has been passed down with them. It's important to identify the problems your childhood upbringing may have caused so you can begin to resolve the ways in which old beliefs keep you trapped. But don't get stuck in blaming others. Blame can become just another trap.

repressed emotion can lead to a depressed immune system. And unprocessed feelings like fear, anger, and resentment keep us bound to a spiritual hopelessness—a particularly threatening place to live. The bottom line: the feelings you don't express must be repressed, causing you to be depressed, and opening the door to be oppressed.

To prevent emotions from building up in an unhealthy way, it is vital to allow yourself to feel whatever feelings are inside and to fight the desire to judge them as good or bad. The feelings are simply a readout on where you are in life. Identifying and revealing your feelings enables you to cut a clear path through inner turmoil and get to your real needs. Even socially unacceptable feelings like anger, sadness, fear, or guilt can be celebrated because they can help you discover the needs they're covering up. And that's important when you're trying to overcome a fixation on food or the couch. If food becomes your life raft in a sea of unmet needs, it prevents you from discovering what can really satisfy and nourish your soul. Unless you know what you need, you will rarely get it.

RELEASING FEELINGS

Rather than keeping feelings in, you can identify them and then choose to express them in an active, positive way. Your feelings do not have to control you; they do not have to dictate your behavior. Being angry doesn't mean you have to scream and hurt someone, nor does it mean that you're a bad person. Feeling rejected doesn't mean you have to withdraw.

You can release feelings in a number of positive ways: writing and lifting up your words in prayer, creating something with your hands, singing, talking, exercising. Permit yourself to feel the feelings and process them. Realize it is normal to have many conflicting feelings, and it takes practice to identify them correctly. Being stressed or upset are not feelings, so continue to dig until you name what you are really feeling. Being "stressed" could be feeling tired, guilty, out of control, afraid. Feeling "bad" could be feeling lonely, sick, or scared. Allow that feeling to come over you—and then watch it fade as you release it. It will, and you can. The next step is to learn to match the feeling with the appropriate need. If you are sad, you may need to cry or talk. Eating is not the answer.

> **SMART WEIGH TIP**
>
> *Look up. Focus on the power that you need to make lasting change.*

This process may seem like a journey into very unfamiliar—even frightening—territory. But it's a vital part of releasing the healing mechanism within you, including your ability to lose weight and keep it off. Quietly and repeatedly asking yourself "How do I feel?" is a way—your own way and at your own pace—to uncover slowly what needs to be brought out into the light.

JOURNALING FEELINGS

The most effective—and freeing—step I took in this area was to begin to keep a journal. In that privacy, I can frankly say whatever I am feeling.

I had been encouraged to keep a journal for quite a while, but I always protested, "That's not for me!" I didn't feel that I had the time, or patience. And what if someone got hold of it?

A loving friend challenged me to look honestly at my protests, asking if they were really excuses. Out of respect for her, I began to write. I found ten extra minutes in my day, and began a miraculous journey to a new kind of freedom. Instead of my age-old pattern of putting off dealing with things until later, I found that by looking at my life's happenings *as they were happening*, I could discover how I really felt about what was occurring. I found that under my "nice and busy " smile, there was often hurt and anger.

Slowly my self-consciousness began to fade, and I was able to write out more and more of the feelings and thoughts that flooded my heart and soul. Through journaling I came to know the reality of the words penned by wise Solomon: "A heart at peace gives life to the body" (Proverbs 14:30).

I've used an inexpensive spiral-bound notebook to record my feelings, and I've used my portable computer. If your journal is not portable, keep a small notebook with you to jot down notes about your appetite, feelings, and the things that affect you throughout the day. Keeping a food diary is often a good place to begin if you want to change your eating habits. A small notebook will allow you to record what you eat and when you eat it at the time you are doing so—it is much more accurate than relying on memory. Add to this journal notes about how you feel physically before and after eating: are you energetic, alert, full, and strong, or fatigued, foggy, starved, unsatisfied, and shaky? You may be so used to feeling bad that you haven't noticed how serious it really is. Recording this information will help you see the connection between what you eat and how you feel physically and emotionally.

You can examine the feelings you've written about during a time set aside to reflect and be strengthened. If possible, be consistent about the time of day for your journaling, a time that best suits who you are. I write early in the morning, almost every morning, because I'm a morning person. Some people write on their lunch break; others before they go to sleep; some once a week; still others just when they feel the need.

Consider choosing a place in your house that has a particular ambiance for you—somewhere pleasant to "go to" when you write. In this room, desk, table, corner, bed, or sitting area, you should feel safe to write about your feelings. If you wonder, "What in the world do I write about?" let me give you a jump-start: I begin every journaling time with "Yesterday, I…" I write about what happened in my yesterday and, more important, I write about how those events made me feel. Journaling gives me a chance to express my fears, inadequacies, regrets, joys, hopes, and discoveries. When I feel happy, I can write about that. When I feel sad or angry or worried, writing helps me identify those feelings. The act of writing also helps me to name vague, free-floating feelings. Believe me, there is enormous power in calling a spade a spade. Once you name how you feel about something, you begin to receive power over it. It is no longer an unknown assailant.

If it is difficult for you just to pull your feelings about a particular situation "out of the air," you may find it helpful to make a list of strong emotion words: ANGRY, AFRAID, SAD, REJECTED, HUMILIATED, LOVED, GUILTY, DEPRESSED. Chose one, then write quickly (without censoring yourself) whatever things, events, people, or thoughts are called up by that word at that moment.

WHEN TO STOP, LOOK, AND LISTEN

WHEN YOU FEEL BAD: angry, sad, afraid, guilty, lonely, hungry, tired, sick, numb, depressed, hostile.

WHEN YOUR THINKING BECOMES A HINDRANCE: thinking about food when you aren't hungry or it's not an appropriate time to eat; thinking about your weight when it's not the real problem; worrying obsessively; thinking about anything too much.

WHEN YOUR CHOICES INVOLVE TOO MUCH: eating, drinking, spending, working, drugs, dangerous overactivity, compulsive sex or pornography, reckless actions.

WHEN YOUR ACTIONS INVOLVE TOO LITTLE: recreation, replenishment, healthy pleasures, sleep, exercise, intimacy, friendship, or social contact.

Don't worry about how strange or bizarre or mean it might sound, and don't worry about your writing skills or grammar. Remember, your journal is just for you.

Feeling an emotion is not a problem—it is what you do with a feeling that takes you toward or away from health and wholeness. As you look at it on paper, you can gain new perspective about the situation that may have caused the feeling in the first place. You can ask, "Why did that person or situation trigger such a feeling?" Did it remind you of something in your childhood? Did it make you feel ashamed or inadequate? Is there tension with another person that needs to be discussed and resolved?

Carve out that soul time for yourself. It may be enough just to feel your emotions and acknowledge them—or you may need to do significant work to resolve deep-seated soul wounds. Letting go of negative feelings opens up space within you for joy, freedom, and health. Your journal can be a powerful vehicle to help you break free of the diet trap.

SPIRITUAL CONNECTION

When I was twenty-four and had all of the trappings of success, I felt empty and without purpose. My relationships weren't working, and even though I was "living well," I wasn't *feeling* well. I was physically tired and emotionally weary. Although I had been raised with religious tradition, that was all I had known—tradition, rules, and rituals. I did not have a personal connection with my Creator.

From this very low point I looked up and came to know a living God who could affect every part of my life. That changed my entire life—and changed how and why I was living it. My new focus on wellness took on a higher significance. I was now interested in the bigger picture: on caring for the magnificently created human being

I knew myself to be so that I could feel well, be well, and do well in gratitude to my Creator. In the years since, I've continued to experience the joy of knowing I am loved by the One who created me, and that has given me the ability to love and care for my body and my soul—and others.

I am convinced that striving for physical wellness and freedom from the diet trap without addressing spiritual and emotional health is a futile exercise—we are a sum of our parts, and spiritual needs cannot be separated from physical ones. The body-soul-spirit connection is an amazing one: the care that we give, or don't give, to our body certainly not only affects our physical energy and well-being, but also our ability to think clearly, to see life through a positive lens, and to connect spiritually and relationally.

Our deepest needs are met through relationships. We fill our souls through connecting with others in positive ways and connecting with ourselves through reflection and recreation. We fill our spirits by connecting and feasting with God. A vital, personal relationship with God and honest relationships with others pave the way to our healing. To thrive, we must be connected physically, emotionally, and spiritually.

Like many people, I have my own definition for what being spiritually "connected" means. My personal religious orientation is the traditional Christian faith, and my use of the term "spiritual" is rooted in the Bible, the Old and New Testament theology. I don't believe that God is a disconnected higher power that I am struggling to reach up to, struggling to perform for and receive acceptance from. I believe that God, in His love, reaches down to humanity—and to me, personally. He empowers me by living within me. By inviting His Spirit to dwell within my spirit, my life has been linked with the unlimited love, power, and wisdom of the Divine. When I view the world, my relationships, and my struggles through the eyes of my Creator, it makes all the difference in my attitude and my personal power.

At some point in our lives, we all experience feelings and circumstances that challenge us, sometimes beyond what we think we can handle. Your struggle with your weight and eating might be one of these points. Tragic circumstances can also change our lives in a heartbeat, seemingly with no explanation. And it is in these most difficult times that feel so out of control that we can allow our weaknesses to be covered by the great power of God. We can connect with that power.

The scientific and medical fields are beginning to identify an incredible current of healing power that comes through spiritual connection. Studies from around the world are emerging suggesting that humanity has been "wired" for God. There is now medical evidence that prayer and other forms of spiritual connection can help significantly to heal the ravages of stress, fatigue, and illness.

The latest revelations about spirituality and wellness emphasize the power of three components of religious experience: (1) personal faith, (2) religious practice, and (3) prayer. One such study, conducted at Duke University Medical Center, revealed that all these were powerful tools in the fight against illness and stress. Another study showed that regular prayer can positively affect a person's heart and respiratory rates, lowering blood pressure and slowing brain waves—without drugs or surgery. Studies have even shown a powerful impact on health even when the ill do not know they are being prayed for.

Choosing to let go of my own vision of personal strength and live empowered by God is my path to living a life of spiritual connection and significance. Rather than trying in all my human power to make things work, I now know, deep in my soul, that I will see change through prayer, not by attempting to control the situations or the people in my life. The energy needed to hold onto—and attempt to accomplish in my own strength—the things that I was never meant to control wears on my body, soul, and spirit. This "wear" shows up clearly in physical messages: fatigue, sickness, and excess weight to carry the burden. These physical and emotional "diseases" are but symptoms—telling me and warning me that I have diverted from my spiritual path of peace.

You might wonder how a mere human being can connect with the Divine. I have connected with God through prayer, through listening to powerful music, through reflecting on the beauty of God's creation, through the quietness of a church or garden, through helping another in need. I've learned to pray about my own needs and the things I'm concerned about, asking for divine guidance and strength. Rather than focusing on specific results and demands, I ask for heavenly perspective about specific problems—an ability to see with clear vision the way my Creator does. The result is renewed strength and power.

It is through this power that I have discovered that personal, long-lasting change is possible. Connecting spiritually nourishes the soul the same way that food and water nourish the body. I must nourish my soul with Spirit-inspired "food"— the truth of who I am and why I was created. Knowing the truth about who I am is critical to my emotional well-being. It's critical to yours as well. It determines how you live, what you accomplish, and how you treat—and are treated by—others.

Many of us are so focused on caring for others that we tend to put our own needs on the back burner. Is it because we get more strokes that way? Or, is it that we don't believe we are worth being taken care of? If you don't feel valuable, taking care of your body seems unimportant and it will be easy to get caught in destructive patterns of eating. If you think you are junk, you will eat junk food.

But once you can see yourself through your Creator's eyes, you will desire new ways to care for yourself.

When you see yourself in a new light, your image of yourself will not depend so much on how others see you—or their response to you. With a correct image of who you are, you will wince at the idea of a binge, cringe at the thought of falling asleep on the couch in a food coma, and wonder "Why would I do that to myself?" You deserve to live free of the diet trap—and you can.

As you move forward on your journey—not just "following a diet" but embracing a new way of living—change begins to occur in every arena of your life. Physically, you are developing new habits, rituals, and routines—and letting go of old ones. Emotionally and relationally, you are choosing new ways of relating to the world and yourself, and processing feelings in differing ways. Spiritually, you are coming more alive and discovering that you are worth loving and caring for in new ways. New beliefs, new thoughts, new feelings, new behavior—all are changes with lasting power.

The results are wonderful—but change never comes easily. Resistance comes clothed in sabotage—often from within, and sometimes from others. To learn to identify and overcome sabotage is to learn a life lesson that will serve you well in all areas of living and loving.

CHAPTER 20 ▪ Overcoming Sabotoge and Setbacks

| | | | | | | | | | | | | | | | | | | | | | | | | | | | | | | | | | | | | |

What lies behind us and what lies before us are tiny matters compared to what lies within us.

—OLIVER WENDELL HOLMES

"I don't know what's wrong with me," Sandy lamented. "I love the new way I'm living. I love the way I'm feeling. I love telling others about my new life. But I started sobbing this morning for no reason I could see. I just don't know what I'm feeling, but I've been depressed all day."

Sandy spoke these words six months after making amazing changes in her lifestyle and perspectives. You may remember reading about Sandy's lifetime struggles with weight in Chapter 1. She was overcoming those struggles, day by day, and she looked and felt marvelous physically. She had lost forty-two

> **SMART WEIGH TIP**
>
> *Know your triggers. You have to know which moods send you to the cookie jar before you can do anything about it.*

pounds and truly knew that she could keep them off for life. Yet clearly, on this day, something was wrong. "Do you know what's going on with me, Pam?" she asked, confusion evident in her eyes.

Yes, I did have a clue about what Sandy was feeling. She was experiencing the challenge of change—and it was threatening to sabotage her new-found freedom. Strange as it may sound, she was grieving, and thereby experiencing a myriad of emotions from a variety of sources. As thrilled as she was with the positive changes in her life, she was sad and mad, panicked and helpless, all at the same time.

It is very natural for lifestyle changes like Sandy's to trigger a sense of loss. She had hated the way she used to eat, but she'd eaten that way for a long time. She loved the new foods and patterns of eating, but she missed regularly indulging in the comfort foods that had meant so much to her for so many years.

Most important, Sandy was seeing some of the patterns that had caused her to fail in her previous diets. Through counseling and team support, Sandy had learned that being overweight had, on a subconscious level, actually helped her throughout her life. The excess weight was her "voice"—it spoke for her without Sandy ever having to say a word.

To her parents, her inflated size spoke silently but loudly: "You can't control me." To men, her larger size said, "Don't touch me." And to her husband, her extra weight said quietly, "I don't want intimacy."

As difficult as it was, Sandy was now finding the words for those silent messages and admitting them to herself. She was no longer willing to keep weight on just to speak for her. But that didn't mean that letting go of the old patterns was easy. Yet, Sandy had to in order to embrace fully the new. And that meant letting go of grief as well.

Sandy's emotional battle symbolizes the battle we all fight any time we enter the process of change. It's a battle we must identify and win—because defeat means imprisonment in the same old self-defeating ways. Often, in the throes of change, we get stuck—in old patterns, old thinking, and old ways of doing things. Let's face it, change stirs up old buckets of fear within us and can be terrifying. But if we cave in to the fear, we remain stuck in old patterns simply because of our own resistance to change—a powerful trap in and of itself. The old, no matter the misery it has delivered, is familiar and less frightening.

Even a life filled with constant chaos may be comfortable and "safe" because it's all we've ever known. Battling weight and fighting food may be exhausting, but if you've only lived in a war zone, making peace can bring a deafening calm. So expect internal resistance. Habits and thought patterns that have been learned through a lifetime require supernatural power and patience to unlearn.

The fact is, real change is most apt to happen—really happen—only when the misery of where we are is greater than the fear of where we might be going. In matters of health, I often see crisis as the wake-up call that tells people it's time to change—or else. It may be a doctor telling you to change your eating habits or go on medication for diabetes, hypertension, or elevated cholesterol. It may be an expensive suit that no longer fits, screaming at you to get in shape. It may be that you are picking up every cold, flu, and virus that's around and you're sick and tired of being sick and tired. The desire to change must rise up and face the fear head-on.

OVERCOMING SELF-SABOTAGE

As you feel your fear or resistance swirling within you, you might ask, "What in the world is there to be frightened of? We're just talking about a different—and healthier—way of living! What's so scary about that?" Actually, there are a myriad of fears that arise as saboteurs of lasting change: fears of failure, commitment, disapproval, even of success.

FEAR OF FAILURE is a powerful force in resistance to change. It may be best expressed in the question I'm often asked by my clients: "What if I try this new way of living, and don't stick with it? I've never stuck with any diet before, so why should I believe I'm capable of changing my whole way of eating and living? Won't I just end up a failure and a laughingstock, like always?" They expect themselves to do everything right from the get-go, miraculously changing lifelong patterns overnight, rather than accepting that they'll need to invest time into a *process* of change. The fear of not being able to change—perfectly, quickly, and once and for all—keeps them from even starting. Or, when they experience the inevitable setbacks inherent in the change process, they use the "evidence" of failure to condemn themselves into staying trapped. When the old inner voices chide, "See, you never could do it right and you never will," self-sabotage is often the next step.

FEAR OF COMMITMENT is another common obstacle to setting firm goals or accomplishing them. People manage to keep postponing what they might like to do with their lives for fear that if they accomplish a goal they will have to hold onto it—and that just seems impossible. After all, how good is their track record—especially in the area of health and self-care? Why start anything, why make *any* improvements, if you're not positive you can sustain them perfectly for life? And what if the goal you set is the wrong one? What if it doesn't meet your needs?

This kind of thinking is similar to that of the alcoholic considering whether to choose sobriety over continuing physical and spiritual demise. If a jittery alcoholic, just admitting she is powerless over her disease and considering her next step, were to believe she had to make a rock-solid commitment *today* to stay sober till the day she dies, she may never choose sobriety. That's simply too big a bite to chew.

That's why in programs like Alcoholics Anonymous, newly sober members are urged to take recovery "one day at a time." Thinking ahead is simply overwhelming—and unnecessary. What matters is what they choose *today*. Only in time do they discover the liberating truth that a good choice today usually leads to a good choice tomorrow, and the next day, and the next. But they only have to live them one day at a time. So don't let fear of committing to your well-being become an obstacle or excuse. Choose *The Smart Weigh—just for today*.

FEAR OF DISAPPROVAL OR REJECTION is another saboteur of positive change. This is a valid concern but it needn't be hindering. A major challenge in any personal process of change is dealing with the reactions of your family and friends. Your change may be as scary to them as it is to you.

When we make changes that are in our best interest, friends and family often say, "I liked you better the way your were!" or "Please don't change any more—I like you the way you are!" Psychologists call this subtle or overt pressure to change back to our old ways "changeback pressure." Those pressuring us often feel threatened by our changes because they are losing someone or something familiar. Often they like the old you a bit better, particularly if the old you met their needs—even at the expense of your own. They may want you to change back to being their "binge buddy," or to one who never shows feelings, or to the person who by "being the one with the *real* problem" could help them deny their own struggles.

Sabotage from "inside the camp" is sometimes very real. Many family members and friends want to see weight loss and success for their loved ones as long as they can control it. If they can take the credit, and if their loved ones do it *their* way, they will help. As badly off as you may have been in your "old ways," it may have been more comfortable for them—especially for spouses.

Husbands often try to motivate their wives to lose weight. But, ironically, they are sometimes the least helpful since they are too personally involved. Some typical "motivators" employed by spouses: "You have such a beautiful face; if you could just lose that weight..." or "I'll pay you ten dollars for every pound you lose." Or, "Get into that bikini, and we'll go on that cruise you've been wanting." All fall short of offering positive assistance.

Why? Subconsciously some husbands fear their wives' success. There is so much at stake: loss of eating as a form of entertainment; new foods being served and old ones disappearing; a more physically attractive wife, causing insecurity in some husbands. The sabotage may take the form of subtle complaints about the new way of eating ("Why don't we ever have anything good to eat anymore? You used to be such a good cook!" Or "Honey, you eat anyway you want, but don't mess with my food—I'm not the one with the problem.") Sometimes the sabotage is more direct—he may bring home ice cream or donuts or boxes of candy to reward you for your success.

Similarly, wives often sabotage their husbands' attempts to change their eating patterns. They start out being supportive, often making the appointment to see me, or buying the book. They go "all out" on the new grocery shopping patterns and cooking techniques. But when the husband shows signs of succeeding in his health goals (slimming down, gaining energy, maintaining an exercise regimen), things can change on the home front. Some wives fear their husbands' growing good looks and the new sense of confidence they exude. The husband's success can actually be a double-edged sword to the wife, who may feel that his improved health is a reproach on the way she was previously feeding her family.

How do you hold your own against the sabotage of a spouse or others who may not even be aware of the harm they are inflicting?

First, anticipate and prepare for your loved ones' possible reactions. By expecting negative actions and comments, you can minimize their effect. Write and seek counsel with a friend or a professional to help you identify how you are feeling—and to learn how to communicate lovingly and effectively with your saboteurs.

Most important, make the decision that you are changing your living patterns for yourself—not to please others or to be rewarded with approval, or a vacation. Gaining your personal freedom is reward enough. And remember that the only person capable of gaining the freedom you desire is *you*. Another person cannot force you to change, nor can he or she prevent you from doing so. You decide what you eat, the way you breathe, the water you drink, the exercise you do.

FEAR OF SUCCESS believe it or not, also prevents many people from making positive changes. We may feel that we don't deserve to succeed, feel good, or live free. Some of us won't allow ourselves to trim down to an attractive size because we fear being a sexual target. Or maybe we've been taught as children that we are being selfish when we take care of ourselves.

> **SMART WEIGH TIP**
>
> *Do it for yourself. As long as somebody else is pushing you, no matter what you do or what you try, it'll never work.*

These fears not only serve as obstacles to change, buy are often the vacuum that sucks us back to the old entrapping behaviors. I love the motivational speaker Zig Ziglar's declaration, "Courage is not the absence of fear; it is going on in spite of the fear." And an exciting thing often occurs when we do go on: we may find that by facing the fear, it evaporates.

How often have you avoided doing a task that you thought would be impossible or particularly embarrasing, such as the first time you drove a car, or attempted to water ski? When you finally did it, it wasn't half as bad as you anticipated, and the joy and freedom—of driving, for example—was surely well worth facing your fear.

One of my clients, Kim, helped begin some of the first aerobic dance classes in our area. At the time she started the franchise, she was carrying fifty extra pounds that she just couldn't drop after a difficult pregnancy. She was attracted to the idea of fun exercise, and out of her own need to start doing *something* to get moving, she organized an aerobics class.

The idea of fun exercise to music stirred lots of excitement and attracted many to come to the first class. But Kim passed on the first class, and the second, and the third. Her fear of others seeing how out of shape she was—and how easily out of breath she became—kept her from fulfilling her dream for quite a while. The day she finally walked into the class, leotard-clad and all, she did so with eyes almost closed and shaky knees. But five minutes later, she was having a great time, dancing alongside others to a new life of wellness. She determined just to look at the class—and not in the mirror.

A few years later, Kim was *teaching* three classes a day—in five locations. Her weight finally fell, but her joy of outfacing fear is what she prizes most. And now she does take a glimpse in the mirror now and then!

THE POWER OF A DREAM

Fear is a natural response to change, but it loses its power when healthy motivation shines brightly. This is why the first best step in overcoming self-sabotage is to identify the *why* of the change you desire. What is your personal dream for wellness? Take a few moments to review pages 234-235, where we explored this issue. Your underlying motivation in living free of the diet trap has to be rooted in a genuine and personal passion for positive change, for the right reasons. The only way to turn a goal into a living reality is through emotionally connecting to it—with passion.

In this process, refuse to look at what you need to do, what you should or should not do, or what you must or must not do. It is impossible to be emotionally connected to or be passionate about a list of rules for very long. This kind of focus keeps your eyes on the behavior you are trying to avoid rather than on the new way of living life you want to embrace.

As I discussed in Chapter 5, having a positive perspective and positive goal is powerful because we are destined to hit whatever we have our eyes on. Instead of keeping your focus on what *not* to do or aim for, look at what you *want* to obtain and how you desire to live. You may want to make a list that looks something like this:

- I want to live a life overflowing with energy and well-being.
- I want to be fit; I want a body that works for me.
- I want to be well; I want an immune system that protects me from sickness and disease.
- I want to be healthy and vital as I age.
- I want to be at peace with my body and with my food.
- I want to treat myself well—and believe I deserve it.
- I want to provide the framework for a healthy attitude about food for my children.

We need to be honest with ourselves and commit to a few, simple, heartfelt goals that are close to our heart. Even if our initial list turns out to take us just partway down the road, it will at least get us *on* the road—and we will learn a lot in the process.

MAKING YOUR DREAM A REALITY

The next step in the process of change is to identify and become educated in the new habits that will help you to realize your desires. This is the "work stage" of change—and many people actually enjoy it. You may take classes, read books (including this one), and gather more information about how to "just do it." There's a sense of personal power in this stage—of working hard to figure out the solution to your problem.

Letting go is the third step of change: we must make room for the new in our lives. And that means we must let go of destructive thought patterns and leave behind self-defeating behaviors. There is a time for everything, and a season for every activity... a time to tear down and a time to build up. There isn't room within you for both the old patterns and the new.

To unlearn habits and thought patterns that have been developing for a lifetime requires motivation, patience, and courage. Whenever you let go of the old—even self-sabotaging behavior and thinking patterns—you experience loss. In every transition, happy or sad, letting go of what was involves grief.

Grieving the loss is the fourth step of change. Yes, this is painful. This is where Sandy was. She was doing the right things, but getting what felt like wrong results. Instead of getting easier, her process of change was getting harder. She was expecting to feel wonderful, but at the moment she was just feeling awful.

As you make changes, you may, like Sandy, feel depressed, lonely, guilty, helpless, angry, panicked, resentful, hopeless, hostile—and perhaps silly about it all—before you finally feel relief. This stage had been a secret agent of sabotage to Sandy in the past. The grieving and letting go of the familiar had always driven her back to seeking comfort in food.

But not this time. As she saw her lifelong weight problem dissolving, she didn't want to go back to the same old defeat. This time she got support to push through her fears and claim her new life of health and vitality. A setback—whether physical, emotional, or spiritual—became merely an inevitable event along the road of change rather than a step off a cliff.

Sandy finally began to learn from her own experience that the pain of loss would be balanced by the joy of change. For the first time in her memory, she felt physically vital and emotionally fulfilled, and connected—spiritually and relationally. She was learning to look in places other than the refrigerator for strength and support.

> **SMART WEIGH TIP**
>
> *Practice early detection—weigh yourself once a month. If you've crept up two pounds, get back on the weight loss track.*

DO YOU NEED SUPPORT?

Like Sandy, you may want to ask yourself if you need support. Learning to reach out for help is a huge step on the road to freedom and overcoming self-sabotage—yet it's one of the more rewarding aspects of healing. Why? Because asking for help undergirds your desire for lifelong progress. I know from my own experience that reaching out can be scary; it reveals my vulnerability and challenges my "old tapes" of "I don't need anything; I can (and should be able to) do this on my own." But, believe me, your success in changing your life for the better is much more likely if you stop trying to go it alone. Isolation and self-reliance are not only symptoms of our old entrapment, they practically guarantee that we'll stay stuck.

Acknowledging a problem to at least one other human being says that you know you need help and that you are worth helping. We were created with a natural need to be understood and accepted. Nonjudgmental relationships—whether with trusted friends, a counseling support group, a small home-care group, or a ministry team—show wounded people that they can trust again. Choose your confidante carefully and prayerfully. I encourage my clients who are dealing with issues such as sexual or alcohol abuse in the family to seek professional counseling. These are deeply painful issues that affect every part of your being. A professional therapist has the skills to help you walk through—and out of—painful memories, family systems, and current traps. Not everyone needs a professional counselor, but a person with whom you can honestly share your soul is vital.

Human support is vital for breaking the back of any dependency and busting out of any trap. It can meet the need for intimacy and build our self-esteem in ways that our family and life-up-till-now may never have been able to do. But realize that while others can care, they cannot fix. Just as food is not your ultimate comforter, neither are people your ultimate source of health and well-being. They will never be able to anticipate your needs quickly enough or understand you fully enough. No one can be there for you twenty-four hours a day. Only God can do that. But putting trust in a tangible relationship and opening yourself up for human support will give you strength for change—especially for the long haul.

The supportive relationships you cultivate can be a beautiful reflection of your Creator's love and hope for you. So find the right kind of support. A nag won't do; neither will a partner in crime. Look for people who can empathize with you, encourage you, and believe in you.

WHEN YOU WANT TO HELP SOMEONE ELSE

We all feel that we have infinite wisdom and the right perspective into someone else's situation. We've spent a lifetime learning from all sorts of mistakes—and it's natural to want to share the wealth.

This is especially true when we have a vested interest in seeing the people we care about change for the better. If we're learning to live *The Smart Weigh* ourselves, we want others to join us. That would make our own journey easier, we think, and may even be *the* difference in our long-term success or failure.

You know what? That's stinking thinking. Remember, *you* are responsible for your own choices; *you* have the power, through your spiritual connection, to stay true to your healthy path without the full support of everyone around you.

But, naturally, we want the people we love to be well and happy, and to benefit, as we have, from positive lifestyle changes. This can be frustrating because we certainly can't control others; but our support, offered in effective ways, can be life-shaping, maybe even life-saving. It requires some innovative strategies and time, but it can make a critical difference in someone's well-being. Supportive spouses seem to be particularly strong motivators. A study by Yale University researchers found that overweight people whose spouses were positively involved in their weight-loss programs lost almost three times as much weight compared with subjects in other studies that focused on the individual alone. Another study from Indiana University found that married couples who joined exercise programs together were more likely to have stuck with it after a year, compared to those who had joined solo.

So what's the right track to take when trying to get a loved one on board the healthful-living bandwagon? Here are some guidelines:

HELP THEM SEE THEIR CURRENT LOCATION. Don't hard sell, but gently nudge them toward the healthy door's threshold. Don't try to nag or push them across it. Next time you get the urge to offer all your wisdom, consider this: Advice, as most people tend to give it, is rarely helpful. Solicited or not, when you make someone's decisions for them, you enable them to remain dependent on you. And if they don't accept your advice, they're likely to feel as if they've disappointed or offended you.

The bottom line is this: No one makes long-lasting personal change unless *they* want to. But gently helping them to see how they *really* feel in their current health situation—how they sleep, their productivity and stamina, their quality of life, the things that are hindering them from enjoying life—might help them to determine *for themselves* where they want to go, and why.

HELP THEM SEE THEIR DESTINATION. The best support is to give concrete reasons and reminders about *why* they should stay the course to better health. A man might need to be encouraged by how well he will hit the golf ball with less weight on his frame. A teenager may need to see how a clearer mind will yield better concentration and studying. A woman may want more energy—what she can do *with* her body when she's fit and well rather than *to* her body to beat it into submission.

HELP THEM FIND DIRECTIONS. Your loved ones may now have recognized the value of change, but don't have the tools or know-how to get there. Helping them to do some research of their options—a fitness class to join, a community health program that's soon to begin, a highly recommended nutritionist to counsel with, a book like this one—will steer them to the right road. Just remember that what they do with the information you give them is their choice—and it may be to do nothing at all.

USE THE EIO TECHNIQUE. That's Empathy, Information, Options. Here's an example: A friend who has been struggling to overcome a poor body image has been invited to join the office volleyball team but is self-conscious about being seen in sports attire. Rather than saying "Don't worry about that—you *need* the exercise!" give (1)

Empathy ("Wow, that's a tough problem"); (2) Options ("What's the worst thing that could happen? How will you feel if you don't? Would it be less stressful to play on a community volleyball team where you don't know and work with your teammates?") ; and (3) Information ("I think if it were me, I'd figure, 'Hey, what have I got to lose? They know me, they want me, they've asked me'"). When you encourage, you're helping your friends to help themselves.

BE THEIR CHEERLEADER. Downsize your expectations, and expect your loved ones to stall, take occasional wrong turns, maybe even drive off the road. Help them to see that long-term change is best achieved by taking it slowly and getting there alive. Cheer them on and assure them that you believe in them, no matter what rate their progress. Just as you cannot be made to feel guilty about your personal healthy choices, you do not have the power to make others feel guilty about their own unhealthy choices. Keep your eyes on your own road.

A journal is a great gift to give your loved one because they can record even the tiniest steps of progress. When they are reminded of how good an accomplishment, even a small one, feels, they may be encouraged to stay faithful to the whole healing journey.

GROWING UP, GROWING FREE

"Just Say No" has been a powerful campaign slogan warning children and teens against drug use. The irony is that we adults often can't even say no to a chocolate chip cookie! And peer pressure didn't die in high school. No matter what your age, you must learn—and remember—to say one simple word that tends to get stuck in the human throat: *No.*

When you are offered a food that doesn't fit into your wellness plan, there's no need to give a reason. Neither is there a need to feel guilty, especially if the other person knows what efforts you are making to change. (If they made the cookie "just for you," then there's another issue going on.) A caring friend or family member will respect your desire for freedom and will understand a simple "No, thank you," or "I don't care for any—thank you." Period. These words communicate strength and decisiveness: the truth is that you *can* eat anything; but some foods you choose not to eat *today*.

When you reach the point where you can make an adult commitment to live and live well, you can break free of the diet trap once and for all. Nonetheless, you may sometimes crave some foods. If so, don't overreact. Good health is not affected by one hot fudge sundae, one piece of birthday cake, or one hotdog at a ball game. Don't try to fast the next day, punish yourself with restrictive eating, or take a laxative. And don't fall into the trap of, "I've blown it now, so I may as well keep going!" Just get back on track.

> **SMART WEIGH TIP**
>
> *Repeat this to yourself:*
> *"I can lose weight—*
> *and I will."*

This is especially important when you are most stressed and most vulnerable to emotional messages that signal you to eat. When feelings and stressful situations get too hot to handle, it may seem simpler to return to your old way of eating than to change your way of dealing with life. Overcoming each difficult time—and learning from the ones that overcome you—will make the next one easier. You will not just change old habits, you will establish new ways of living that really work.

WILLPOWER DOESN'T WORK

Once understood, the secrets of *The Smart Weigh* are relatively simple. But, embracing these principles and making genuine change will require more than education alone. Information does not change lives; only revelation promotes lasting change.

Information can be received as head knowledge and may give momentary inspiration, but revelation is received in the heart. It is not just a good idea or something we "should" do. We begin to change our way of eating and living only when we see—truly see— the difference it makes in our personal lives.

BECOME A STUDENT OF YOUR SETBACKS

There will be times when your momentum with healthy eating and living will get seriously off track—but that doesn't mean you have failed, or that *The Smart Weigh* "doesn't work." It does mean that you are human and you were not designed to be the Master or Mistress of your Universe.

If you encounter some rough waters, use journaling as a tool to help you study the setback and see what's going on—*really*. Reflect and write on the past hours and days and ask yourself:

1. *Have I gotten off track in taking care of myself?* Am I tired, hungry, or stressed? Did I go long hours without eating? Am I missing the balance in nutrients? Have I been getting too little sleep?

2. *How do I feel—really?* Anxious? Discouraged? Depressed? Afraid? Sick of focusing on weight loss? Mad at my wife, husband, mother, or boss?

3. *What do I need?* A break? To be less of a perfectionist? Someone to say "good job" or notice how well I'm doing?

4. *What am I expecting?* To lose weight more quickly? Not to have cravings? Never, ever to have a setback?

5. *Is that reasonable?* No.

6. *What is reasonable?* To lose one pound a week—and to expect to have hard times. That's how life is sometimes.

7. *What could I say to myself that would be positive?* That I don't have to be per- fect; *progress* is great. That I'm doing the best I can with what I have to work with, and that I feel *so* much better.

8. *What can I do to get back on track?* Eat a power snack this afternoon, and go for a walk when I get home. Journal everything I'm feeling this evening. Talk to my spouse about how I've been feeling at work. Call a friend and ask for some encouragement.

Yet, once envisioned, our tendency is to rely on our own strength or willpower. The problem is, it's just not enough—and never has been. It's not natural to "control" eating; it's unrealistic to think that any of us can muster up enough willpower to control it for a lifetime. We need to receive help from a greater power than we can "conjure up" ourselves.

But for many people, willpower and self-reliance are the goals—they are going to do it the right way, in their own way, or not at all. Yet, research shows that people who successfully shed bad habits actually have the same number of slip-ups in the first month as those who ultimately fail to change. The difference is that those who succeed don't let a lapse become a collapse. They don't aim for perfection because they accept that it's impossible. Instead, they accept that they will make "less than best" choices occasionally, and accept "progress" as enough. With this mindset, a slip-up does not seal their fate; instead they study their setbacks and simply move on.

I believe that the final and winning step of change is a life principle: Each day we must decide whom to believe about our habits and hang-ups, our successes and our slip-ups. I believe we have a very real enemy—one who will ceaselessly attempt to cast a pall of hopelessness over us. The voice may say, "You can never change. Just count how many times you've failed. Look at the life you've had, what you've done, what's been done to you. You could never live another way."

This enemy attempts to steal our hope and self-worth and to detach us from the spiritual connection we were created for. When we lose our spiritual connection, we lose our vision and purpose for our life. Hating ourselves, hating our bodies, and living in a self-destructive manner not only prematurely takes our life, but takes the life out of us. The unspoken message we too often follow is: eat, drink, and be merry, for tomorrow you die.

But I believe there is another power in this battle. This is the Voice of truth—my Creator—speaking into my life. His voice tells me that I have been created to be a mighty winner, that I am loved, that I need only to receive and trust. The Voice says that I am to value myself because I am of infinite value to God, and that by choosing to live life well I can continue to receive a power that is greater than I.

Each of us has the deciding vote. You and I break the tie; we decide with whom we will side. I chose many years ago to cast my vote with God—the genuine transformer of my life.

STAYING THE COURSE

Over the course of these past seven weeks you've done what few people do—you've followed through on a vision and a commitment. Research tells us that it takes twenty-one days to break a habit, and thirty days to establish a new one. It takes forty days to start feeling comfortable with your new way of living. So your efforts during these seven weeks have worked to start sealing your new behavior of eating, exercising, resting, and self-care into lifetime patterns. As you continue to live free of the snare, you will need to keep putting into daily practice what you now believe.

May your journey be one that leads you to a fulfilled life—body, soul, and spirit. May you be filled with good food, good health, and great joy!

SAMPLE FOOD DIARY

YOUR NAME: _Lynne_   WEEK BEGINNING _3/2_

	BREAKFAST	LUNCH	DINNER	COMMENTS AND EXERCISE
FRIDAY	PROTEIN: 6:35 am _2 eggs_ COMPLEX CARB: _whole wheat toast_ SIMPLE CARB: _1 orange_ ADDED FAT: SNACK★: _6 crackers, 2 string cheeses_	PROTEIN: 11:30 am _1 chicken breast_ COMPLEX CARB: _1 large baked potato_ SIMPLE CARB: _1 side veggie, dish of strawberries_ ADDED FAT: _1 Tbsp. sour cream_ SNACK★: _1/2 of a turkey sandwich_	PROTEIN: 7:00 pm _salmon steak_ COMPLEX CARB: _wild rice_ SIMPLE CARB: _1 orange_ ADDED FAT: _salad dressing_ SNACK★: _cereal and skim milk_	_up at 5:45 am – 6oz apple juice, walked 40 mins._ _4:45 pm afternoon snack_ ☑☑☑☑☑☑☑ CHECK YOUR WATER AS YOU DRINK
SATURDAY	PROTEIN: COMPLEX CARB: SIMPLE CARB: ADDED FAT: SNACK★:	PROTEIN: COMPLEX CARB: SIMPLE CARB: ADDED FAT: SNACK★:	PROTEIN: COMPLEX CARB: SIMPLE CARB: ADDED FAT: SNACK★:	☐☐☐☐☐☐☐ CHECK YOUR WATER AS YOU DRINK
SUNDAY	PROTEIN: COMPLEX CARB: SIMPLE CARB: ADDED FAT: SNACK★:	PROTEIN: COMPLEX CARB: SIMPLE CARB: ADDED FAT: SNACK★:	PROTEIN: COMPLEX CARB: SIMPLE CARB: ADDED FAT: SNACK★:	☐☐☐☐☐☐☐ CHECK YOUR WATER AS YOU DRINK

★ REMEMBER TO HAVE A CARBOHYDRATE AND A PROTEIN AS A POWER SNACK.

WEEKLY FOOD DIARY

YOUR NAME: _____WEEK BEGINNING_____

	BREAKFAST	LUNCH	DINNER	COMMENTS AND EXERCISE
MONDAY	PROTEIN: COMPLEX CARB: SIMPLE CARB: ADDED FAT: SNACK★:	PROTEIN: COMPLEX CARB: SIMPLE CARB: ADDED FAT: SNACK★:	PROTEIN: COMPLEX CARB: SIMPLE CARB: ADDED FAT: SNACK★:	☐☐☐☐☐☐☐ CHECK YOUR WATER AS YOU DRINK
TUESDAY	PROTEIN: COMPLEX CARB: SIMPLE CARB: ADDED FAT: SNACK★:	PROTEIN: COMPLEX CARB: SIMPLE CARB: ADDED FAT: SNACK★:	PROTEIN: COMPLEX CARB: SIMPLE CARB: ADDED FAT: SNACK★:	☐☐☐☐☐☐☐ CHECK YOUR WATER AS YOU DRINK
WEDNESDAY	PROTEIN: COMPLEX CARB: SIMPLE CARB: ADDED FAT: SNACK★:	PROTEIN: COMPLEX CARB: SIMPLE CARB: ADDED FAT: SNACK★:	PROTEIN: COMPLEX CARB: SIMPLE CARB: ADDED FAT: SNACK★:	☐☐☐☐☐☐☐ CHECK YOUR WATER AS YOU DRINK
THURSDAY	PROTEIN: COMPLEX CARB: SIMPLE CARB: ADDED FAT: SNACK★:	PROTEIN: COMPLEX CARB: SIMPLE CARB: ADDED FAT: SNACK★:	PROTEIN: COMPLEX CARB: SIMPLE CARB: ADDED FAT: SNACK★:	☐☐☐☐☐☐☐ CHECK YOUR WATER AS YOU DRINK

★ REMEMBER TO HAVE A CARBOHYDRATE AND A PROTEIN AS A POWER SNACK.

	BREAKFAST	LUNCH	DINNER	COMMENTS AND EXERCISE
FRIDAY	PROTEIN: COMPLEX CARB: SIMPLE CARB: ADDED FAT: SNACK★:	PROTEIN: COMPLEX CARB: SIMPLE CARB: ADDED FAT: SNACK★:	PROTEIN: COMPLEX CARB: SIMPLE CARB: ADDED FAT: SNACK★:	❏ ❏ ❏ ❏ ❏ ❏ ❏ CHECK YOUR WATER AS YOU DRINK
SATURDAY	PROTEIN: COMPLEX CARB: SIMPLE CARB: ADDED FAT: SNACK★:	PROTEIN: COMPLEX CARB: SIMPLE CARB: ADDED FAT: SNACK★:	PROTEIN: COMPLEX CARB: SIMPLE CARB: ADDED FAT: SNACK★:	❏ ❏ ❏ ❏ ❏ ❏ ❏ CHECK YOUR WATER AS YOU DRINK
SUNDAY	PROTEIN: COMPLEX CARB: SIMPLE CARB: ADDED FAT: SNACK★:	PROTEIN: COMPLEX CARB: SIMPLE CARB: ADDED FAT: SNACK★:	PROTEIN: COMPLEX CARB: SIMPLE CARB: ADDED FAT: SNACK★:	❏ ❏ ❏ ❏ ❏ ❏ ❏ CHECK YOUR WATER AS YOU DRINK

WEEKLY COMMENTS _____

_____

_____

_____

_____

GLOSSARY

ADENOSINE—a brain chemical that produces a sedative effect. The production of adenosine is blocked by caffeine.

ADRENALINE—a chemical produced in the adrenal system when the brain puts the body on alert for survival. Adrenaline surges during the stress response, heightening the alerting and protective systems in the body that stimulate the fight or flight reaction.

AMINO ACID—the units comprising protein. Some are essential, meaning that the body can neither make them nor store them. A complete protein is one that supplies all eight of the essential amino acids.

ANTIOXIDANTS—substances that trap wayward oxygen and prevent the process of cellular oxidation, the equivalent of cellular "rusting." Antioxidants can target and neutralize damaging free radicals in the body.

BLOOD SUGAR—the level of glucose in the blood. Blood sugar levels have a powerful influence on our health and well-being—affecting our energy, moods, concentration, appetite, and disease risk.

CAROTENOIDS—phytochemicals that serve a strong antioxidant function, protecting against disease. Found primarily in dark green leafy and bright red or orange fruits and vegetables.

CARBOHYDRATE—an essential nutrient that comes mostly from plant sources. The energy carbohydrates provide for vital body functions is critical, as are the essential vitamins, minerals, phytochemicals, and fibers it contains.

> **COMPLEX**—commonly called starches and found primarily in grains and starchy vegetables, these carbohydrates require a longer time to be digested into sugars and taken into the system as energy. In their unrefined form, these foods are a source of much-needed fiber.

> **SIMPLE**—commonly called sugars and found primarily in fruits and nonstarchy vegetables, these carbohydrates contain a wealth of fiber, vitamins, minerals, and phytochemicals and are digested and released into the system as energy much more quickly than the complex type.

> **REFINED**—complex carbohydrate (starch) that has been stripped of its natural fibers and most of its vitamins, minerals, and phytochemicals. These carbohydrates break down quickly during digestion and are rushed into the bloodstream to be metabolized.

> **WHOLE**—carbohydrates that have been prepared without destroying their nutritive value or fiber. These carbohydrates are broken down more slowly in digestion, gradually and steadily releasing glucose into the system to be burned for energy.

CHEMICAL GYMNASTICS—wide fluctuations in body chemistries. These occur when the body is thrown out of balance because of overconsumption of food, increased emotional or physical stress, or inadequate fuel or sleep.

CHOLECYSTOKININ—a hormone with practically the opposite action of galanin—it promotes the feeling of satiety and fullness. This hormone is triggered into production by a moderate intake of fat.

CHOLESTEROL—a fatty, wax-like substance produced by the body and present in all animal products. Cholesterol is necessary for hormone production, for digestion, and to form cell membranes. But, when cholesterol accumulates in excess levels in the blood, it can deposit and harden in blood vessel walls, causing atherosclerosis, which can increase the risk of stroke and heart attacks.

> **HDL CHOLESTEROL**—high-density lipoproteins. Considered the "good guy" form of cholesterol that protects the vessels from building fatty deposits and decreases risk of cardiovascular disease.

> **LDL CHOLESTEROL**—low-density lipoproteins. Considered the primary culprit in increased heart disease risk. It is the substance that builds up as plaque in the arteries.

CORTISOL—a hormone produced by the adrenal system in response to chronic stress. Cortisol exerts great influence on immune function, blood pressure, pulse rate, metabolism, and fat storage. It also inhibits the production of testosterone and increases the production of insulin.

DOPAMINE—a vital chemical neurotransmitter that brings high levels of energy, alertness, and arousal. Abnormally high levels of dopamine result in high anxiety—to the point of aggressiveness and paranoia. Excessive "brain alert" stimulates production of hormones that contribute to fat cell lock-down.

ENDORPHIN—a morphine-like brain chemical that kills pain and contributes to feelings of self-esteem, euphoria, and emotional well-being. Endorphins are natural calming agents that release you from the stress response and are responsible for what is termed "runner's high."

ESTROGEN—a hormone that serves to regulate the menstrual cycle. It also acts as a mild antidepressant and gives protection against diseases such as osteoporosis and cardiovascular disease.

FAT—an essential nutrient found in animal products and plant oils. Fat is vital for growth, lubrication, hormone production, and the absorption of certain vitamins. It is also a concentrated source of calories that is easily stored as fat on the body.

> **SATURATED FAT**—found in dairy and meat products, including milk, cheese, ice cream, beef, and pork. It can also be found in coconut and palm oils, nondairy creamers, and toppings.

> **TRANS FAT**—formed when vegetable oils are hardened into solids, usually to protect against spoiling and to maintain flavor. Examples include stick margarine and shortening, deep-fried foods such as French fries and fried chicken, and pastries, cookies, doughnuts, and crackers. Read the ingredient list of any processed foods you buy. If you see the words "partially hydrogenated," look for a different product—especially if it is one of the first three ingredients. Hydrogenation is a manufacturing process that converts a polyunsaturated or monounsaturated oil into a saturated fat.

> **MONOUNSATURATED FAT**—found in olive, canola, and peanut oils. These fats increase good HDL cholesterol and decrease bad LDL cholesterol, and thus the risk of disease.

> **OMEGA-3 FATTY ACIDS (EPA AND DHA OILS)**—found in all fish and seafood, particularly cold-water fish such as salmon, albacore tuna, swordfish, sardines, mackerel, and hard shellfish. The only

plant source is flaxseed. Omega-3 fatty acids decrease triglycerides and total and bad LDL cholesterol. They reduce the tendency of the blood to form clots, stabilize blood sugars, improve brain function, and reduce inflammation.

POLYUNSATURATED FATS—found in corn oil, cottonseed oil, safflower oil, sesame oil, and sunflower oil, as well as avocado, sunflower seed kernels, sesame seeds, almonds, walnuts, and pecans. These fats decrease both bad LDL and good HDL cholesterol, so aren't the best choice.

FAT CELL CODE—an intricate communication system in which the body's production of hormones and chemical neurotransmitters determine how the body processes fat. Fat will either be burned, or stockpiled into the fat cell for storage.

FAT CELL LOCK-DOWN—a state in which the fat cells are stockpiled with fat, which causes the cell doors to slam shut and prevent the body from naturally releasing fat. The fat cell becomes resistant to insulin's ability to unlock it and allow the natural fat-burning capacity to be released.

FAT STORAGE FORMULA—when stress, a lack of self-care (sedentary lifestyle, sleep deprivation, erratic or over eating), and states of imbalance (illness, hormone dysfunction, depression, or worry) put the body into a survival mode of energy storage through the slowing down of the metabolism.

FREE RADICALS—unstable compounds produced in the body that can damage vital cell structure. Many chronic diseases and premature aging are linked to the damage caused by free radicals circulating in the body.

GALANIN—a brain hormone that regulates the fat that you store as well as your body's desire for fat. The higher your galanin level, the higher your propensity to seek and find high-fat foods, and the more fat you store. Galanin is released when the body breaks down body fat (as it does in dieting), when the diet is high-fat (over 30 percent of calories), or when several hours have passed between meals, allowing a fall in blood sugars or insulin levels. Eating more frequently, eating less fat (20 to 25 percent of calories), and eating adequate low-fat protein lowers galanin production.

GLUCAGON—a hormone that serves to balance insulin levels. The higher your glucagon level, the lower your levels of insulin. Glucagon levels are increased with an adequate and frequent protein intake.

GLUCOSE—a simple sugar that is the building block of starch. In the small intestine, digestive enzymes break down large molecules of complex carbohydrates (starch) into smaller molecules. These and simple carbohydrates (sugars) are then broken into simpler monosaccharides (glucose, fructose, and galactose) to be absorbed into the bloodstream where they are available as a source of energy to the cells. Glucose is the most critical of these monosaccharides, because it is the source of fuel used by the brain, central nervous system, and lungs. It is so important to your body that if your diet doesn't provide enough carbohydrates to supply glucose, the brain will signal a shortage, and muscle tissue will be broken down to supply the shortfall. That means you lose body muscle (not fat) to feed your brain.

GLYCEMIC INDEX—A measure of the glucose-loading power of a food. The index ranks foods from 0 to 100, estimating whether the food will raise blood sugar levels dramatically and quickly (fast release), moderately (quick release), or just a little (slow release). Carbohydrate foods that break down quickly during digestion have the highest glycemic values—the blood sugar increases rapidly and the rise is fast and high. Carbohydrates that break down slowly, releasing glucose gradually into the bloodstream, have low glycemic ratings.

GLYCOGEN—the body's readily available storage supply of glucose— stored in the liver and muscle. The body maintains a certain level of glucose in the blood to serve the brain, lungs, and central nervous system. To ensure an easily accessible supply of glucose, the body stores it in the muscles and the liver. This stored glucose is called glycogen.

INSULIN—a hormone produced by the pancreas that is necessary for carbohydrate metabolism. It serves as the "key" to unlock the body's cells to allow carbohydrates to enter the cell to be burned for energy. Insulin influences the way you metabolize foods, determining whether you burn fat, protein, or carbohydrates to meet your energy needs—and ultimately determining whether you will store fat.

KETONES—a waste product of abnormal fat metabolism. Ketones are produced when carbohydrate intake is inadequate and the body is insulin-deprived. Fats instead of carbs are broken down to be used as an inefficient energy source.

KETOSIS—a dangerous state of inbalance wherein the body is circu- lating high levels of acidic ketone waste products. Symptoms of ketosis can include bad breath, frequent urination, interrupted sleep, constipation, nausea, general edginess, and lightheadedness. In clearing ketones, the body excretes sodium and potassium, which can result in dehydration and abnormal heart rhythms. The body also retains uric acid, which can trigger gouty arthritis, gout, and kidney stones.

LEPTIN—a hormone produced in the body to give a sense of satiation and hinder the amount of insulin released. Leptin targets and blocks neuropeptide Y, a brain chemical that increases appetite for carbohydrates and increases insulin production.

LIPOPROTEIN LIPASE (LPL)—an enzyme that enables fat to enter muscle cells to be burned for energy and enter fat cells for storage. Saturated fats, a too low fat intake, and high insulin levels suppress LPL at the muscle cell and activate it at the fat cell-directing fat to the fat cell to be stored.

MUSCLE—a complex body system that uses energy to propel the body and body functions. Muscle stores glycogen and essential fatty acids to be used as energy.

MELATONIN—a hormone produced by the pineal gland in the body that contributes to the regulation of circadian rhythms—the wake and sleep cycles.

METABOLISM—a measure of how many calories we burn per minute for body functions. This includes automatic, involuntary functions like breathing, heart beat, digestion and blood circulation, as well as voluntary activity and movement. The largest amount of calories used (70 percent) are those burned to maintain our basic body functioning.

MICRONUTRIENTS—essential vitamins and minerals that are needed by the body in minute quantities, yet have critical functions. These nutrients are often found in foods in trace amounts, requiring a variety of foods to be eaten to meet the body's needs.

MINERALS—inorganic compounds that serve as building blocks for structures such as bones and teeth, and work with fluids and electrical transmissions. Over thirty minerals are crucial to good nutrition and fat release.

NEUROTRANSMITTERS—brain chemicals responsible for sending specialized messages from one brain cell to another. Examples are serotonin, endorphins, dopamine, and adenosine.

NUTRACEUTICALS—compounds in foods that go beyond the nutrients alone. They carry preventative and healing properties against disease.

PHYTOCHEMICALS—powerful plant compounds filled with detoxifying enzymes and antioxidants. Phytochemicals help to protect the body from diseases and aging—along with powering the immune system for wellness. Only a few hundred have been identified, and it is estimated that plants contain hundreds more. They can be received only by eating plant foods.

PROGESTERONE—a hormone that, like estrogen, is involved in regulating the menstrual cycle and works to prepare the lining of the uterus for pregnancy. Progesterone is thought to be the hormone culprit for PMS-related symptoms due to its suppression of the brain chemical dopamine.

PROTEIN—an essential nutrient that comes primarily from animal products and legumes. Protein serves as a vital building block for the body's growth, healing, and repair. It can be used as a more efficient energy source than fat when carbohydrate intake is deficient.

SEROTONIN—a chemical neurotransmitter that brings calm, increased well-being, a bright perspective, a sense of satiety, and appetite control. Serotonin is called the natural feel-good chemical and master weight control drug. It suppresses the tendency to binge and controls increased appetite triggers.

TRIGLYCERIDES—a body fat that serves to transport nutrients throughout the body. Triglycerides often rise to a high level in the blood when there is a nutrient overload (too much food at one time), a high intake of refined carbohydrates, or excessive intake of alcohol.

VITAMINS—organic molecules that the body does not produce on its own, but cannot do without. Vitamins do not give energy, but as chemical catalysts for the body they contribute to its production and allow the body to use it correctly. They make things happen! Vitamins A, D, E, and K are fat-soluble; B and C vitamins are water-soluble.

RESOURCES

BOOKS AND TAPES
BY PAMELA M. SMITH, R.D.

THE ENERGY EDGE

If you are like millions of Americans who allow fatigue to control their lives. Pam's best-selling book, *The Energy Edge,* is for you! The 300 pages of this, deluxe hardcover book are filled with Pam's blueprint for life—giving you the energized tools you need to outsmart the energy "vandalizers" that drain your energy supply. The simple strategies and high octane meal and snack ideas laid out for you will allow a river of energy and stamina to be released from within. (Also available in soft-cover.)

THE GOOD LIFE—A HEALTHY COOKBOOK

A wonderful feast of Pam's most savory recipes. This cookbook offers complete meals for breakfast, lunch, and dinner, plus scrumptious desserts and power snack ideas. Cooking techniques and plate design are presented easily and practically. Food that is good for you tastes great! For the novice or gourmet cook, this book is designed for every-one to enjoy—and it's beautiful! It's a deluxe hardback edition with full-color photography.

EAT WELL—LIVE WELL

A bestseller, this is Pam's nutrition guidebook for healthy, produc-tive living. This large, hardback edition presents "The Ten

Commandments of Good Nutrition" in detail, along with directions for menu planning, grocery shopping, and dining out—from fast food to gourmet. The large cookbook section contains innovative, time-saving recipes. Meal plans for weight loss and weight management are included.

THE SEVEN SECRETS TO LIVING THE GOOD LIFE
A video and audio tape series
In this dynamic four-tape series (audio or video), you will learn how to fit healthy living into your busy schedule, turbo-charge your metabolism and your immune system, seal all the "energy leaks" in your body, and recharge and refuel while you lean down. Pam demonstrates her healthy and delicious cooking techniques and gives easy tips for traveling and dining out healthfully. Available in: 4–tape video series or 4–tape audio series.

FOOD FOR LIFE
More than a nutrition guide and cookbook, *Food for Life* shows how to eat smart and walk in abundant life. It presents Pam's secrets for staying fit, fueled, and free—helping you to explore your relationship with food and yourself. You will discover how to choose the best food, manage weight, and develop a proper perspective for feeding yourself emotionally and spiritually. Meal plans, recipes, and specific action steps are included. Available in: deluxe hardback edition or softcover edition.

FOOD FOR LIFE: A-DAY-AT-A-TIME
This thirty-day devotional guide will equip and empower you to break free from the food trap—forever!

COME COOK WITH ME

This is the kid's cookbook! A wonderful way to teach children nutrition through the basics of healthy cooking. Great for picky eaters! Includes kid-proven recipes, how to set a table, and some great lessons on manners. Handwritten and fun.

ALIVE AND WELL IN THE FAST LANE

A lighthearted and informative nutritional guidebook for the whole family—in a fun, handwritten, and illustrated format. Includes tips for healthy eating on the run.

HEALTHY EXPECTATIONS

This is the expectant mother's handbook with the latest information for nourishing mom and baby. It includes an extensive question and answer section with a proven, natural technique for overcoming morning sickness. This book is filled with love and wisdom. Meal plans and tips for direction before, during and after delivery are included. (An optional mom's journal is available to complement this beautiful book.)

FOR ORDERING INFORMATION ON PAM'S BOOKS AND MATERIALS, SPEAKING AND WORKSHOPS, PLEASE CONTACT:

LIFE COMMUNICATIONS
PO BOX 541115 • ORLANDO, FL 32854
800–896–4010

LifeLine
Press
202–216–0600
VISIT PAM'S WEBSITE AT WWW.PAMSMITH.COM

INDEX